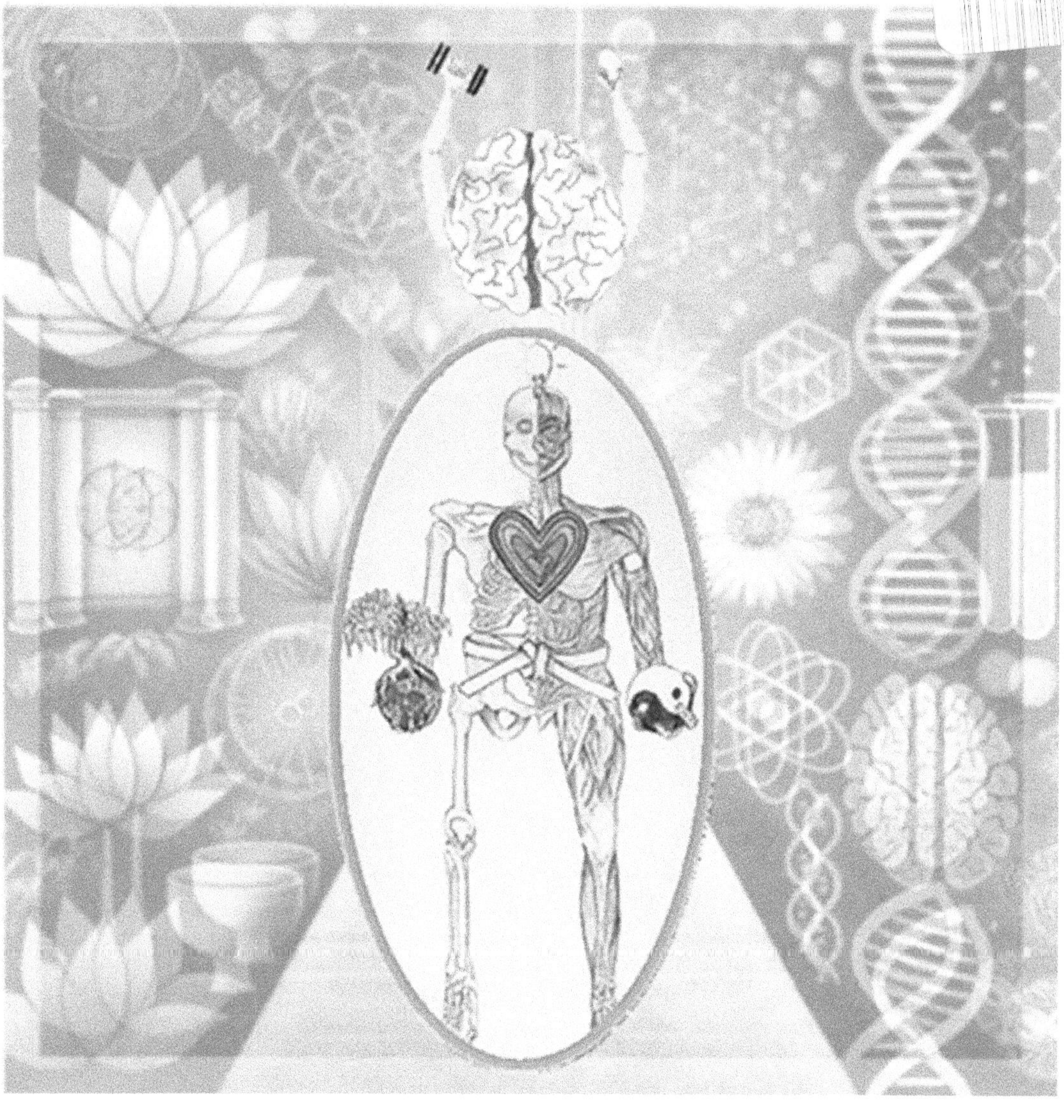

Shayne T Pattie

Eclectic Human Body: The Interplay of Western Centric and Eastern Centric Human Health Sciences, the Differences and their Integration.

2nd Edition.

Author: Shayne T Pattie

Cover Illustrator: Angela Pattie

Editors: Peta-Jane Pattie, Dr. Shellee Franssen, Phillip Deguara

Indigenous Advisor & Contributor: Gayle Roe

Music & Learning Contributor: Claire Dickson

Other Contributors: Chris Bovey, Brittney Bogotto

2025

In loving memory of Fiona.

Contents

Contents _____ 4

Preface _____ 8
   Why the 2nd Edition _____ 8

Human Body Basic-Complex from a Western Centric ____ 10
   Introduction & Brief History _____ 10
   Body Systems _____ 13
      Body Systems Introduction _____ 13
      Circulatory (Cardiovascular) System _____ 14
      Respiratory System _____ 17
      Skeletal System _____ 19
      Muscular System _____ 24
      Nervous System and the Brain _____ 26
      Known Brain Differences in Autism (ASD) and Attention Deficit Hyperactivity Disorder (ADHD) _____ 32
      Endocrine System _____ 35
      Digestive System _____ 38
      Genitourinary and Reproductive System _____ 42
      Integumentary System _____ 45
      Immune System _____ 48
      Fascia _____ 52
      Mitochondria _____ 54
      Summary and the System Interplay _____ 57
   Western medicine's focus on disease and symptom management _____ 59
      The role of specialists, primary care physicians, and allied health professionals _____ 60
      Counselling Psychology and Psychiatry _____ 61
      Psychology of Human Body Brain Connection Introduction _____ 62
      Stress and Trauma Brain and Body changes _____ 68
      Psychology of Sensory Systems _____ 72
      Enteric Nervous System (nutrition and mental health) _____ 76
   The Microbiome Revolution: Modbiotics, Prebiotics, and Probiotics for Optimal Health _____ 77
      Brief Microbiome Explanation _____ 77
   Very Brief Introduction to Molecular Biology: The Building Blocks of Life _____ 82
      DNA, Genes, and the Blueprint of Life _____ 82
   Extra Information to discuss with a medical or allied health professional _____ 85
   Technology, Artificial Intelligence and Surgical Interventions _____ 86
   Pharmaceuticals: Role of Drugs in Targeting Specific Symptoms or Pathogens _____ 88
   Revisiting role of diet, exercise, and lifestyle changes in preventing chronic diseases _____ 94

- Nutrition Information 96
  - Mental Health and Nutrition revisited 103

Brief Dip into Physics, Psychology and Physiology — 111

Psychology and learning — 113
- Defining learning 113
- Memory Summary 115
- Learning Across the Lifespan 117
- Pre-learn, learn and drill Theory 120
- Kolb's Experiential Learning Model 121
- Transformational Leadership and Learning 123
- Learning Styles 123
- Sensory Impacts/Barriers for Learning 127
- 5E Model of Instruction 129
- Illusion of learning 133

Psychology Specific Learning Frameworks and Ideas — 135
- Journey vs Destination 136
- Motivational Interviewing 137
- Positive Thinking 138
- Neuroplasticity 140
- Conditioning 141
- Observational/Social Learning 145
- Dunning Kruger Effect & Johari Window 147
- Stages of Change 149
- FAIL, FAILURE & SUCCESS 152
- Proficiency and Becoming Great 154
- Change is a Direction & Not a Destination 157

Other Learning & Achieving Frameworks — 159
- Aboriginal 8 Pedagogy Framework 160
- Goal related frameworks 162
- Goal Summary 170

Types of intelligence IQ/EQ/AQ — 172

Defining motivation and "the Why" — 175
- Motivation Types 176
- 3 Forgotten Motivation Areas 177
- Identifying Obstacles 178
- Awareness of the Treacherous Trio 179
- Music, Sound, & learning 181

Neurodivergence & Learning Introduction — 187
- Autism and ADHD learning brain 188
- Trauma brain learning differences 191
- Learning Disorders 192
- Irlen Syndrome 194

Human Body Basic-Complex from a Eastern Centric ____ 196

- Traditional Medicine ____ 197
- Limitations ____ 198

Tai Chi Practice for Health ____ 199
- What is Tai Chi ____ 199
- Common Types of Tai Chi ____ 201
- Dr. Paul Lam's Tai Chi for Health ____ 202

Qi Gong Understanding ____ 204

Yoga Understanding ____ 212
- Yoga and Body Systems ____ 213
- Yoga Breath Work, Chakras, and more ____ 214

Herbalist Understanding ____ 216
- Separating Herbs into Basic Function ____ 217

The Mind in Eastern Thought ____ 227

Human Body Basic-Complex Integration of Western Centric and Eastern Centric   228

Recap ____ 228

Holistic Health ____ 229
- Sleep, Thought and Our Brain ____ 229
- Chakras and Neurology ____ 233
- Human Health and Earth ____ 234
- Immune and Allergies ____ 235

Psychoneuroimmunology Understanding ____ 236

Psychology Tools as examples of the Integration between Western and Eastern Centric ____ 240

Ethical Considerations ____ 248

Brief Dip into Health and Martial Arts ____ 250

Brief Introduction ____ 250

Physical Health benefits of Martial Arts ____ 251

Mental Benefits of Martial Arts ____ 252

Community, Belonging, and Social Support ____ 254

Examples of Martial Arts ____ 255
- Itosu Shito Ryu Karate ____ 256
- Rhee Tae Kwon Do ____ 257
- Wing Chun Kung Fu ____ 258
- Muay Thai (Bob Jones – BJC) ____ 259
- Zen Do Kai Karate ____ 260
- Pressure Point Knowledge ____ 261

Importance of Exercise and Physical Fitness — 263

Defining Exercise and Fitness — 263

Pilates Understanding — 264

Resurgence of Calisthenics and its Advantages — 266
- Brief History of Modern Calisthenics — 266
- Review of the Basic Science of Calisthenics — 267
- Suggestions to Improve Skills – Scaling — 269

Strengths and Weaknesses of Modern Gyms — 270
- Strengths of Modern Gyms — 271
- Weaknesses of Modern Gyms — 272
- Fitness Across the Lifespan — 273

Integrating Technology, Data and Virtual Coaching into Health and Fitness — 275

Fitness Exercises – Pilates, Gym, Calisthenics and Yoga — 278
- Exercise Overview — 278
- Pilates Exercises — 280
- Gym — 285
- Body Weight, Calisthenics & Gymnastic Rings — 290
- Yoga — 302

Deidentified Case Studies regarding Western and Eastern Integrated Care — 305

Person 1 — 305

Person 2 — 308

Appendix/References — 309

Formal References — 309

Relevant Course/Degree/CPD References — 323

Informal References — 324

Previous Influential Professionals — 326

Preface

Why the 2nd Edition

The first edition was a great tool for me to have all my human body-related knowledge in one area for me to help myself, my clients and hopefully share it with the world in book form. I wrote the first edition through a story/journey lens but found that the audience who wanted to read this type of non-fiction, wanted more information, better structure and less journey focus.

As a person I am always looking to improve and found areas in the first edition that I felt was lacking, and some areas that didn't need to be in this edition. As such this edition will attempt to fill these gaps and provide an even more eclectic resource about the human body. This book is still written for adults and older teenagers to understand the human body from multiple perspectives.

I have also added majority of the contents from my second book I wrote titled 'Learning Understanding Oneself and Improving How We Learn', because I felt health and learning effect each other bidirectionally.

This edition will more overtly attempt to include the differences and interplay between Western and Eastern scientific traditions and information and more overtly discuss the role of physics in health, mental well-being, and the philosophical underpinnings that tie these concepts together. I strongly believe that the integration of diverse fields can lead to a more complete understanding of the human nature.

This edition will maintain the martial arts section of the first edition, but again expand on this, and expand the fitness and movement related sections from the first edition.

As with all books I write, I have not directly linked the references used in the book text but have included a list of references and influences at the end of the book. I understand that this can be frustrating when trying to track a source, however, since the information in this book is from a variety of sources, courses and professional knowledge, it was too difficult in tracking where each area of information originated.

There are many useful resources in the reference section, and I strongly recommend anyone who finds this book useful, explore this section.

I believe that books still have a place in the modern world. In a fast-paced world, slowing down can be a good thing. As an author, psychologist and fitness and martial arts nerd, I strongly believe there is still a place for books. Books can provide an opportunity for structured learning. They present the information in a structured and logical progression allowing the reader to follow, absorb and then question the material at their own pace and without online distractions.

Books also serve as a reference tool both for the period it is written serving as a long-term resource that can be revisited for guidance and reinforcement of information and ideas, and can serve as an information progression marker for future readers. Reading books has also been found to improve the retention of information when compared to reading digital media. This is believed to be because the focused engagement helps the reader better understand and retain the material.

Human Body Basic-Complex from a Western Centric

Introduction & Brief History

This Western Centric section will provide a brief overview of human body, and current practices and information from the Western Centric viewpoint. It will discuss the body's various systems that are important to understand separately and together and provide other relevant information such as the biomedical model, use of pharmaceuticals and other areas. The idea of East vs West is not a new one, however, I have chosen to use this as the overarching framework for this edition to exemplify the strengths of both systems of understanding the human body. This subsection will include a very brief history regarding "Western Science".

What is currently conceptualised as "Western Science" has a long history that involves most of the world including Egypt, China, and many Arabic countries. The Ottoman empire, Egyptian empires and Chinese empires (such as the Qing Dynasty) had entire centres of learning and a cultural focus on learning. Technical arts such as ballistics, engineering and medicine formed important societal practices. These centres of learning did not focus on an idea of science as a standalone field, rather improvement across the spectrum. The need to express and to please deities, ward off evil spirits and please divined rulers also led to advancements in art and indirectly technology. One of the most famous examples is Chinese gun powder used for firework displays (it took approximately 500yrs for the Chinese nation of the time to use this for war with the invention of the "Chinese Fire Arrow). Chinese Languages have also told a story about how science was considered "investigating things and extending knowledge" as per the translation of 'gezhizue'. Following European influence during the interwar period, the new translation of science became 'kexue', meaning "classified learning based on technical training".

The idea of the state first and religion second also led to more technocratic states and leaders, further increasing the speed of technological innovation. The Ottoman-Khedival state went through a rapid process of military and bureaucratic reform with rapid advances in medicine, music, geography and translation skills leading to better control and training of its military. This empire employed people from various nations including France, Italy and England which allowed for not just technological advancements for the Ottoman-Khedival state, but also incidental cultural and science exchange.

The Ottoman Beirut slowly changed their language to add specificity when discussing information and learning. They went from an idea of factual and spiritual knowledge having similar meanings to slowly adding specificity by separating knowledge and spiritual understandings into 'ilm', 'ma'arifa' and 'hikma' (science, knowledge and wisdom). Knowledge became associated with fact, representing a higher order truth involving the systemisation of facts through the derivation of natural laws.

Closer to what is considered "Western roots", various Greek and Italian cultures such as Athens had leading philosophers and artists who were discovering scientific breakthroughs (such as Pythagoras, Davinci, etc.), just under different headings. What is now considered modern science involves a strong emphasis on categorisation that has strong ties to the ancient Greek emphasis on categorisation.

This categorisation emphasis was evident in Europe during the Scientific revolution starting in 1500 CE, followed through the renaissance period and solidified the idea behind many scientific practices of today. The idea and later the term "Western Science" is rooted in more modern history. By the 'Interwar' era (1918CE – 1939CE) science was being used as a tool to bridge the worlds of the "East and West", however, the term slowly became used by historians to differentiate the two. This differentiation was strongly encouraged by many European countries as a political tool rather than a science tool, and before the end of the 20th century, the term "Western Science" became synonymous with scientific structures that use a basic concept of experimental learning and falsifiable structures and language.

This very structured understanding of scientific thought led to the separation of mind and body and reinforced the individual human being separate from the environment. This type of thought was popularised by various influential people such as Descartes and Fraud. This popularisation spread throughout the European and later the "Western" world, quick scientific advances were made, many specialisations arose leading to an even greater understanding of many different but 'silo-like' understanding of the human body. This improved understanding came perhaps at the cost of the previous eclectic understanding of the human and human health, leading to the current accepted model of human health in the Western countries.

The Western Centric view established processes behind how the information is gathered and what makes it a fact. This process is known as the scientific method. This involves careful observation coupled with rigorous scepticism, because a person's cognitive assumptions can distort their interpretation of the observation. Scientific inquiry includes creating a hypothesis through inductive reasoning (a method of drawing conclusions by going from the specific to the general), testing it through experiments and statistical analysis, and adjusting or discarding the hypothesis based on the results. A scientific hypothesis must be falsifiable, implying that it is possible to identify a possible outcome of an experiment or observation that conflicts with predictions deduced from the hypothesis; otherwise, the hypothesis cannot be meaningfully tested. The purpose of an experiment is to determine whether observations agree or disagree with hypothesis.

The eight principles of the Scientific Method include – defining a question, gathering information and resources (observing), forming an explanatory hypothesis, testing the hypothesis by performing an experiment and collecting data in a reproducible manner, analysing the data, interpreting the data and drawing conclusions that serve as a starting point for a new hypothesis, publish results and lastly having the information retested (often completed by other scientists). In psychology this scientific model is used in research, procedural implementation, group program design and even in counselling. The only difference in psychology counselling the scientific model, is the person being seen by the professional would be represented as N=1, and the various psychological theories and tools would therefore have to be customised for effective counselling assistance.

The Western Centric specialisation has led to a "symptoms focus" in many medical and health fields throughout the Western world which has had many short-term benefits but also led to longer term consequences.

As a side note, many Arabic cultures including the Islamic culture have practiced their own versions of medical models that incorporated ideas from both Western and Eastern models. This would be an interesting area to explore further for readers who finish this book to investigate the similarities and differences.

Only recently has previous eclectic understandings begun to re-influence how professionals assist people in the health fields. This eclectic view will be explored later in the book, first in the "Eastern" centric view, and then in the 'Integration' section.

Body Systems

Body Systems Introduction

There are multiple different body systems that all have important roles and work together in an adaptive way. The idea of "body systems" is a way to simplify the very complex human body. The body's organs and systems communicate with each other multi directionally (through chemical signalling and electric signalling), with the kidneys, stomach and brain communicating with all our organs multi-directionally. The body systems discussed here include Circulatory System (also called the Cardiovascular System) including Lymphatic, Respiratory System, Skeletal System, Muscular System, Endocrine System, Digestive System, Nervous System, Genitourinary System including the Reproductive System, Integumentary System and Fascial System.

This 'body systems' section is focusing on male and female anatomy only and not intersex or other sexual combinations for simplicity purposes. A lot of the information presented in this book is relevant for most sex combinations that humans can be born with and present with, however, I felt I would not do the combinations justice.

Circulatory (Cardiovascular) System

The Circulatory System (also called the Cardiovascular System) includes aspects of our Lymphatic system. It relies on a healthy and rapid transport system in the body to – deliver nutrients and oxygen to our cells, carry away wastes, toxins, and carbon dioxide, and allow for the chemical messengers such as hormones to move around the body. When there are fatty deposits in the arteries it can lead to high blood pressure and other serious outcomes, and a blood clot can cut off blood supply to a vital organ or brain.

The average healthy adult heart can be measured as approximately two adult fists and sits close to the centre of the chest. It is protected by our thorax, sits between the two lungs and is known as a muscular pump. The heart is split into halves by the septum and each half contains two chambers separated by a cusped valve. The first chamber is known as the Atrium and leads into the second chamber called the Ventricle. The atria (two atrium) are fed into by large veins. The body's veins hold approximately 70% of the body's total blood supply and contain valves which help the blood travel in the correct direction.

Into the right atria is the inferior vena cava, where deoxygenated blood from our head and upper body is delivered. Blood from the veins fill the right atrium and then during the first part of a heartbeat known as the Atrial Systole, the blood is pumped through into the right ventricle through the Tricuspid valve. During the part of the heartbeat known as the ventricular systole, the right ventricle (which is now full of blood) contracts and forces blood out through an artery called the Pulmonary Artery, which branches off and takes the deoxygenated blood to the lungs, where the lungs will draw out the carbon dioxide and flood it with oxygen. The oxygenated blood from the lungs is then transported to the left side of the heart, entering the left atrium via the Pulmonary Veins. The oxygenated blood is then pumped into the left ventricle during atrial systole via the mitral valve and from this ventricle, it passes into the artery known as the Aorta. The aorta then branches out several times into increasingly tiny vessels and the vessel transports oxygenated blood throughout the body.

Due to the heart processes, it is vital that the two parts are kept apart. However, when a hole in the heart forms, the person doesn't receive enough oxygen and becomes exhausted and may appear blue. In the womb, the heart isn't fully formed until the end of pregnancy with some babies being born with the septum still not completely sealed, but in most cases, this is remedied soon after birth either naturally or via surgery.

Arteries have a strong muscular wall and contain elastic fibres that are used to stretch as they receive new blood from a heartbeat. The smooth muscle fibres can relax or contract, increasing or decreasing their inner hollow tube, which the blood flows through. This process explains the potential fluctuation of blood pressure. Lifestyle habits can increase a person's blood pressure due to a decrease in elasticity within the arteries. Negative habits may include smoking, eating a poor diet, and not getting enough exercise. These negative habits can make it harder to lower blood pressure within the artery because the person can't increase the size of the hollow inner tubes. The lack of stretch also means the heart must forcefully push the blood along, which can escalate to heart disease.

Large arteries branch off into smaller versions called arterioles and from there they branch off to form tiny capillaries. Networks of capillaries form the capillary beds that feed tissues and cells from head to toe. The total length of capillaries in the skeletal muscle of an average human is estimated to be between 9,000 and 19,000km long. This disproves the previous number of 100 000km estimated by August Krogh who miscalculated the density of capillaries in humans and had based his estimate on a 143kg body building male who had a minimum of 50kgs of muscle mass. This estimation from 1922, was then extrapolated and accidently turned into a fact by the science community until 2021-2024 when various studies began to debunk the previous number. Whilst arteries are muscular tubes, capillaries are tiny, featuring a layer of Endothelium made of flat small cells which can become drawn apart when the capillary dilates, which increases permeability. This is vital as it allows for the easy transfer of molecules. It is only in the capillaries where blood can release molecules and take up molecules. Certain capillaries are even more permeable than others, such as in the digestive tract and kidneys. There are also leaky versions of capillaries known as Sinusoids, which occur in the liver where the leakiness functions to allow the liver total access to the contents of the blood.

Veins branch out to form venules in the same way that arteries branch out to form arterioles, but veins and arteries are structurally different, with veins having less muscle in their walls and one-way valves. These valves open to allow blood to flow through towards the heart. If the blood starts flowing back towards our feet, the valves close off to stop this. Veins and venules are not exposed to the same sort of blood pressure as arteries and arterioles and they rely on the blood entering veins from the capillary beds to start pushing the blood along, combined with a suction motion at their other end. During an inhalation, the pressure changes in the chest, drawing blood into the heart. The contraction of skeletal muscle also helps to get the blood moving through the veins. As the muscles contract, veins which the muscles surround are squeezed, and blood up if forced up. This means people need to move around to get the venous blood moving.

Red blood cells, also known as Erythrocytes, account for nearly half our blood's volume. The term Haematrocrit refers to this percentage and you may see it mentioned on blood tests. Males have a slight haematrocrit at 42-52 percent while females have 37-47percent. Red blood cells are made in the red bone marrow and live for around 120 days, before popping at the pressure of tiny vessels becomes too much for them. Packed with haemoglobin (250 million haemoglobin molecules per red blood cell) our red blood cells can carry up to a billion oxygen molecules each. The iron molecules in the haemoglobin bond to the oxygen. This is why people with low iron can be impacted, and how it has a marked impact on how nourished our cells and tissues are by oxygen.

White blood cells (monocytes and later macrophages) form part of our immune system, and unlike red blood cells which have lost their nucleus by the time they enter circulation. White blood cells are fully equipped with their nucleus and are very useful and move around the body. The monocytes also play a secondary role with emotions and research has found that every neuropeptide receptor that could be found in the brain is also on the surface of the human monocyte. Human monocytes have receptors for opiates, PCP, and other peptides such as bombesin. These emotion-affecting peptides, then, appear to control the routing and migration of monocytes, which are very pivotal to the overall health of the human body. White blood cells only account for around 1percent of the total volume of blood and a healthy white blood cell count is between 4800 and 10800 per cubic millimetre of blood.

Platelets, also known as Thrombocytes, are the fragments of what used to be rather large cells called Megakaryocytes. They come into use when we are bleeding with their fragments becoming sticky, forming a plug to stop the blood leaking. Sometimes their ability to form clots can cause problems, such as when the blood doesn't clot well (Haemophilia and other clotting disorders) meaning a risk of someone bleeding to death. Another clotting issue can arise when a clot forms, when and where it shouldn't form, leading to Thrombosis (blocking of a vessel). The position of thrombosis will greatly influence the health outcome. The most common place for thrombosis occurring is the legs, but if they reach the brain, they can cut off the blood supply and cause a stroke.

The Lymphatic System assists the Circulatory System by draining excess fluids and proteins from tissues back into the bloodstream to assist in preventing tissue swelling and protects the Circulatory System from foreign invaders. There is also a newer known body system known as the Glymphatic system which works with Glial cells and connects with the Lymphatic system at the Dura to help clear waste from the brain.

Some common cardiovascular related issues include Hypertension, Arteriosclerosis, Angina, Varicose Veins, and Hypotension.

Respiratory System

The Respiratory System's primary role is to supply our blood with oxygen so it can be delivered to all parts of the body. Normally we breathe in through our nostrils. From here the inhaled air will move deep into the bony cavities behind the nose, all of which feature smaller bones called Turbinates. Their function is to churn the inhaled air so that it communicates with the mucous membranes within the cavity. The sinuses are connected to the nasal cavities by little tubes, and these are prone to congestion when we have an upper respiratory tract infection. The sinuses are lined with mucous membranes which normally help to trap the dust and microbes, but during an infection, all the mucous can trigger annoyance and other emotions.

The nasal cavity communicates with the throat via the Pharynx. The pharynx houses the Epiglottis which functions to close off the windpipe from food and drink. The pharynx divides into the Oesophagus at the back leading down to the stomach and into the larynx at the front for inhaled air. The larynx becomes the trachea, and this is a strong smooth muscle structure supported by horseshoe shaped cartilage coated with more connective tissue.

The inside of the traches is lined with hairy epithelium. Two bronchi emerge from the trachea, which are strong, and made of smooth muscle and cartilage, with each one leading to a lung. Within the lung, the bronchus divides and subdivides into increasingly smaller tubes. The smallest tubes are called bronchioles and have no cartilage.

The smallest bronchioles terminate in grape-like structures called alveoli. Alveoli features an elastic membrane, allowing them to fill with air. The alveoli walls are composed of two different types of cells – type 1 alveoli cells (site of gas exchange) and type 2 alveoli cells (septal cells which secrete alveolar fluid). Wandering phagocytes called dust cells patrol the alveoli, and their role is to deal with any dust that makes it deep into the lungs. Alveoli are surrounded by pulmonary capillaries, that have deoxygenated blood run through them from the right ventricle of the heart. The type of alveolar cells assists the alveoli with gas exchange in the lungs. The air that has filled the little alveoli is rich in oxygen and this high concentration of oxygen compared to the low concentration of oxygen in the pulmonary capillaries drives the movement of oxygen molecules out of the air sacs and into the bloodstream. All the oxygenated blood is then transported and used to nourish cells throughout the body. During this the pulmonary capillaries have a high concentration of carbon dioxide, while the lungs should have only a low concentration. This forces the carbon dioxide out of the blood into the alveoli, down the concentration gradient via the diffusion process. We then exhale the carbon dioxide as we breathe out. This exchange occurs over the respiratory membrane comprising the single cell wall of alveoli and the single cell capillary wall.

When diseases such as pneumonia occur, the lungs can become consolidated with fluid which thickens the respiratory membrane, making it much more difficult for the gas exchange to take place. In emphysema, the little alveoli become merged together which decreases the surface area for gas exchange. With milder respiratory illnesses which feature large amounts of mucous, the flow of air into the alveoli is reduced, and cancers and other areas of inflammation can physically block the passage of air. This leads to less oxygen and more carbon dioxide in the body, leading to a more acidic environment in our body.

The lungs themselves are wrapped in two layers of serous membrane (parietal and visceral pleura) known as the pleural membrane. The space between the two membranes is known as the pleural cavity and this is home to a small amount of lubricating fluid, preventing the two membranes from sticking to each other. Inflammation of the pleural membrane can lead to accumulations of fluid in the cavity known as a Pleural Effusion. When air gets between these two membranes, it's known as Pneumothorax. The lungs are divided into lobes by fissures. The left lung has a superior and inferior lobe only (due to the location of the heart and smaller lung size) whilst the right lung also has a middle lobe.

The two important muscles involved in the process of breathing in and out are the diaphragm and the intercostal muscles. When we inhale, the diaphragm muscle contracts, flattens out and elongates the thoracic cavity; at the same time the intercostal muscles contract and pull the ribs up and out to further expand the thoracic cavity. Due to the change in pressure within the thoracic cavity, the little alveoli in the lungs experience a drop in pressure and air floods into them down a concentration gradient. When we exhale, the diaphragm relaxes and springs back into its original shape. And another set of intercostal muscles draw the ribs back in, which squeezes air up and out of the lungs. The process is known as pulmonary ventilation. For the lungs to perform their job, they need a degree of elasticity, and the bones need a good amount of movement, however, there are illnesses which reduce this elasticity such as Fibrous Lungs Disease, or bone illnesses such as Arthritis, which leads to breathing becoming laboured.

Common issues regarding the respiratory system include Colds and Flus, Sinusitis, Sore Throats, Asthma, COPD (Chronic Obstructive Pulmonary Disease), Chest Infections and Hay Fever.

Skeletal System

Skeletal System – There are approximately 206 bones in the adult human body. This section will again focus on the bones and joints that have been and are currently relevant to my professional and personal knowledge. The Skeletal System has many roles – it supports our body weight, allows for movement, produces blood cells, supports immune system, protects and supports organs and stores minerals in the body. In summary bones are a type of living tissue and are responsible for more than just holding us up.

The human skeleton can be broken into eight sections – the Skull, Spine, Chest, Arms, Hands, Pelvis, Legs and Feet. The main bones that make up the Skull are the: Frontal Bone, Parietal Bones, Temporal Bones, Occipital Bone, Sphenoid Bone and Ethmoid Bone. The Skull has a Tendon known as the Galea that sits over the dome of the Skull. There are 33 bones in the Spinal Column and are often separated into 5 sections – the Cervical, Thoracic, Lumbar, Sacral and Coccyx. There are seven Cervical bones, twelve Thoracic bones, five Lumbar bones, five Sacral bones and the Coccyx made up of four fused bones. There are three main Ligaments that connect along the Spinal Column including the – Ligamentum Flavum, Anterior Longitudinal Ligament and the Posterior Longitudinal Ligament. The Joints along the Spinal Column are referred to as Facet Joints. Joints have often been thought to be passive, but research is now finding that joints are very active in our body and can be strengthened the same way as our muscle – through appropriate training. Our bones are also changeable as will be discussed, but briefly speaking our bones also include the fibrillar part of our bone known as the collagen part, which is often not taught or seen when learning about the skeletal system.

The main bones that make up the Chest are the Thoracic Vertebrae, seven of the twelve pairs of Ribs, and the Sternum. The main Tendon in the chest is called the Pectoralis Tendon, and the seven pairs of ribs connect to the Sternum via their own Costal Cartilage.

The main bones that make up the Arms are the – Humorous, Radius and Ulna bones. The main Ligaments that connect to this area are the – Ulnar-Collateral Ligament, Lateral Collateral Ligament and the Interosseous Membrane. The main Joints that connect to this area are the – Humeroradial Joint, Proximal Radioulnar Joint and Distal Radioulnar Joint.

The main bones that make up the Hands are the – fourteen Phalanges, five Metacarpal Bones and eight Carpal Bones. The main Ligaments that connect to this area are the – Dorsal Intercarpal Ligaments, Palmar Intercarpal Ligaments, Interosseous Intercarpal Ligaments, Pisohamate Ligament and the Pisometacarpal Ligament. The main Joints that connect to this area are the Proximal Interphalangeal Joints and Distal Interphalangeal Joints.

The main bones that make up the Pelvis or Pelvic Girdle are the – Hipbones (Ilium, Ischium and Pubis fused together in adults), Sacrum and Coccyx. The main Ligaments of males and females that connect to this area are the Sacrotuberous, Sacrospinous and Iliolumbar. Females' Pelvis also contain the Broad Ligament and Ligaments of the Ovaries and Uterus. The Joints that connect to this area are the – Sacrococcygeal, Lumbosacral, Pubic Symphysis and Sacroiliac.

The main bones that make up the Legs are the Femur, Tibia, Fibula and Patella. The main Ligaments of the Legs are the Anterior Cruciate Ligament, Posterior Cruciate Ligament, Medial Collateral Ligament and Lateral Collateral Ligament.

The main bones that make up the Feet and Ankle are the – Talus, Navicular, Cuneiform, Calcaneus, fourteen Phalanges and five Metatarsals. The main Ligaments in the Feet and Ankle are the – Plantar Fascia Ligament, Plantar Calcaneonavicular Ligament, Calcaneocuboid Ligament and Lisfranc Ligaments. The main Joints of the feet and ankle are the – Subtalar Joint, Midtarsal Joint, Tarsometatarsal Joint Complex, Metatarsophalangeal Joints and Interphalangeal Joints.

There are at least six different types of bone – the Long Bone, Short Bone, Flat Bone, Irregular Bone, Pneumatic Bone and Sesamoid Bone. The Long Bones have a long thin shape and work as levers to permit movement with the help of muscles such as the Tibia and Femur. Short Bones have a cubed shape and allow movement of areas such as the Wrist, and the Tarsal Bones of the Feet. Flat Bones have a more flattened, broad surface and are made up of a layer of sponge-like bone between two thin layers of compact bone and their main purpose is to protect internal organs such as the Brain, Hips and Pelvic organs. Irregular Bones do not fit the above three types and perform various functions in the human body including protecting nerve tissue and providing support for the Pharynx and Trachea. Pneumatic Bones can also be classified as a subset of Irregular bones but contain large air spaces lined by Epithelium. Sesamoid Bones are the bony nodules that are found embedded in the tendons or joint capsules and assist the body through resisting pressure, minimising friction, altering the direction of the pull of the muscle and maintaining local circulation.

The outer layer of the bone is called the periosteum and tendons and ligaments attach to our bones via our fibrous connective tissues (fascia) to facilitate and respond to movement. Under the periosteum is the compact bone, a thin layer, and beneath this is the spongy (cancellous) bone. The spongy holes are full of red bone marrow, the site of blood cell formation. Inside the cavities of our long bone, we find yellow bone marrow, which serves as a fat storage facility. Therefore, our bones' secondary roles include making blood cells, storing fats and are a reservoir of calcium and phosphates.

Ossification is the process of bone forming. In the mother's uterus, the tiny bones start out as little cartilaginous forms which eventually undergo ossification. The process of ossification requires calcium, which we originally receive from our mother via the placenta. This calcium is laid down in concentric circles, hardening the structure. At the centre of these circles is the Haversian canal.

There are two ossification processes – intramembranous ossification and endochondral ossification. Intramembranous ossification is where the bone is formed within the fibrous connective tissue membranes by condensing mesenchymal cells. Endochondral ossification is where the bone is formed within hyaline cartilage which is then made into bone. As we mature, our bones grow in length and diameter and undergo remodelling. The main elements of bone formation include osteoblasts which secrete bone ingredients, osteocytes which are mature bone cells that help maintain the daily activity of bone tissue and osteoclasts which breakdown and resorb bone tissue.

When a bone is broken, it heals via a process known as calcification. The first event is the formation of a fracture haematoma (blood clot) which occurs when the blood leaks from vessels ruptured in the break. An inflammation response then occurs where the capillaries grow into the blood clot and white blood cells flood the area, with this first stage lasting several weeks. The second stage is the formation of the fibrocartilaginous callus. As granulation tissue fills the site, a procallus is formed and fibroblasts and osteogenic cells move in. Collagen fibres are then laid down to connect the two ends of the broken bone. The osteogenic cells transform into chondroblasts which then start to produce fibrocartilage, and this stage can last around three weeks. Next the bony callus forms which involves the replacement of the fibrocartilage callus with bone material. This happens as osteogenic cells transform into osetoblasts, which then start to produce spongy bone trabeculae, which then join portions of living and dead bone. This stage lasts three to four months. The final stage is bone remodelling and involves osteoclasts actively doing their job of breaking down bone cells, so they can be replaced by new compact bone around the periphery of the fracture. Bone healing is important and benefits from its piezoelectrical properties.

Bones are a multidirectional and anisotropic piezoelectric material that exhibits an electrical microenvironment. The electrical signals play a very important role in the process of bone repair, which can effectively promote osteoblast differentiation, migration, and bone regeneration. Piezoelectricity can be defined as the electric charge that accumulates in solid materials such as bone, DNA and various proteins in response to applied mechanical stress. Our bones are seventy percent inorganic hydroxyapatite and 30 percent organic type one collagen, and most of our body is Piezoelectric or has properties of this.

The bones' Osteoblasts that are used to regenerate bone, also release a chemical known as Osteocalcin that has been linked to memory improvement through hippocampus activation. As such bone loss in older adults, has also been found to increase the risk of dementia, currently thought to be directly connected to the loss of Osteocalcin. Osteopontin is another chemical communicated by the bones, which communicates to the body to boost immunity. Bones also release signals that have been found to improve reproductive health in men's testes and muscular stamina. Bones communicate with the body's organs, and bone health directly influences our cognitive age through the regulation of specific hormones.

Bone Density is important for everyone and become more important as we age. The factors that work together to ensure the health of our Bone Density include – dietary calcium, vitamin D from the sun and from diet, healthy diet with vitamins and minerals, naturally occurring hormones, and regular weight bearing exercise. Regular weight bearing exercise has been studied and a theory known as 'Wolff's Law' discusses this. According to Wolff's Law naturally health bones will adapt and change to the stress they are subjected to, with heavier loads (within realistic parametres) leading to stronger bones. Wolff's Law was created by German anatomist and surgeon Julius Wolff in the 19th century and has been found to be accurate in most cases but did not discuss how bones can become stronger through changes in our bone geometry. Bone messaging directly increases risk of osteoarthritis when too much sclerostin is available which blocks bone repair and indirectly increases ageing. Exercise that involves mechanical loading such as resistance training or running, reduces the sclerostin, allowing for bone repair. This recent research further supports previous research, involved in Wolfe's law.

Tendons act as connectors between muscle and bone and allow for movement, whilst Ligaments connect bone to bone and usually hold structures together for stability. They are made out of connective tissue that have a lot of strong collagen fibres. Joints are complex and are often made up of Cartilage, Synovial Membranes, Ligaments, Tendons, Bursas, Synovial Fluid and Meniscus. The four types of Joints are – Ball and Socket Joints such as shoulder and hip, Hinge Joints such as fingers and knees, Pivot Joints such as the neck and Ellipsoidal Joints such as the Wrist.

The three basic categories of joints are fibrous, cartilaginous, and synovial. Fibrous joints fix together adjacent bones with tight fibres and are almost immovable. Cartilaginous joints have some movement and are made of cartilage. Synovial joints are freely movable joints which feature a joint capsule, with a synovial membrane, articular cartilage, ligaments and in some sites a menisci and bursae. The synovial fluid is a gloopy like substance and lubricates the joint. The more we move the more synovial fluid we make and the less we move the less we make. When a joint is starting to stiffen, it can often be due to less synovial fluid. The cartilage at either end of the articulating bones has no blood supply and relies on synovial fluid to nourish it. Pain, stiffness, and inflammation often are caused by the synovial fluid not reaching the cartilage and the cartilage being damaged as a result. Also, if a muscle around a joint becomes too tight, they can compress the cartilage producing similar symptoms.

Adding to what has been discussed about the skeletal system so far, it is noted that until recently it has been taught that the skeletal system is mostly a continuous compression structure, like a brick wall with the head resting on the 7th cervical vertebra, the thorax resting on the 5th lumbar and so on, down to the feet. However, more recent research into the human body has instead suggested that tension (tensegrity) and compression work together. In this model the bones are seen as spacers, pushing out into the soft tissue and the tone of the tensile myofascia becomes the determinant of the balanced structure, where tension and compression work together to constantly try and achieve a balance.

Common issues in the Skeletal system can include Osteoarthritis, Rheumatoid Arthritis, Gout, Fractures and Fibromyalgia.

Muscular System

Muscular System – There are over 600 muscles in the human body. In the fitness world, we first learn about the six muscle groups, and later the core. From there we slowly begin the journey through the complexity of the muscles and become more specific with our own and other people's exercise prescription. The six main muscle groups are the Chest, Back, Arms, Shoulders, Legs and Calves. The core is often included in most exercises as it the powerhouse and should be used with most if not all exercises. This section will also include several Tendons as often the Muscles and Tendons are discussed together with fitness related training or recovery.

Bundles of muscle cells can look stripy and make up the fibres that are bound together to form a muscle. Their stripes are created by the actin and myosin filaments which slide across each other on an ATP (Adenosine Triphosphate) fuelled reaction that causes muscle fibres to shorten, contracting the muscle. Each muscle cell is wrapped in a fibrous connective tissue sheath and the bundles are then further sheathed. A whole muscle is also sheathed in a connective tissue known as fascia. This fascia extends at the end of muscles to form the tendons that attach to bones.

There are two main types of muscle twitch fibres, known as 'Fast-Twitch' and 'Slow Twitch'. Fast twitch fibres are helpful in giving a person sudden bursts of energy which can be helpful in lifting heavy weights, sprinting, etc. Fast twitch fibres are known as Type 2 and there are two subtypes known as 2a and 2b. Slow twitch fibres are helpful in endurance or longer-lasting activities such as long-distance swimming or running. The most common balance at birth is 50% fast twitch and 50% slow twitch. However, genetics and lifestyle choices such as the types of exercise and muscular-skeletal stress a person puts on their body, can influence this this balance as we age. Common examples can be found in the different athlete types (power lifter, marathon runner, football player, etc.) with variances ranging from 10 to 90% of one type or the other, with the distribution also being highly dependent on the muscle. As with most areas of human health, it the genetics a person is born with and the epigenetic expression (environment/life choices) influencing each other bidirectionally.

When training the chest and shoulders the main muscles discussed are the: Pectoralis Major, The Pectoralis Minor, Sternocleidomastoid, Supraspinatus, Trapezius and the Deltoid Muscle.

When training the Back, the main muscles discussed are the: Sternocleidomastoid, Trapezius, Deltoid, Teres Minor, Teres Major, Latissimus Dorsi, Supraspinatus, Rhomboid Major, Rhomboid Minor, Quadratus Lumborum, Serratus Anterior, Serratus Posterior and Erector Spinae. The Gluteal muscles can often be placed in this category dependent on exercise focus, as can many of the other core muscles.

When training the Arms, the main muscles discussed are the: Deltoid, Pectoralis Major, Pectoralis Minor, Biceps Brachii Short and Long Heads, Subscapularis, Teres Major, Latissimus Dorsi, Flexor Carpi Radialis, Triceps Brachii,

Brachioradialis, Flexor Carpi Ulnaris, Extensor Carpi Ulnaris, Extensor Carpi Minimi, Extensor Carpi Radialis, Abductor Pollicis, Extensor Pollicis and Pronator Teres.

When training the legs (upper half) the main muscles discussed are the: Semitendinosus, Biceps Femoris, Semimembranosus, Gluteus Maximum, Gluteus Minimus, Gluteus Medius, Iliopsoas, Psoas Major, Adductor, Abductor, Sartorius, Tensor Fasciae Latae, Rectus Femoris, Vastus Medialis, Vastus Lateralis, Iliotibial Tract, and Piriformis.

When training the calves or lower legs the main muscles discussed are the: Gastrocnemius, Soleus, Tibialis Anterior, Tibialis Posterior, Peroneus Longus, Achilles Tendon, Extensors, and Flexors.

When training the core, the main muscles discussed are the: Rectus Abdominus, Transverse Abdominus, Serratus Anterior, Serratus Posterior, External Obliques, External Intercostal, Internal Obliques, and Erector Spinae. There is a long and unresolved debate about how much of the body should constitute the core. For beginners the focus is normally an unofficial band that could be covered by a small towel width around the stomach and lower back. For more advance fitness people and athletes the core can include as little as the towel area, and as much as the Gluteal muscles to the Latissimus Dorsi from behind and from the Transverse Abdominus to the Lower Pectoralis Major from in front. This is because more difficult body weight exercises such as the Human flag, require the person to have muscle control over most of their body.

There are at least three categories of muscles in the body – Skeletal Muscle, Smooth Muscle, and Cardiac Muscle. Skeletal Muscles are referred to as Voluntary Muscles as they can be consciously controlled. Skeletal Muscles are connected to our bones via tendons, and within each muscle there are thousands of muscle fibres. The Skeletal Muscles are the muscles responsible for movement. Smooth Muscles are detected in the stomach, intestines, and blood vessels, and are referred to as Involuntary Muscles. The primary purpose of Smooth Muscles is to cause the organs to contract to transport chemicals out of the organs. Cardiac Muscles refer to the muscles in the heart and are important for blood pumping and is also considered Involuntary Muscles.

Common issues in the Muscular system can include muscular dystrophy and muscle injuries often caused by sport or ageing.

Nervous System and the Brain

The Nervous System is divided into the CNS (Central Nervous System) and PNS Peripheral Nervous System). The CNS is comprised of the brain and spinal cord and the PNS are all the bundles of nerve fibres that run down through the body from the CNS. The PNS is divided up on a functional basis with the Somatic Nervous System in charge of our special senses and conscious decisions such as movement, the Autonomic Nervous System in charge of the unconscious and visceral activity in our body such as digestion.

Neurons are our nerve cells, and they transmit and receive information. Some send messages to the brain, some from the brain to other areas of the body. There are different types of neurons including: Motor, Sensory, Inter and Pyramidal cells. Each neuron has a cell body with branch like projections called Dendrites and a long tail called an Axon. The Axon conveys a nerve impulse away from the cell body, whilst the dendrites convey a nervous impulse towards it. An axon communicates with another nerve cell, or with a glandular cell or a muscle cell (causing it to secrete or contract). Some axons are covered in a white fatty insulating layer called Myelin which helps to transmit impulses faster.

Nerve impulses travel from neuron to neuron, or from neuron to gland or muscle cell and this is known as an action potential. Sodium and Potassium ions drive the process through a concentration gradient. Because a cell membrane is selectively permeable, there won't be a completely balanced concentration of these ions on either side, which allows for the use of concentration gradient to transmit an impulse. Within neuron cell membranes there are sodium-potassium pumps which pump out three sodium ions for every two potassium ions that it brings in. When a neuron is not doing much, there is a slightly increased positive charge of sodium ions outside the cell. These positive ions form a line on the outside of the cell membrane which then attracts a line of negatively charged ions within the cells against the internal side of the cell membrane. This then creates an electrical charge across the membrane called the Resting Membrane Charge.

When part of the cell membrane becomes excited, that part of the membrane becomes more permeable to sodium ions and the positively charged ions outside the cell suddenly all rush into the cell so that the cell is more positive on the inside compared to the outside. This process is called Depolarisation of the membrane. In response the next section of the membrane becomes excited, and the same thing happens, which excites the next bit and so on in a wave effect. Just as the sodium channels open, so do the potassium channels, but not as quickly. As they allow potassium ions out of the cell, flowing down its concentration gradient, they decrease the number of positive ions inside the cell, restoring the membrane to its resting state. This is known as repolarisation of the cell membrane.

When one of the action potentials reaches the end of a neuron it triggers the release of a neurotransmitter and these cross a gap if it exists between one neuron and the next, and then bind to receptors on the next neuron. These are synapses (where one neuron meets another). Neurotransmitters may have to cross the gap, and this gap is known as the synaptic space. Neurotransmitters are peptides or amino acids and with the CNS they may be either inhibiting or excitatory. Once it binds to a receptor it prevents any other neurotransmitter from binding and asserting its effect. The effect of the bound neurotransmitter ends when the neurotransmitter is either actively taken back into the neuron (reuptake), when it's broken down by enzymes or when it diffuses away passively from the receptor and out of the synaptic cleft.

The process of nerve impulses travelling down one neuron, potentially hopping over a gap, to continue over to the next neuron, is how most of the body's information is moved around. An impulse may be sending sensory information to the brain, or it may originate in the brain and pass all the way down to our big toe, which causes it to wiggle by contracting muscles.

The CNS consists of the brain and the spinal cord, protected by Meninges which are a special membrane. There are three meningeal layers – the Dura, the Arachnoid Mater and the Pia Mater. The Dura is the tough outmost layer. The middle Arachnoid layer is rich in blood vessels and fibres. The innermost layer, the Pia Mater is soft and communicates directly with the brain. Between the middle and inner layer is a layer of Cerebrospinal fluid. This fluid helps to cushion the CNS structures, acting as a shock absorber.

The brain is an organ composed of billions of nerve cells. Some areas of the brain appear grey because of the neuron cell bodies and unmyelinated axons. Some parts look white because of the myelinated axons. Neurons in the brain have the potential to grow many dendrites and this allows for an incredible number of potential connections between neurons. The different parts of the brain include the Cerebrum, Cerebellum, Thalamus, Hypothalamus, Hippocampus, Amygdala, Brain Stem and Spinal Cord.

Cerebrum is the site of our higher functions such as special senses, speech, conscious movement, and awareness. Within the cerebrum is the motor cortex which controls voluntary movement and the sensory cortex which receives information about sensations from the skin muscles and joints. The outer layer of the cerebrum is called the cerebral cortex and contains four lobes – the Frontal lobe (speech, emotions, planning, problem-solving, movement and reasoning), Parietal lobe (movement, orientating ourselves in space, stimuli perception and stimuli recognition), Temporal lobe (speech, memory, hearing, and emotions), and Occipital lobe (visual processing).

The Cerebellum is involved in coordination of movement and balance. The Thalamus receives vast amounts of sensory data and is involved in motor functions, and our emotions. The Hypothalamus is the body's thermostat. It is responsible for the increase in temperature during a fever and plays a role in the function of the autonomic nervous system and the endocrine system and is the conductor of the pituitary gland. The Hippocampus is involved in our learning and memory and converts short-term memories to permanent memories. Amygdala is involved in fear, emotion, and memory. Working with the Thalamus, Hypothalamus and Hippocampus, it forms the Limbic system, also known as the seat of our emotions. Brain Stem extends from the base of the brain and houses the control centres for the respiratory system and heart and is involved in vasomotor control. Spinal Cord continues down from the brain stem, travelling through the spinal column (protected by the vertebra) where it is also protected by the cerebrospinal fluid and meninges. From the spinal cord sprout nerve fibres in bundles known as Sensory ascending and Motor descending tracts that branch off to innervate the whole body

The PNS is comprised of nerves and sensory receptors. Nerves are bundles of nerve fibres wrapped in a connective tissue sheath and are big enough to be seen with the naked eye. They transmit information from the brain and spinal cord to other areas in the body via the wave effect of the action potential. The majority of the PNS includes the 43 different segments of nerves – 12 pairs of Cranial Nerves and 31 pairs of Spinal Nerves. Thirty-one pairs of spinal nerves exit from the spinal cord, and they innervate the skin and muscles on our trunk, arms, and legs.

There are two types of nerves present in the PNS – Motor (transmitting information from the CNS to elsewhere in the body) and Sensory (receive information from sensory receptors and transmit this information back up to the CNS). Since the PNS includes all the parts of the Nervous System outside of the Brain and Spinal Cord, there are many pathways and subsections including the – Somatic Nervous System, Sensory Nervous System, Sensory Receptors, Motor Nervous System, Autonomic Nervous System, Sympathetic Nervous System, Parasympathetic Nervous System, and Enteric Nervous System. Most of these systems interact either directly or through another system.

The Somatic Nervous System can be found throughout the human body. The nerves in this system deliver information from our senses to the brain and involves the voluntary control of body movements via the use of the skeletal muscles. It consists of Afferent (Sensory) and Efferent (Motor) nerves, is responsible for the Reflex Arc, uses Interneurons (connects Spinal Motor and Sensory Neurons) to perform reflexive actions, and interacts with the various other nervous systems.

There are different types and classifications of sensory receptors including Visceroceptors, Proprioceptors, Exteroceptors, Mechanoreceptors, Nociceptors, Photoreceptors, Thermoreceptors and Chemoreceptors. Visceroceptors are found within internal organs and tubes/vessels, and these let the brain know about internal changes such as blood pressure fluctuations. Proprioceptors are found within joint capsules and tendons, and these give the CNS information about where the body is in space. Exteroceptors detect external sensory information, and they are also part of the special senses. Mechanoreceptors are sensitive to touch and pressure. There are four types of Mechanoreceptors including Meissner corpuscles, Merkel cells, Ruffini corpuscles and Pacinian corpuscles. Nociceptors are sensitive to damage to tissues such as pain, extreme heat and extreme cold. Photoreceptors in the rods and cones of the retina are sensitive to light. Thermoreceptors are sensitive to temperature changes. Chemoreceptors are sensitive to chemical changes and include receptors for taste and smell as well as visceral receptors that are sensitive to changes in the plasma level of oxygen.

The Autonomic Nervous System is a section of the nervous system that controls our vital functions including breathing, circulation, heart rate, digestion, etc. It is divided into two further divisions the sympathetic (fight/flight) nervous system and the parasympathetic (rest and digest) nervous system.

The Sympathetic Nervous System is involved in the fight/flight response to perceptions of danger. The sympathetic nerve stimulation communicates with the heart to make it beat faster and more forcefully and it raises the blood pressure. It also makes breathing more rapidly and moves blood away from areas like digestion and the reproductive system and diverts it to the skeletal muscles and the brain. It dilates our pupils to allow for more light, so we can see more clearly, and triggers the release of adrenaline. It also liberates glucose and fat stores. It can also cause low appetite and low libido as side effects of the Sympathetic nervous system response. This stimulation is preparing the body for a short, sharp burst of activity, whether it is a genuine physical threat or a perceived stress. This leads to issues when the perceived stress is longer lasting.

The Parasympathetic nervous system is a strand of the nervous system that is for a healthy state of being, known as rest and digest. The parasympathetic nerves slow the heart rate and breathing and divert blood flow back to the areas that have previously been abandoned.

Lastly, the Enteric Nervous System contains approximately 500 million neurons and many variations of neurons and is often referred to as the second brain. Changes with our nutrition can have a direct impact on our primary brain's functioning via communication from our gut to our brain via the 'Gut-Brain Axis'. The Enteric Nervous System assists the body's other nervous systems in controlling motor functions, local blood flow, mucosal transport and secretions, modulating immune and endocrine functions and assisting with sensory modulation and control. When the Enteric nervous system is negatively impacted by stress and poor nutrition it can cause various other health related issues in the brain and body.

Common Nervous system related issues include prolonged stress, neurological tension, Muscular tension, poorer mental health including anxiety, mood swings, reduced dopamine and GABA production, reduced serotonin synthesis, reduced melatonin production and subsequent insomnia, impaired absorption of important nutrients, gut inflammation and brain inflammation, inaccurate hunger and craving signalling, dysregulations in the brain, poorer memory, headaches, migraines and neurological disorders such as Alzheimer's and Epilepsy.

The Brain is very complex and every time scientists think they are getting close to understanding how it functions, new discoveries and understandings are made. Some other areas of the brain not yet discussed include Broca's area, Wernicke's Area, the Corpus Callosum, the Basal Ganglia and the Pineal Gland.

Broca's Area was first described by the French physician Pierre Paul Broca in 1861. It is located in the frontal lobe and is involved in speech production and language processing. Like most areas of the brain, this is directly impacted when the CNS is overloaded. This overloading can appear as a selective speech impediment and/or as poorer memory regarding language.

Wernicke's Area was first discovered by German neurologist Carl Wernicke 1874. It is located in the temporal lobe and is involved in the comprehension of speech and written language. When this area is overloaded, the person might experience focus difficulties both with reading and auditory information.

Both the Broca's Area and Wernicke's Area work together for language processing. For example, when you hear someone speak, Wernicke's area processes the meaning, and if you decide to respond, Broca's area formulates the words and sends signals to the motor cortex to move the muscles required for speech.

Corpus Callosum

The corpus callosum connects the left and right hemispheres of the brain, allowing them to communicate and share information. The Corpus Callosum can be thought of as the brain's bridge. For instance, if you see something with your left eye (processed by the right hemisphere), the corpus callosum allows the information to be shared with the left hemisphere, which might be responsible for language processing, enabling you to describe what you see.

Basal Ganglia and Cerebrum

The basal ganglia work with the cerebrum to regulate movement and procedural learning. When learning a new skill, like riding a bike, the cerebrum plans the movement, while the basal ganglia help in fine-tuning and making the movements more automatic over time.

Cerebrum and Pineal Gland

The cerebrum, particularly the hypothalamus, influences the pineal gland's production of melatonin based on light exposure, regulating sleep patterns. For instance, as it gets dark, the hypothalamus signals the pineal gland to release melatonin, making you feel sleepy.

Prefrontal Cortex

The Prefrontal Cortex plays a major role in higher-order thinking, decision-making, and planning. It is responsible for generating and evaluating new ideas, problem-solving, and goal setting. When a person is calm, eating enough and sleeping enough, it is easier for them to utilise their prefrontal cortex's ability and improve their general decision making.

Default Mode Network

The Default Mode Network (DMN) is a network of structures in the brain crucial for imagination, daydreaming, and the ability to form spontaneous ideas.

Anterior Cingulate Cortex

The Anterior Cingulate Cortex allows individuals to switch between different ideas or solutions. It helps manage conflict and error detection, supporting the ability to think in novel ways and combine unrelated ideas into creative solutions.

Known Brain Differences in Autism (ASD) and Attention Deficit Hyperactivity Disorder (ADHD)

Both ASD and ADHD involve differences in brain structure, connectivity, and function. The specific patterns vary between the two disorders and are different for everyone. ASD is more associated with atypical social brain networks and sensory processing, while ADHD is characterised by deficits in executive function and attention networks. These differences help explain the distinct behavioural and cognitive profiles seen in individuals with these conditions.

Identified ASD Brain Differences

Cortical Thickness – recent studies have shown differences in cortical thickness in individuals with ASD, particularly in the frontal and temporal lobes, which are associated with social communication and sensory processing. These differences can lead to benefits in hyperfocus and fixated thinking as well as leading to greater difficulties regarding the rigidity in thinking and sensory sensitivities.

Amygdala and Hippocampus – The amygdala, which is involved in emotion processing, is often enlarged in children with ASD but may normalise or decrease in size in adulthood. The hippocampus, involved in memory and navigation, may also show structural differences. Again, these difference can improve some aspects of memory and reduce other memory types (an example might be better factual memory and poorer interpersonal memory).

Corpus Callosum – Reduced size and connectivity in the corpus callosum, the bundle of nerve fibres connecting the two hemispheres of the brain, have been observed in ASD. This might negatively impact emotion regulation but might improve brain dominance linking to hyperfocus.

Hyperconnectivity in Local Networks – Individuals with ASD often show increased connectivity within local brain networks but decreased connectivity between different regions. This may contribute to the intense focus on specific interests and difficulties with broader, integrative cognitive functions.

Default Mode Network (DMN) – The DMN, which is active during rest and involved in self-referential thoughts, often shows atypical connectivity in ASD. This may relate to difficulties in social cognition and perspective-taking.

Glutamate and GABA – Imbalances in excitatory (glutamate) and inhibitory (GABA) neurotransmitters have been observed in ASD. This may affect brain excitability and contribute to sensory sensitivities and other symptoms. Understanding individual nutrition needs can help regulate some of the difficulties that arise.

Serotonin – Some studies suggest altered serotonin levels in individuals with ASD, which could impact mood regulation and social behaviour.

Social and Communication Regions – Brain regions involved in social communication, such as the superior temporal sulcus and fusiform face area, often show atypical activity in ASD. This means that traditional social activities might be more difficult, however, many ASD brains can socialise, but often this looks different to the neurotypical presentation.

Sensory Processing – Over or under-reactivity to sensory stimuli in ASD is linked to differences in how sensory information is processed in the brain. This often leads to sensory sensitivity and/or sensory seeking behaviours that might appear atypical.

Identified ADHD Brain Differences

Prefrontal Cortex – The prefrontal cortex, which is responsible for executive functions like decision-making, attention, and impulse control, is often smaller or less active in individuals with ADHD. This can lead to poorer emotion regulation but may also improve a person's adaptability.

Basal Ganglia and cerebellum – Differences in the basal ganglia, particularly in the caudate nucleus, have been observed in ADHD. These structures are involved in motor control and behavioural regulation. This might lead to a person appearing "clumsier" and might be linked to poorer proprioception.

Hypoconnectivity in Large-Scale Networks – ADHD is often associated with reduced connectivity in large-scale brain networks, such as the frontoparietal network, which is involved in attention and executive function.

Default Mode Network (DMN) Dysregulation – In ADHD, there is often an issue with the DMN not deactivating properly when a person needs to focus on a task, leading to distractibility.

Dopamine and Norepinephrine – ADHD is closely linked to deficits in dopamine and norepinephrine signalling, particularly in the prefrontal cortex. These neurotransmitters are crucial for attention, motivation, and impulse control, which are typically impaired in ADHD.

Stimulant Medications – The effectiveness of stimulant medications, which increase dopamine and norepinephrine levels, supports the role of these neurotransmitters in ADHD. Stimulants in neurotypical people often stimulate the brain. However, in ADHD brains some stimulants will have the same effect, whilst other stimulants will have a relaxing effect. This can lead to difficulties and confusion with medically assisting a person experiencing ADHD related difficulites.

Attention Networks – Brain regions involved in sustaining attention, such as the dorsal attention network, often show reduced activity in ADHD.

Reward System – The brain's reward system may be underactive in ADHD, leading to difficulties with motivation and a preference for immediate rewards over delayed gratification.

Developmental Trajectories and Sensitivities in ASD and ADHD

Early Brain Overgrowth – Some studies suggest that infants and toddlers with ASD and ADHD may experience early brain overgrowth, particularly in the frontal and temporal lobes, followed by a slower rate of growth in later childhood.

Stabilisation or Decline – Over time, some of the structural brain differences in ASD may stabilise or even decline in adulthood.

Delayed Cortical Maturation – Individuals with ADHD often show a delay in the maturation of the cerebral cortex, particularly in regions associated with attention and executive function. This delay may gradually catch up in late adolescence or early adulthood.

Both ASD and ADHD involve atypical sensory processing, but the nature and impact of these sensitivities may differ between the two conditions. The difficulty with any neurodivergent differences is that there is a very large overlap between the two populations with approximately 20-70% of people with diagnosed ASD also meeting the diagnostic criteria for ADHD, and approximately 30-80% of people with diagnosed ADHD meeting the diagnostic criteria for ASD. ASD is often characterised by more extreme and varied sensory responses, while ADHD is associated with distractibility and difficulties with sensory modulation. Understanding these differences and overlaps is important for developing effective interventions and support strategies for individuals with either condition.

The sensory processing areas of the brain, particularly the somatosensory cortex and auditory cortex, often show hyperactivity in response to stimuli. The amygdala (involved in emotional responses) may also be more reactive to sensory overload, contributing to anxiety and distress.

Sensory Processing Disorder (SPD) – Some individuals with ASD symptoms may also be diagnosed with Sensory Processing Disorder (SPD), characterised by extreme responses to sensory experiences, such as strong aversions to certain textures or an inability to filter out background noise. At the time of writing, SPD is still not accepted by psychologists and psychiatrists, but this is likely to change in the near future.

Endocrine System

The Endocrine System is a series of glands that secrete hormones directly into the blood and it works as a team with the nervous system to manage many different bodily functions. The Neuroendocrine hormones are secreted by neurons into the circulating blood and influence the function of target cells at another location in the body. The Endocrine system has many purposes including – controlling and coordinating the body's metabolism, energy levels, reproduction, growth and development and assisting in the response to injury, stress and mood. There are normally eight important parts of this system including the – Hypothalamus, Pineal Body, Pituitary, Thyroid & Parathyroid, Thymus, Adrenal Gland, Pancreas and Ovary for Women and Testis for Men.

Hormones are mostly peptide molecules that act on specific target cells in other tissues. Steroid hormones are made from cholesterol. By bonding to target cells, a hormone changes the activity of those cells (increasing or inhibiting activity). The hormone responds to negative feedback in the body when there's a raised level of a hormone circulating in the blood, the receptors then feed the information back to the gland which then responds by lowering the output of the hormone.

The Pituitary gland is a pea-sized endocrine gland that is attached to the hypothalamus in the brain, that is made up of two glands – Anterior and Posterior pituitary glands. The pituitary glands are known as the Master Gland as they control or strongly influence many of the body's other glands. Its many jobs including Growth hormone production (which is important throughout life, as it assists in tissue replacement and in the metabolism of fats, proteins, and carbohydrates), Prolactin production (responsible for triggering the production of breastmilk), Thyroid stimulating hormone, Gonadotrophic hormones, Adrenocorticotrophic hormone (triggered by the hypothalamus and stimulate the release of adrenal cortex hormone and is one of the principal stress hormones) and Melanocyte-stimulating hormone (stimulates the skin's melanocytes, which release pigment/melanin).

The hypothalamus produces hormones and then these migrated down into the pituitary gland, these include – Oxytocin (helps to eject milk from the breast, is involved in uterine contractions, and is a powerful "bonding" hormone) and Anti-diuretic hormone (increase the reabsorption of water in the nephron, forming a more concentrated urine and conserving water for the body).

The Thyroid gland lies in the front of the neck below the larynx. The gland has "wings" with one on either side of the Isthmus, across the throat. It releases thyroxin and triiodothyronine which stimulates the metabolic rate in cells and stimulates growth. It also releases Calcitonin which reduces the amount of calcium in the blood.

The Parathyroid glands are four very small glands which are sunken into the thyroid gland. They release parathyroid hormone which works alongside Calcitonin to regulate calcium levels in the blood. It promotes calcium absorption in the intestines as well as increasing reabsorption of calcium from the bones. It is the counterbalance to the thyroid. When the parathyroids don't secrete enough of their hormone the lack of calcium in the blood can cause intense, excruciating muscle spasms (tetany) and convulsions.

Adrenal glands sit atop the kidneys. The middle part of the gland (medulla) secretes adrenaline (epinephrine) and noradrenaline (norepinephrine), and these are known as the fight/flight hormones. The outer part of the gland (cortex) secretes steroid hormones called glucocorticoids including cortisone. These hormones are involved in glucose, protein, and fat metabolism, promoting the mobilisation of energy stores so that the body has enough glucose to meet its needs. They also depress the immune system and inflammatory responses to divert energy away to other processes. The cortex also secretes mineralocorticoids such as aldosterone and androgens. Women post-menopause convert the androgens to oestrogen.

An excess of cortex hormones can lead to conditions such as Cushing's disease which presents with hypertension, a moon face, weight gain on the trunk, emaciated limbs, thin skin, and diabetes. A deficiency of the steroid hormones can lead to conditions such as Addison's disease which presents with fatigue, diarrhoea, and cardiovascular disease.

The fight/flight response continues, and in our modern life this can become unhelpful. When stress doesn't pass in minutes or seconds the hypothalamus directs a releasing hormone to the pituitary which in turn secretes an adrenocorticotrophic hormone (ACTH). ACTH tells the adrenal cortex to release cortisol, and this hormone primes the body to handle the perceived stress, making sure that the stored energy within the body is moved back into the bloodstream as sugar.

Cortisol is an anti-inflammatory hormone, but when the parasympathetic system doesn't start, then it can lead to the body adapting to stress. Symptoms of this include tiredness, weepiness, anxiety, agitation, poor concentration, exhaustion, tired immune system, and mental fatigue.

Gonads in women are called ovaries and their hormones are oestrogen and progesterone. Whereas male gonads are called testes and their hormone is testosterone. The pancreas is an exocrine gland within the digestive system, but it is also an endocrine gland because it has groups of cells called the Islets of Langerhans which secrete the hormones insulin, glucagon, and somatostatin into the blood. These hormones are involved in the regulation of our blood sugar levels. The thymus gland sits behind the sternum and secretes thymopoietin and thymosin, both are involved in the development of T-lymphocytes. As we age the thymus gland slows, and this leads to physical atrophies. The pineal gland helps with our circadian rhythms and is located in the roof of the third ventricle of the brain in the diencephalon. It receives information about light from our retina, and when we receive less light, it starts to secrete the hormone melatonin, contributing to our sleep patterns. Another hormone secreted by this gland is serotonin.

Common issues in the Endocrine system include Hypothyroidism, Hyperthyroidism, hormonal imbalances and Diabetes.

Adipose tissue (fat) is slowly being recognised as its own system, but for now it is recognised as part of the Endocrine System section. It utilises the blood vascular system as an information highway for the Leptin and 600 other types of messengers. Body fat sends signals to the brain, bones and other organs to regulate eating and optimise energy intake and consumption, through the use of hormones such as Leptin; and our genetics, medical conditions, Interoceptive health and other factors influence how we respond to these signals. Overeating to obesity levels can trick the immune system into thinking that the excess lipids being released in the body are intruders. The immune system then tries to do its job, becomes whelmed, bursts and then releases toxic substances into the blood vessel walls leading to various medical difficulties such as heart disease and stroke. Exercise produces a chemical known as IL-6 which can reduce the incorrect messaging, thereby reducing the accidental immune response damage.

Digestive System

The Digestive System can be said to start in the mouth with the teeth breaking down food and also includes many other body parts including the lips, mouth, pharynx, epiglottis, oesophagus, cardiac sphincter, stomach, pyloric sphincter, duodenum, bile duct, pancreatic duct, jejunum, ileum, ileocaecal valve, caecum, appendix, ascending colon, transverse colon, descending colon, sigmoid colon, rectum and anus. This system can be aided by some simple behavioural practices including eating when as relaxed as possible, chewing food until almost liquid, ensuring sufficient digestive enzymes, eating a variety of pre and probiotic foods and ensuring sufficient glutamine. Chewing food until almost liquid also allows for the rest of the digestive system to be better prepared. Saliva is released in response to the Sight and Smell of food, after taste, more is released by the Parotid, Submandibular and Sublingual Glands – The Salivary Amylase starts the Enzymatic Breakdown of Starches. Saliva is created under Autonomic control and is stimulated by the Parasympathetic nerves and inhibited by the Sympathetic nerves. Saliva production is slowed during stress states via the Sympathetic Nervous System, which can then lead to digestive difficulties as a side effect.

Swallowing food once chewed, initiates the Autonomic swallowing reflex leading to waves of Peristalsis, which in turn help move the food down the Oesophagus. The Oesophagus is lined with Epithelium and a gooey coating of Mucous to help it withstand the potential abrasive state of food. Food then moves into the Stomach via the Oesophageal Sphincter. When the Oesophageal Sphincter is working well, it stays shut unless food is entering or unless vomit is exiting. When there is a Leak, the Acidic contents can cause reflux and other issues. Food then enters the Mucous Lined Balloon shaped stomach, and then closed off at the top by the Oesophageal Sphincter and at the bottom by the Pyloric Sphincter.

When food enters the Stomach, the Hormone Gastrin (made by G-Cells) is released which triggers the release of Gastric Juice (composed of highly acidic Hydrochloric Acid, with a pH of 1 and is made by the Parietal Cells). Food is then mixed with the Gastric Juice, Mucous, Gastric Lipase, Water, and Intrinsic Factor. Gastrin also makes the Stomach Churn more to allow for the mixing of the food with the Gastric Juices. Due to the Hydrochloric Acid, the Pepsinogen is converted into Pepsin, which is the Enzyme that starts the breakdown of Proteins. Pepsinogen is inactive until it is converted into Pepsin, which is a positive, as if the Pepsinogen was always active, it could digest our body's own structural proteins.

Hydrochloric Acid also assists immune function by destroying potentially dangerous microbes. It also triggers the release of Cholecystokinin in the Duodenum, which then triggers the release of Bile and Pancreatic Juice, making the Hydrochloric Acid and important trigger for the cascade of digestive secretions. Some medications that suppress the acidity in the stomach may lead to a weakening of the digestive tract.

After Protein digestion has begun, the food is churned into a more liquid state and is now known as Chyme. After several hours, the Chyme enters the Duodenum of the Small Intestine via the Pyloric Sphincter. This may take from 1-6 hours depending on the level of fat in the meal.

The Small Intestine has 3 parts – the Duodenum, the Jejunum, and the Ileum. The Small Intestine is approximately 6-7 metres long, and squeezes the Chyme by Segmentation, which is where the small segments are closed off at a time to force food along the path. As well as digestion, the Small Intestine is also designed for absorption. The walls of the tubes are covered in Tiny Projects called Villi, which increase the surface areas available for the process of absorption. Each Villi contacts Lacteal (lymph duct), and the Lacteal is where the fat is absorbed and sent into the Lymphatic Circulation. Each Villus is covered in its own Microvilli, which further increases the surface area.

The Duodenum secretes Secretin and Cholecystokinin (as above). The Secretin triggers the release of a Bicarbonate-Rich fluid from the Pancreas which then neutralises the acidic Chyme. Secretin also has an Inhibitory effect on the Stomach, telling the Stomach it can slow down. Cholecystokinin promotes Bile Release from the Gallbladder and activates the Pancreas to release Pancreatic Juices, and these two digestive aids enter the Duodenum through the Sphincter of Oddi. Cholecystokinin has other actions. It inhibits hunger (Neuropeptide that communicates with the brain), and it also interacts with Immune receptors across the body. This leads to a dampening of the Immune System.

Pancreatic Juices continue the process of starch, fat, and protein digestion while the Bile gets busy Emulsifying fats, allowing for easier digestion from the Lipase Enzymes. Pancreatic Juices contain Proteases which are an inactive form of a protein enzyme which need to be converted by Enterokinase to prevent self-digestion. They also contain Lipases and Nucleases and Amylases.

Bile is made in the Liver by Hepatocytes and stored in the Gallbladder. Hepatocytes draw Molecules from the blood to make the Bile including Water, Bile Salts (made from Cholesterol), Inorganic Salts and Bile Pigments (derived from the breakdown of Haemoglobin from our old Red Blood Cells. Bile Pigments give our Urine and Faeces their distinctive colour. If Bile can't enter the Duodenum, we may see evidence of – poor fat absorption (Steatorrhoea/fatty faeces leading to a lighter pigment in the faeces), Yellowing of the skin/Jaundice caused by the building up of Bile Pigments in the Blood and can cause darker Urine.

Chyme passes on from the Duodenum down into the Jejunum and then into the Ileum where the Digestive process is completed. It is this process that allows our body to breakdown and use the healthy vitamins and minerals it needs from good food choices.

Malabsorption can arise for various reasons – lack of Acidity in the Stomach, lack of Pancreatic Juices or Bile entering the Duodenum, or from issues with the lining of the Intestines. This then leads to a lack of nutrients reaching the bloodstream and a lack of nutrients reaching the tissues and cells of the body. This then leads to several symptoms such as general fatigue, through to nutritional deficiencies.

Leaky Gut Syndrome suggests that the damage to the lining of the Intestine allows for large molecules such as Proteins, toxins and allergens (which normally can't cross the Epithelium of the Intestines whole) to squeeze between gaps, and entering the bloodstream triggering an immune response as they are recognised as foreign. It has many other possible causes including low dietary fibre, excess of harmful microbiota, excess alcohol, age, Crohn's disease, Cystic Fibrosis, Rheumatoid Arthritis, Atopic Eczema, HIV, NSAIDS and antibiotics, stress, Small Intestinal Bacterial Overgrowth (SIBO) (measured with specific breath test), and for people with gluten sensitivity, the Gluten Protein may trigger Zonulin (protein that increases the permeability between cells of the wall of the digestive tract). Leaky Gut can cause allergies, auto immune disorders, inflammation, neurological functioning issues, gut bacteria issues, and increase risk of mental health difficulties.

When digestion occurs correctly, the remnants of the absorbed food will now pass down through the Large Intestine (Colon). If there is prolonged stress, the Ileocecal valve and other valves may be impacted, increasing the risk of constipation, haemorrhoids, colitis and IBS. The Colon is divided into the initial Caecum (from which the enigmatic Appendix protrudes), the Ascending Colon, Transverse Colon, Descending Colon, and Sigmoid Colon. A lot of water absorption happens in the Colon and any remaining nutrients will also cross the Epithelium into the bloodstream.

However, sometimes digestion doesn't occur properly for many reasons. One of these reasons includes the liver not being able to assist the body in detoxification process well enough as the natural process of the liver turning fat-soluble toxins into water-soluble toxins is interrupted. If a person is having symptoms of nausea, morning headaches, bloodshot eyes, constipation, poorly formed stools, pain in the upper shoulders and under the rib cage or dull skin with boils and infections, it may be related to poor liver functioning. In these instances, various lifestyle changes often need to be made, and some people believe that there are detoxification methods a person can implement to assist the body's natural process. Examples of this includes use of saunas, water therapies, specific enemas, vegetable and specific vegetable juice combinations, skin brushing and hydrotherapy.

If all goes well to this stage, when the Faeces moves down to the Rectum, it stretches the walls and triggers the defecation reflex. Soluble fibres can be Prebiotic, meaning they benefit from the bacteria in your gut. When their balance is changed from – antibiotic use, medications, hormone therapy, illness, or poor diet, we can become vulnerable to a variety of digestive issues and system-wide health issues. Probiotics are helpful short term, but in the longer term, Prebiotic fibres are a very successful method for establishing a good bacterial population.

Common issues that arise regarding the digestive system and poor digestions include Diarrhoea, Constipation, IBS (Irritable Bowel Syndrome), an increase risk of insomnia, Chron's disease, Indigestion, Excessive Acid,

Inflammatory Bowel Conditions, Food Allergies, Food Intolerances and Haemorrhoids. Digestive problems are also strongly correlated with poor mental health – bidirectionally and with the most common including stress related mental illnesses such as PTSD, Anxiety and Depression, as well as various other mental health related difficulties. Our digestion requires, or at the very least, benefits from the parasympathetic nervous system being active during digestion.

Genitourinary and Reproductive System

The Reproductive System is part of the Genitourinary System, and is different for men and women, and some people are born intersex where they may have one or parts of both reproductive systems. The female reproductive system is a group of organs including the – Ovaries, Fallopian Tubes, Uterus, Cervix and Vagina, also contains the Clitoris which extends inside and outside the body. Ovulation cycles, menstruation cycles and puberty changes make the female Reproductive System more complex than the more simplified male Reproductive System. The male reproductive system includes the external organs of the Penis, Scrotum and Testicles and the internal organs of the Vas Deferens, Prostate and Urethra.

The female reproductive system is orchestrated by the hormones produced by the ovaries. Oestrogen is an important hormone for the reproductive system and there are several types including Oestradiol (very strong), Oestrone (weaker form) and Oestriol (made by the kidneys from other types of oestrogen and is the weakest). The different types of oestrogen are responsible for promoting the female secondary sex characteristics (including – breasts, soft skin, female body hair patterns and female fat distribution), maturation of ovarian follicles, contributing to skin structure, contributing to blood vessel structure and contributing to bone strength. Oestrogens stimulate the cells that have receptors for the hormone, such as breast cells and uterine cells, so that they can increase in number. Oestrogen also stimulates these cells to make more oestrogen receptors, rendering them more sensitive to the hormone.

Each month, women who are of "reproductive age" (which can vary depending on the individual person) have the potential to experience menstruation, which is a cyclical loss of the lining of the uterus. During the first half of a cycle, the ovarian follicles develop and midway through the cycle a mature follicle exits its ovum and ovulation occurs. The ovum is released by the abdominal cavity and most make their way to the safety of a fallopian tube; however, some go astray and can lead to an ectopic pregnancy. At the halfway point in the cycle, luteinizing hormone released by the pituitary, then triggers the empty follicle to mature into a structure called a corpus luteum. A corpus luteum secretes progesterone and this then supports a pregnancy if one occurs by preparing the uterus for the arrival of a fertilised egg. Should fertilisation not occur, then the thickened walls are shed, and this is lost as menstrual blood.

Menstrual and Fertility issues are common, and the cycle progresses in a rough pattern (although, every person is different and may therefore follow their own cyclic pattern). Day 1-4 is the follicular (proliferative) phase, and this is where the follicle stimulates the hormone and a small amount of luteinising hormone trigger the ovary to develop its ovarian follicles. The developing follicles produce oestrogen, and this oestrogen then encourages maturation of the ovum. On Approximately day 14 the blood oestrogen level reaches a certain level; the positive feedback mechanism causes a surge of luteinising hormone. This luteinising hormone surge causes an oestrogen surge which pushes forward the maturation of an egg cell and its subsequent release from the follicle (ovulation).

If all goes well, the egg will be taken into the fallopian tube by the wafting of the ciliated epithelium in the tubes. Approximately day 14-28 is when the secretory (luteal) phase, the luteinising hormone continues to stimulate oestrogen production and transforms the empty follicle into a corpus luteum. This secretes progesterone which prepares the lining of the uterus (endometrium) to accept a fertilised egg. The rising levels of progesterone and oestrogen inhibit the hypothalamic-pituitary gonadotrophic system. This inhibition reduces the levels of follicle stimulating and luteinising hormones. If sperm hasn't met the egg, the corpus luteum degrades and the ovarian hormones fall to their lowest point in the cycle. The ischaemic phase occurs where the blood supply to the endometrium is cut, and the lining starts to shed. And finally, on days 1-5 the Menstruation occurs where if an egg was not fertilised two weeks after ovulation, the ischaemic phase will see the start of a period. The first day of the period is day 1 of the cycle.

The male reproductive system often focuses on the prostate. The prostate is a gland, and its secretion is the fluid which is released with sperm upon ejaculation via the urethra. The prostate is located on top of the urethra and is the size of a chestnut. If it becomes enlarged, it can push on the urethra and block the flow of urine from the bladder to the urethra.

The urinary system serves a vital purpose filtering our blood and excreting urea, wastes, and surplus water. The system includes the kidneys, their ureters, the bladder, and its urethra. Each kidney is situated on either side of the spine and has a ureter which runs down to the bladder. The bladder sits in the bottom of the abdominal cavity and when it is full of urine it swells enough to be findable above your pubic bone.

The kidney filters 125ml of blood each minute, and within an hour, all your blood has been filtered through the kidneys. Within a kidney are units called nephrons, which are windy little tubules, and approximately a million exist between both kidneys. Each nephron contains Glomerulus (small spherical structure that contains glomerular capillaries), Proximal Tubule (convoluted tube that transfers the filtered substances down to the loop of the Henle), Loop of Henle (U-shaped portion of the tubule which continues from the proximal tubule and draws out more water and salt from the remaining filtrate), Distal tubule (continues from the loop of Henle and is the site of further pH management) and the Collecting duct (near the end of the process).

By the time the filtrate reaches the Collecting duct, all fluids and molecules that can be reused have been passed back into the blood and only toxins and waste remain, and this filtrate is now known as urine. The antidiuretic hormone increases the reabsorption of water in the collecting duct, concentrating the urine. In the absence of antidiuretic hormone, more urine is produced. As levels of this hormone rise, the collecting ducts become more permeable to water and more water passes back into the blood. The collecting ducts channel urine out of the kidney through the renal pelvis via the ureters (the peristalsis moves the urine) and the urine flows down into the bladder for storage. As the bladder fills, its elastic muscular walls stretch. When we urinate, the urine passes through an internal and then an external sphincter down the urethra and out of the body. The kidneys also influence lifespan via the regulation of phosphorus and communication of phosphorus levels in and with the bones.

Common genitourinary system issues include Urinary Tract Infections, Kidney Stones, four different categories of Premenstrual Syndrome (PMS-A, PMS-D, PMS-H and PMS-C), Menopause, Prostrate issues, Infertility and Endometriosis.

Integumentary System

The Integumentary System is our body's outer layer and includes the – skin, nails, hair and skin nerves and glands. It has many roles with the primary role being to act as a physical barrier to protect our body from bacteria, infection, injury and sunlight. The other roles the Integumentary System has includes – Heat Regulation, Secretion, Excretion, Sensation, Absorption and Synthesising Vitamin D.

The skin is the barrier between our internal and external environment and is one of our first lines of immune defence. The skin has It has several layers including the Epidermis, Stratum Corneum, Stratum Lucidum, Stratum Granulosum, Stratum Spinosum, Stratum Germinativum and the Dermis.

The Epidermis is the outer layer that is constantly shedding and regrowing. About 60million dead Keratinised cells from the outmost layer of the epidermis are shed each day. Blood nourishes the epidermis to fuel this high rate of renewal, and the capillaries come via the dermis. The bottom portion of the epidermis undulates (the papillae) allowing for a greater surface area for the blood supply and for nerve endings. It's the papillae that gives the skin a swirling appearance and our fingerprints.

The Stratum Corneum is known as the horny layer and is the tough outmost layer of the epidermis. These are the dead cells that a full of keratin. This layer adapts to external forces which is why the stratum corneum is tougher on the feet. The Stratum Lucidum is the clear layer that is beneath the stratum corneum and is made of cells that are almost completely broken down. The Stratum Granulosum is the granular layer and is beneath the stratum lucidum. This is where the cells are broken down, while the nuclei are still intact. Stratum Spinosum is the prickle cell layer made of living cells with membranes intact, with interlocking fibrils extending from the membranes. If the layer is subject to continued pressure, the cells undergo mitosis leading to a growth of new skin in that spot. This leads to calluses. Stratum Germinativum is the germinative layer and is the deepest layer of the Epidermis and is where the cells germinate. As well as epithelial cells, this layer also contains keratinocytes and melanocytes (which pigments the skin).

Finally, we have the Dermis. This is a layer of connective tissue which contains various structures including: blood and lymphatic vessels, hair follicles, sebaceous glands (connect to the hair follicles and the sebum that they secrete, keeps the skin waterproof and prevents it from becoming dry), sweat glands, and in the ears, there are ceruminous glands (which make wax as a defence strategy). The dermis also contains sensory nerve endings such as Merkel's cells, Meissner's corpuscles, and Pacinian corpuscles.

The skin functions as a barrier between our body and the outside world and supports the immune system. The keratinocytes make an anti-viral called Interferon, and the Langerhans cells protect us against microbes that make it through the top layer of the epidermis. The skin is waterproof and stops liquids and germs permeating the tissues beneath and locks moisture and nutrients within us.

The skin also communicates through changes in skin colouring when embarrassed, stressed, shocked or frightened. The skin also plays an important role in thermoregulation and uses the nerve endings in the touch organ (skin).

There are at least two kinds of skin healing – Epidermal healing (superficial injuries) and deep wound healing (penetrates through to the dermis or subcutaneous layer). Epidermal wound examples include grazes, abrasions, and mild burns. When the skin detects epidermal injuries, the basal cells from the stratum germinativum of the epidermis start to enlarge and move across the wound with cells from each side of the wound moving across until they meet in the middle. This meeting of the cells triggers a response called contact inhibition which stops the basal cells from enlarging and moving further. Meanwhile a hormone called 'epidermal growth factor' is released, triggering the division of basal stem cells to replace the basal cells in the stratum germinativum that originally moved up into the wound. This makes sure there is a solid base beneath the wound.

Type two injuries require a lot more healing because multiple layers are involved. There are four phases to deep wound healing including the Inflammatory, migratory, proliferative and maturation phases. The Inflammatory Phase is when a blood clot forms to seal off the gap/wound. Vasodilation of blood vessels in the vicinity of the wound allows a flood of blood that brings white blood cells to battle infection and mesenchymal cells that will develop into fibroblasts. The Migratory Phase is when the blood clot turns into a scab and epithelial cells move beneath the scab to form a bridge of cells. The fibroblasts originating from those mesenchymal cells delivered during the initial inflammatory response then begin to create scar tissue made up of collagen fibres and glycoproteins. The broken blood vessels now start to regrow, and the wound cavity is filled with a tissue known as granulation tissue. The Proliferative Phase is when a proliferation of epithelial cells underneath the scab form new skin under the scab. Lots of collagen is still being laid down to provide stability and the blood vessels continue to grow. Finally, the Maturation Phase is when the scab is lost, and the epidermis is now back to the thickness it should be. The collagen fibres become more organised and there are fewer fibroblasts present. Deeper wounds are more prone to infection and prolonged inflammation. Other common skin issues include Acne, Eczema and Psoriasis.

Our Hair has several purposes including protecting our eyes from dirt and water, keeping heat in our body, assisting in the cooling response (sweat on hair), and protecting the skin from other damage such as sun damage. The Hair consists of three parts – Hair Shaft (hair we can see), Hair Follicle (keeps hair in skin) and Hair Bulb (responsible for hair growth).

The Integumentary System has four main Glands – the Sudoriferous Glands, Sebaceous Glands, Ceruminous Glands and Mammary Glands. The Sudoriferous Glands secrete sweat through the skin through the pores and hair follicles; the Sebaceous Glands produce natural body oil; the Ceruminous Glands secrete ear wax; and the Mammary Glands are the glands on the person's chest and in female they produce milk after giving birth.

Common integumentary system issues include skin disease, hair loss, poor scalp, nail infection, Eczema, Psoriasis and skin cancer.

Immune System

The Immune System (including the Lymphatic system again) is immensely complex as it has interactions with most, if not all our body systems. As such only the basics of the Immune system will be discussed here.

The body has specific and nonspecific immune responses (cell responses). Nonspecific Immunity cells and structures do various other jobs including immunity. The skin physically protects our internal environment from any substance, particle, or microbe, and has Keratinocytes that produce interferons to protect us from viruses, as well as Langerhans cells that lie deeper in the skin that combat potential microbes or debris that penetrates the outer layer. We have the mucous membranes that act as a barrier with their sticky mucous trapping particles debris and microbes. It becomes a liquid when heated so when our body temperature rises during a fever, the mucous liquefies and then runs freely from the body (such as a runny nose) to expel the trapped microbes from the body. When we suppress the mild to moderate fever with medication, we stop the body's natural response which leaves the mucous sticky and congestion elevates, obviously more serious fevers need to be brought back under control.

Tears are another example of nonspecific immunity, washing away particles that have landed on our eye. Tears are filled with powerful disinfectant Lysozyme. Earwax also contains this, and both physically trap and chemically deal with microbes. Vomiting, defaecating, sneezing and coughing help to get rid of unfriendly particles and microbes. The stomach's Hydrochloric acid destroys microbes.

The white blood cell known as the Macrophage, performs nonspecific phagocytosis on several particles and microbes. They appear as groups at sites where microbes are likely to enter the body such as in the tonsils, in the liver sinusoids (called Kupffer cells) and in our alveoli in the lungs. Their cells change shape so that they can physically engulf whatever they are unhappy with, to seal it off completely and break it down. Neutrophils also carry out phagocytosis.

Once the body is away from the infecting microbe, the hypothalamus tweaks the thermostat, and our temperature rises. The body then feels cold and shivery as the blood from the peripheries is drawn to the core to heat up the core. You may look pale because the peripheral vessels have constricted to bring the blood to the core. Following this, you start to feel hot as the body tries to make it inhospitable for the microbe so that the microbe can't replicate as quickly. The higher temperature also tells our immune system to hasten its action. To help the body then cool down so it doesn't do damage, the body will start sweating and you look flushed, to cool the body as quickly as possible. Sweat also helps rid the body of any toxins that may have accumulated. Only when a fever fails to break, especially in young children, that intervention is required.

The immune system also coordinates a more specific/targeted immune response to specific microbes and toxins which involves the white blood cells called Lymphocytes. There are two types known as B-Cells (made and mature in the red bone marrow) and T-Cells (made in red bone marrow but mature in thymus). The neuropeptide receptors on the white blood cells communicate with the other lymphocytes, by interacting through peptides called cytokines, lymphokines, chemokines, and interleukins and their receptors. Some professionals believe that the thymus can be assisted by gently tapping the sternum for approximately twenty repetitions, three times a day. It is believed that the vibrations assist in "awakening" the immune cells.

Each lymphocyte is active against one specific antigen. An antigen is a marker found on a microbe, particle or toxin and the lymphocytes have receptors for the antigens. When a lymphocyte encounters a microbe, toxin or particle which has the antigen that fits its specific receptor, the lymphocyte activates and the body recognises the activation and initiates the fever, fatigue, and other symptoms such as rashes, spots, sneezing, coughing, and vomiting. Once they are active the B-cells and T-cells differentiate into both Effector Cells (go to work against intruder) and Memory Cells (to allow for a quicker response in future exposures of the same antigen).

Effector B-cells make immunoglobulins and antibodies. Antibodies are carefully synthesised protein molecules that have been built to bind specifically to the antigen that triggered the B-cells that made it. These antibodies then bind to the antigen on the microbe or foreign body and this binding renders the invader to be more vulnerable to further immune attack. The effector T-cells are divided into two groups – Killer cells (directly attack antigens) and Helper cells (support the activity of B-cells by secreting Interleukins).

Inherited immunity is the immunity we are born with due to our genetic history and genes. There are two types of acquired immunity – natural and artificial. Naturally acquired immunity occurs when our body responds to an antigen and produces antibodies at the same time producing memory cells which remember that antigen, or through breastmilk, or through placenta. Artificially acquired immunity occurs through vaccinations and immunisations, where the vaccine delivers a measured quantity of dead or deactivated pathogenic particles so that the immune response is triggered without the development of the disease. Immunisation introduces an amount of artificially produced antibodies into the bloodstream, and this infers short term immunity.

In response to infection or damage in a tissue the immune system triggers an inflammatory response. Neutrophils are sent first and are followed by Granulocytes, and both these white blood cells release chemicals such as Prostaglandins and Histamine which ensure the continuation of the inflammatory response. Local capillaries dilate and increase in permeability to allow more blood to an area and to allow the necessary cells needed to repair the damage or to fight the infections. The tissue swells due to this fluid accumulation and the swelling serves a purpose – to help contain the infection, discouraging it from spreading and to protect the area. The fluid in the tissue is turned into a gel by clotting factors, further helping to trap the infection. Physiology signs of inflammation include Swelling (fluid leaking into tissues from capillaries), Heat (influx of blood and activity in the area), Redness (influx of blood to the area), Pain (squashing of nerve endings by the swelling tissue) and a Loss of function (swelling and the pain).

The body's immune system has hopefully now kept the infection under control, and now the tissue can begin to repair. Many phagocytic white blood cells enter the area and start a cleaning operation, tidying the debris from the repair job. Neutrophils, then Basophils then Macrophages undertake this job. When the tissue is tidied, the white blood cells leave, and we enter the period of resolution. If resolution isn't achieved, it leads to chronic inflammation such as arthritis.

The Lymphatic system's main role is drainage (channelling away fluid and preventing too much storage of the fluid), and it also cleans this fluid and acts as element of the immune system by neutralising potential harmful particles and microbes. The Lymphatic system is best at removing larger particles such as proteins and particulate matter from tissue fluid. The lymphatic process starts within the tissue as tiny capillaries and then become increasingly large, passing through lymph nodes, and emptying into the systemic circulation via the subclavian veins (deep vein that is the major venous channel that drains the upper extremities).

The lymphatic vessels are extremely permeable, which allows for the easy uptake of interstitial fluid. The lymphatic capillary networks "snake" into tissue spaces, draining away the interstitial fluid, and this is where cells empty their waste products. Once within a lymphatic vessel that fluid becomes known as lymph. Lymph contains molecules that are too large to enter the blood through blood vessel walls, like proteins, and if there has been cellular repair occurring the lymph might contain pus, dead cells, bacteria, or even cancerous cells that are all taken up from the interstitial fluid. The nodes will help to filter out and deal with this debris so that it won't end in the blood. When fats are broken down in the digestive tract, they enter the lymphatic ducts called lacteal, which then turn the lymph a milk colour.

Lymph moves slowly through the vessel as it relies on our veins upon the squeezing action of muscles. The more we walk and move, the more we promote our lymphatic circulation. If there are issues with lymphatic drainage, it can cause Oedema. Lymphatic vessels have a good capacity for regrowth into an undersupplied area, so if lymph vessels have become damaged or blocked, drainage will be resumed once the new vessels grow.

Lymph nodes are also known as glands, and we often are more aware of these when we are unwell. Hundreds of tiny bean-shaped nodes are scattered around the body. Some areas of the body have clusters of these nodes such as the groin, behind the knee, in armpit and in neck. If they're swollen, we notice them and may feel the need to massage this area, which may spread an infection. Within each lymph node is lymphoid tissue, with reticular fibres, connective tissue, and many lymphocytes. Lymphatic vessels enter a node at one end, and the lymph is filtered through the fibrous lymphatic tissue. The lymphocytes engulf the cell fragments, microbes, cancerous cells, and other foreign bodies. This is known as Phagocytosis, where a white blood cell such as a lymphocyte swallows a potentially harmful foreign body, dissolving it into harmless fragments. If the lymphocytes find a particle they can't break down, it's stored within the node to stop it from spreading in the body.

Common immune system issues include fever, autoimmune diseases and deficiencies (such as Multiple Sclerosis), an increase in allergic responses, chronic fatigue syndrome, minor infections increasing in frequency, less tolerance, less ability to recover and poorer health across the entire body.

Fascia

Fascia is its own system, as it has a large influence on multiple other body systems, with some scientists calling fascia "the largest sensory organ in the body". Modern yoga instructors also appreciate this and reportedly incorporate the fascia theory as part of the instructor course or recommended readings.

A basic definition of fascia is – the thin casing of connective tissue that surrounds and holds every organ, blood vessel, bone, nerve fibre and muscle in place. It can be found throughout the body and people as far back as DaVinci were discussing this. There are at least seven fascial lines in our body connecting everything together as part of the fascial web including the – Superficial Front Line, Superficial Back Line, Lateral Line, Spiral Line, Arm Line, Functional Line and Deep Front Line. Some scientists and surgeons suggest that the cerebral membrane should also be included in the fascia conversation.

Fascia is the Connective Tissues involved in the movement system, nervous system, immune system, and digestive system. It is the collagenous/fibrous/connective tissues body wide and provides a tensional force distribution network. It helps compartmentalise and separate body areas and assists with communication of strength, force and tension. It also contains mechanoreceptors that respond to mechanical pressure and formation change. For example, the spinal disks are considered fascia and healthy movement of the spine helps strengthen spine fascia.

Fascia also plays a role in the coordination of movement and communicates with our Autonomic Nervous System and Sympathetic Nervous System. Regarding movement, fascia is covered in nerve endings including Proprioceptors and Interoceptors. It also disperses impacts as a tensegrity structure within the body allowing for constant feedback that allows all the muscles to contract and react appropriately. As well as this, fascia also conveys force between muscles and is capable of reforming itself in response to common movement patterns in order to strengthen along specific lines (completed by our fibroblasts). This allows for our movement choices to influence our fascia and is an important part of our movement and overall health including our postural control.

Fascia consists of Cells called Fibroblasts which produce Collagen and other materials needed for the connective tissue that are part of the body's healing process (however, too many Fibroblasts means stiffer movement). There are 2 types of fibres (Collagen and Elastic Fibres), Hyaluronic Acid and Glycosaminoglycan (thickening agent that helps bind to water) and Water (three quarters of fascia is made up of bound water) that make up fascia. Hydration of the fascia is important for overall body health. Active and passive movement helps the fascia replace the bound water like a sponge, and gravity squeezes fluid out of the fascia while moving. Heat improves movement in the fascia and body and a well hydrated fascia allows for decreases in inflammation. Acidity in the fascia, thickens fluid and reduces movement and tightens fascia.

Like most of the human body, fascia is very efficient at adapting. This is positive when we have healthy movement behaviours but becomes unhelpful in examples such as poor posture where the fascia will assist in holding the poor posture. Mobility becomes stuck if positions are held for too long due to fascia supporting how we hold the body. Approximately 40% of our muscle load is distributed to other body functions via the fascia and the majority of musculoskeletal injuries relate to fascial damage. Clumped fascia can also lead to nerve pain by pushing against the nerve areas whilst simultaneously restricting movement further. This can make pain management more difficult than it already is for people with back injuries and other complicated injuries. When one of the larger fascial areas known as the thoracal-lumber fascia which connects the shoulders to the hips is immobilised for too long due to injury, it restricts the sliding ability of fascia and can also increase nerve pain from overproduction of the collagen from the fibroblasts. Stress also has been found to have negative side effects on fascial health such as thickening, tightening and increasing the amount of TGF (Transforming Growth Factor) material.

Specific manual manoeuvring (fascial related massage and specific acupuncture approaches) can assist in releasing some of the tightness and improve mobility, and in some cases, reduce pain. When improvement does occur, it can take up to one year of regular fascial massage (and potentially acupuncture) and appropriate movement activities.

Another interesting idea regarding fascia is that it unofficially has two main different rhythms when it comes to adaptation and change. The first rhythm is the play of tension and compression that communicates around the body as a mechanical vibration, so that it travels at the speed of sound (approximately 1100kph), which is more than three times faster than the nervous system. An example is when a person steps from one room to another where there is an unexpected drop or rise. The nervous system, setting the springs of responsive muscles to the expected level of floor is unprepared for the sharp shock that comes. This is then absorbed instead almost entirely by the fascial system over a fraction of a second, as every nuance of changing mechanical forces is noticed and communicated along the fabric of the fibrous fascial net. The second fascial rhythm is the compensatory speed which can slowly adjust over many years and the body's fascial adjusts and pulls other areas to compensate for injury or weakness. The fascia can also move independently with these rhythms (without muscle stimulation).

Recent research into fascia has found there is approximately an 80% correlation between the sites of traditional acupuncture meridian points and lines and fascial plane locations and fascial lines. The idea of meridians will be covered in the Qi Gong section of the book. Research has also found potential pain receptors within the fascia itself. Fascia Surrounds almost everything in the body. The traditional idea of the classroom skeleton has now been scientifically disproven by fascial related research. The tensegrity understanding of the fascia clearly demonstrates that the previous rigidity associated with the skeleton is incorrect and that future research into fascia is warranted. This research can assist with treating and preventing various muscular, immune, skeletal and other medical diseases that currently have poor treatment outcomes.

Mitochondria

Mitochondria are responsible for most of the useful energy derived from the breakdown of carbohydrates and fatty acids, which is converted to ATP for use as the body's energy at the cellular level. Most mitochondrial proteins are translated on free cytosolic ribosomes and imported into the organelle by specific targeting signals. Mitochondria have their own DNA, which is separate from the cell's nuclear DNA. Until recently, mitochondrial DNA was thought to be inherited maternally only and codes for proteins essential for the mitochondrion's function. However, the most recent research has strongly suggested that mitochondria DNA is transmitted/inherited biparentally.

Mitochondria are central to the functioning of nearly every system in the body, and their health is critical to overall well-being. Nitric Oxide usually acts as a signalling molecule and assists to 'tie the cell's different commitments to its metabolic budget'. Nitric Oxide promotes the formation of mitochondria and enhances the cell's capacity for oxidative metabolism, so disturbances in signalling can lead to mitochondrial damage and may result in neurodegenerative diseases and dysfunction.

Mutations in mitochondrial DNA can lead to a variety of genetic disorders, often affecting organs and tissues that require a lot of energy, like muscles and the brain. Dysfunction in mitochondrial processes can lead to a wide range of diseases and health issues such as increased ageing, cardiovascular diseases, neurodegeneration, metabolic syndrome, oxidative stress, mitochondrial diabetes and cancer. This highlights the importance of maintaining mitochondrial health through proper nutrition, exercise, and lifestyle choices.

Structure &Function Summary of Mitochondria:

Mitochondria are bonded by a double-membrane system, consisting of inner and outer membranes separated by an intermembrane space. The outer membrane is relatively permeable and contains proteins known as porins, which allow molecules to pass through which form channels that allow the free diffusion of molecules smaller than about 6000 daltons. These molecules can enter the intermembrane space, but most of them cannot pass the impermeable inner membrane. whereas the intermembrane space is chemically equivalent to the cytosol with respect to the small molecules it contains, the matrix contains a highly selected set of these molecules. The inner membrane is highly specialised. Its lipid bilayer contains a high proportion of the "double" phospholipid cardiolipin, which has four fatty acids rather than two and may help to make the membrane especially impermeable to ions. This membrane also contains a variety of transport proteins that make it selectively permeable to those small molecules that are metabolised or required by the many mitochondrial enzymes concentrated in the matrix.

The matrix enzymes include those that metabolise pyruvate and fatty acids to produce acetyl CoA and those that oxidise acetyl CoA in the citric acid cycle. The principal end-products of this oxidation are CO_2, which is released from the cell as waste, and NADH, which is the main source of electrons for transport along the respiratory chain—the name given to the electron-transport chain in mitochondria. The enzymes of the respiratory chain are embedded in the inner mitochondrial membrane, and they are essential to the process of oxidative phosphorylation, which generates most of the animal cell's ATP. The inner membrane forms numerous folds called Cristae, which extend into the Matrix of the organelle. These convolutions greatly increase the area of the inner membrane, so that in a liver cell, for example, it constitutes about one-third of the total cell membrane. The mitochondrial matrix contains the mitochondrial DNA, ribosomes, soluble enzymes, small organic molecules, nucleotide cofactors, and inorganic ions.

The primary roles of Mitochondria include energy production, regulation of metabolic activity, apoptosis (assisting in the management of programmed cell death), calcium storage, heat production and the generation of Reactive Oxygen Species (ROS) which assist in cell signalling and homeostasis. Like almost everything in the human body, Mitochondria work with the various body systems to achieve the complex functioning and homeostasis.

Summary of Mitochondria's relationship with the Body Systems

The mitochondria work as part of our body's systems.

For the circulatory system and the muscular system, the mitochondria provide energy that is required for the continuous contraction and relaxation of the heart muscle which relies on the ATP produced by the mitochondria to pump blood effectively throughout the body, and contribute to the regulation of vascular tone and blood flow through the production of ROS and NO.

For the respiratory system the mitochondria use oxygen in the electron transport chain to produce energy, and supply energy needed for the muscles in the diaphragm to contract and facilitate respiration. For the skeletal system the mitochondria are again involved in the energy metabolism of the osteoblasts and osteoclasts.

For the nervous system the mitochondria supply the ATP required for synaptic transmission, action potential propagation and brain function. It is also involved in the regulation of ROS which are critical for neuron signalling and protection against neurodegenerative diseases.

For the endocrine system the mitochondria are involved in the synthesis of steroid hormones in the endocrine glands and is crucial for the production of hormones such as cortisol, testosterone and oestrogen. Mitochondria also help to regulate energy balance through its involvement in the thyroid hormone pathway.

For the digestive system the mitochondria provide energy that is required for the active transport of nutrients across the intestinal lining. In the liver it assists in the detoxification process and the metabolism of fats, proteins and carbohydrates.

For the integumentary system the mitochondria assist skin health by supplying energy for the repair and regeneration of skin cells and help in the production of collagen. Mitochondria are also involved in the body's response to UV radiation by managing oxidative stress and assisting in the repair of damaged cells in the skin.

For the immune system the mitochondria provide the energy needed for the activation and function of immune cells and are involved in the regulation of the inflammatory response. Finally, for the fascia system, the mitochondria supply the energy required for the synthesis of collagen and other extracellular matrix components.

Summary and the System Interplay

Since the body is a complex organic machine, our various systems all have different roles, but communicate with each other either directly or via other systems. The human body is very complex and our knowledge of it is improving and changing almost daily. Many different cultures have different paradigms they use when investigating and understanding the human body as will be seen in some of the next sections. I also note here that the modern "western" scientific approach is very good at understanding the depth and complexities of one specific area of the human, leading to fantastic specialists. However, the body doesn't work in silos (isolation), and there is still plenty of room for other health approaches to assist in this "western" scientific model as these other approaches are often more eclectic and incorporate multiple body systems, but often do not have the specialist knowledge of any one system.

An example of this interconnectivity can be seen when discussing posture, emotions, and perception. The motor cortex of the brain indirectly communicates with our nervous system (often via the hypothalamus). A drastic change in the motor cortex will have parallel effects on thinking and feeling. A practical example of this is when a person changes their posture from having pronated shoulders to opening the chest and gently drawing the shoulders back. This muscular postural change leads to changes in the motor cortex which leads to changes in conscious thought and emotional perception of self. These changes may include subconsciously changing from feeling downtrodden to feeling more confidence. Another brief example of the body's interconnectivity is the physical outwards expression of emotions. All emotions are expressed through both visceral motor changes and stereotyped somatic motor responses, especially movements of the facial muscles. The social and cultural influences often determine what emotions are encouraged or supressed, however, the physical expression of emotions is similar across most cultures.

Emotions also directly influence our body's ability to heal. As will be discussed later, stress increases inflammation and not only increases risk of various medical conditions and difficulties but also reduces the rate of healing and recovery. Alternatively, positive emotions such as calm, relaxed or happy, can directly increase the rate of healing and recovery. This has been shown in many studies over the last fifty years, with perhaps the most famous being from the 1980's. Patients recovering from surgery who looked at nature, and felt calmer as a result, healed faster than patients who looked at a traditional blank hospital wall.

The body's job is to find homeostasis, meaning finding a balance. This is not the same as being as healthy as possible. Our behaviours, emotions, genetics, internal psychology and other environmental factors all determine what our body's homeostasis is.

Key Points & Relevant Personal/Professional Experiences

Western medicine's focus on disease and symptom management

Western medicine's approach is often known as 'The Medical Model'. Whilst prevention is the best option for health, we cannot prevent all disease and degeneration. When disease or degeneration occurs, the medical model can be very helpful in recovery. The many specialists available within the medical model allows for targeted treatments that assist in recovery and often management. The medical model emphasises the diagnosis, treatment and prevention of specific conditions and symptoms, often under strict scientific and evidence-based practices. It focuses on specific organs, tissues, known pathogens, symptoms and body systems to provide specialist and targeted care. The medical model emphasises measurable and observable changes which when combined with utilising technological advances makes understanding the disease or degeneration easier.

Symptom alleviation and treatment often involves addressing the symptoms directly, providing immediate or fast relief through medications, surgery and similar interventions. Chronic diseases and conditions are often managed the same way with the assistance of more intense medications that are used to manage the symptoms but may not address the root causes.

Another key area of the medical model includes the acute and emergency care area. This area is involved in handling acute presentations including illness and injury and can often involve medication, surgery and use of advanced technology such as MRI (Magnetic Resonance Imaging), CT (Computed Tomography) scans, blood tests and X-Rays.

One of the strengths but also limitations of the medical model is its reliance and sometimes overreliance on the use of pharmaceutical medicine. The reliance allows medical professionals and the people being treated a simplified approach to management and recovery. However, when the focus is on symptom management and the person presents with multiple illnesses and symptoms (known as comorbidity), they can be prescribed pharmaceutical medicine for the symptoms of each illness and difficulty, and sometimes even prescribed medicine for the symptoms caused by other medicine. This is often known as 'Polypharmacy' and has led to some people being prescribed more than fifteen different medications by various medical practitioners, which drastically increase the risk of adverse side effects for the person being treated and is unfortunately still supported by the medical model. Another risk of the medical model is that by pharmaceutically treating the symptoms the person is presenting with; it can often lead to other health issues across the various body systems leading to an increased for more medication. As a psychologist, I have seen many clients who were prescribed more than ten different medications simultaneously leading to the effective management of symptoms, but not addressing the root cause of the person's health difficulties.

However, with the rise of improved blood tests, genetic testing such as pharmacogenomics and other advances, it is hoped that the practice of Polypharmacy will reduce or at least be monitored more effectively.

The role of specialists, primary care physicians, and allied health professionals

The medical model has a brilliant framework with a strong reliance on specialists which can include specialist medical doctors and nurses, as well as various other health workers and allied health workers who are designed to work as a team. When the specialists and professionals work as a team, the management of disease and degeneration symptoms often have positive outcomes, which is the primary benefit of the medical model. However, financial resources, individual malpractice, lack of note sharing, professionals overvaluing their input and undervaluing other professionals' input, and political pressures, often lead to poorer practice and poorer outcomes. Too often as a psychologist, I see professionals overvaluing their opinion and not working as a team, leading to poorer health outcomes for the people they are supposed to be helping. However, governing bodies such as AHPRA (Australian Health Practitioner Regulation Agency) in Australia, exist to limit these negatives and allow professionals and people being treated, formal pathways to report negative practices.

There is an ever-increasing number of specialists a person can see to improve their health and wellbeing under this medical model. Examples of medical specialists include Anaesthetists, Cardiologists (General, Interventional, Pediatric) Dermatologists, Emergency Medicine Physicians, Endocrinologists, Gastroenterologists, Geriatricians, General Practitioners, Haematologists, Infectious Disease Specialists, Nephrologists (Kidney Specialists), Neurologists, Obstetricians/Gynaecologists (OB-GYNs), Oncologists (Medical, Radiation, Surgical), Ophthalmologists, Orthopaedic Surgeons, Otolaryngologists (ENT Specialists), Paediatricians, Plastic Surgeons, Psychiatrists, Pulmonologists, Radiologists (Diagnostic, Interventional), Rheumatologists, Surgeons (General, Cardiothoracic, Neurosurgery, etc.) and Urologists.

Examples of allied health professionals that are important in the medical model include Art Therapists, Chiropractors, Dietitians/Nutritionists, Exercise Physiologists, Medical Laboratory Scientists/Technicians, Music Therapists, Occupational Therapists, Pharmacists, Phlebotomists, Physical Therapists, Psychologists, Radiologic Technologists (MRI, CT, X-ray), Respiratory Therapists, Social Workers, Sonographers, Speech-Language Pathologists and Youth Workers.

Examples of Nurse professionals and medical support roles important to the medical model include Clinical Nurse Specialists (CNSs), Emergency Medical Technicians (EMTs), Medical Assistants, Nurse Educators, Nurse Managers, Nurse Midwives, Nurse Practitioners (NPs) (Acute Care, Family, Neonatal, etc.), Paediatric Nurses, Paramedics, Pharmacy Technicians, Registered Nurse Anesthetists (CRNAs) and Surgical Technologists.

Counselling Psychology and Psychiatry

The most common confusion for clients in mental health is the differences between psychology and psychiatry. Simply discussed Psychology studies the mind and behaviour, focusing on cognitive processes, emotions, and social interactions, as well as detailed quantitative and qualitative assessments. Psychiatry is a branch of medicine specialising in diagnosing and treating mental health disorders, often using medical and therapeutic interventions. However, in practice there is often a large overlap between the two. In Australia, a psychologist cannot prescribed medication, but a psychiatrist can, and the psychiatrist is often called upon by other medical professionals to prescribe medication for more complex mental illness presentations such as schizophrenia.

A counselling psychologist in Australia has often completed their undergraduate degree and postgraduate degree in psychology (also known as psychological science at some universities). Following this they will either complete their master's degree to be recognised as a clinical psychologist or complete an internship of 3000 practice hours to be recognised as a general psychologist. This process can take between six and seven years in total. A psychiatrist often completes their medical degree, then their rotations and finally their specialisation and this process can take eleven to thirteen years.

Psychology of Human Body Brain Connection Introduction

The theme of this book has been how interconnected the body is, and this chapter will continue this theme. The human body is ridiculously connected, making both healing and injury more complex. Counselling psychology is considered mental health, but the brain is physical; thought and emotion changes produce physical changes in the body, and life experiences affect us physically. This chapter will attempt to summarise this idea of mental health being physical, and will look at the effects of stress, trauma, substance misuse, and poor nutrition on mental health. This chapter won't be specifically focusing on therapy frameworks for several reasons. Firstly, my summaries would not do the frameworks justice, and secondly there is too much overlap between the frameworks, despite what some passionate single framework practitioners may believe.

Many health professionals understand mental health is just as physical as a broken arm but with several important differences – the physical changes often happen in the most complex organ in our body (the brain), we can't touch or readily observe the brain so it is harder for the individual and treating professional to understand (and even when we see the brain through FMRIs, MRIs and PET scans, there is still a lot of guess work), and the research into understanding the brain is still only in its infancy. We also know now that we store stress all over our body, with some of the main skeletomuscular related areas including the trapezius, sternocleidomastoids (SCM), temporomandibular joints (TMJ), head, chest, psoas, pectorals, scapula region, diaphragm, pelvis, and iliotibial band.

Some of the things we have strong evidence for, regarding mental health and it's physical nature include – ASD may be organic with recent research suggesting a 70-90% genetic component, Schizophrenia may be strongly linked to dopamine (as evidenced by schizophrenia medication and Parkinson's disease studies), brain injuries can change an entire personality of an individual, ASD, ADHD, Bipolar Disorder, Major Depression, and Schizophrenia have a strong genetic component (with at least 2 genes being found to be responsible for regulating the flow of calcium into neurons and impacting their efficiency), poor nutrition not only affects cognitive functioning and maturation but also affects endocrine health and maturation in young people, and nutrient imbalances such as Copper overload, Vitamin B-6 deficiency, Zinc deficiency, Methyl/folate imbalances, Oxidative stress overload and Amino acid imbalances are risk factors for developing antisocial personality disorder, clinical depression, anorexia, obsessive-compulsive disorder, and schizoaffective disorder.

As stated, trauma can influence our gene expression, and not only increases a person's risk of developing mental and physical illnesses but becomes a genetic risk factor for the next four generations if the gene expression occurs prior to reproducing. Some of our genes are turned off or on at birth depending on who the carrier is (male through sperm or female through egg) for example eye colour, height, etc. Whilst there are approximately 80 known imprinted genes, the research is not clear as to which ones are specific to the father or mother and how the genes choose which to express or recode. The complexity of our genetics, combined with professionals no longer being allowed to do direct genetic experimentation on human trials (due to ethics and morals), means we can only discuss risk factors. The research from the Minnesota Twin study strongly suggested that genes played a very strong part in behaviour expression, psychopathology, substance abuse, divorce, and leadership when comparing maternal twins. Epigenetics explains why people such as maternal twins who have the same genetic start (99% the same) can look and behaviour differently by late childhood.

Once we think of mental health as more than thoughts and behaviours, but physical changes or differences, it become easier to understand the importance and relationship between epigenetics and mental health. Research by Harvard university has supported this idea. They found that positive influences such as supportive relationships and opportunities for learning and negative influences such as environmental stress or toxins leave a unique epigenetic signature on the genes' methyl markers, and this can increase the chances of the person and their future generations developing mental illness or other medical illnesses. The importance of movement and or exercise is also becoming discussed more frequently in mental health settings. More mental health professionals are starting to understand the importance of looking at the whole body and not just the mind in a silo. For some people formal exercise is too difficult, and for these people the idea of moving more may be sufficient. A research group developed an acronym known as NEAT standing for Non-Exercise Activity Thermogenesis, meaning to move more.

A detailed example of mental health impacting our physical health is discussed in the 'Anatomy Trains' book. 'All negative emotion', says Feldenkrais, 'is expressed as flexion'. Hunch of anger, the slump of depression, or the cringe of fear many times and in many different forms. They all involve flexion. Among the quadrupeds, as we have noted, only humans put all their most vulnerable parts literally 'up front' for all to see. Subtly or obviously, people protect those sensitive parts: a retraction in the groin, a tight belly, a pulled-in chest. It is natural enough that when they feel threatened, humans should return toward a younger (primary foetal curve) or more protected (quadrupedal) posture.

As well as flexion in the body as an emotion response, negative emotion regularly produces hyperextension of the upper neck, not flexion as seen when the mastoid process is brought closer to the pubic bone. This not only protects the organs along the front, but also retracts the neck into hyperextension, bringing the head forward and down. The total posture, then, of the startled person involves rigidity in the legs, plus trunk and arm flexion, coupled with upper neck hyperextension. The problem comes when the startled posture is maintained (due to prolonged stress or perceived threat). This posture and its variants can affect nearly every human function negatively, though breathing in particular is restricted by shortening of the SFL (Superficial Front Line). When discussing posture it is important to remember that our posture is not static, rather it is a dynamic counterbalance that is in constant change. Understanding this, can be beneficial as it allows a person to frame their posture as changeable rather than feeling stuck in a poor posture triggered by negative emotional, behavioural and environmental experiences. Our posture, like our cognitive functioning and overall health is changeable.

Easy breathing depends on upward and outward movement of the ribs, as well as a reciprocal relationship between the pelvic and respiratory diaphragms. The shortened SFL pulls the head forward and down, requiring compensatory tightening in both the back and the front that restricts rib movement. Shortening in the groin, if the protective tightness proceeds beyond the rectus abdominis into the legs, throws off the balance between the respiratory and pelvic diaphragms, resulting in over-reliance on the front of the diaphragm for breathing. The real, original startle response is marked by an explosive exhale; the maintained startle response shows a decided postural tendency to be stuck on the exhale side of the breath cycle, which in turn can accompany a trip through depression. This highlights the importance of having the body and the mind assisted together, where possible, such as in somatic psychology (i.e., Paired Muscle Relaxation).

Environmental influences such as trauma as well as life choices and/or life opportunities directly impacts our health and functioning, including our own gene expression (epigenetics). These environmental influences can then have the ongoing side effect of influencing future generations (up to four generations) if the gene expression occurs prior to reproducing. This means trauma can genetically be passed on, and positive life choices can also genetically be passed on. If a mother has PTSD the trauma can be passed through epigenetics impacting birth weight, and other physical stress responses such as metabolising cortisol. If a father has PTSD the trauma can be passed through epigenetics increasing rate of depression in the child.

What we call stress is often our cortisol and adrenaline response, which can be expressed physically as discussed, and can even be smelled by animals with dogs/cats/horses having the most research to back this up. Stress ages our DNA, increases the epigenetic expression of harmful responses, weakens our immune system, (often causing or being strongly correlated with various medical difficulties such as Fibromyalgia, heart failure, mitochondrial dysfunction, etc.) and lessens our cognitive resources (people when stressed, often report feeling like they have lost their memory or intelligence). I will briefly discuss the stress response in this subchapter including what is known as the fight and flight response. Fight, Flight, Freeze, Fawn, Feint, Flag, Flop and Fidget are all variations of the stress response a person can experience. The research history behind the terms influences how they are explained and which ones a professional may choose to use in a therapeutic setting.

The freeze response can be seen when a deer is caught in the headlights. It involves the orienting reflex, an inborn impulse to turn your sensory organs towards a source of stimulation. Here the goal is to "stop, look, and listen" to better understand the situation and to determine if there is a threat. Your pupils will dilate as you turn your head towards the sound or sights that sparked your interest or concern. Most importantly, freeze occurs in preparation for action and is short lived.

The flight and fight stress responses are maintained by the sympathetic nervous system. This process involves initial attempts to flee danger; however, if it is impossible to escape you will resort to the fight response. The sympathetic nervous system increases blood flow to the heart and muscles of the arms and legs accompanied by faster and deeper breathing. Simultaneously, skin will grow cold, and digestion is inhibited.

The fright response is a stress or trauma response that we see when flight or fight do not restore safety or there is no escape. The fright response may take over with feelings of panic dizziness, nausea, light headedness, tingling, and numbing. According to Schauer & Elbert (2010), this stage is considered to have "dual autonomic activation" seen in abrupt and disjointed alternations between sympathetic and parasympathetic nervous system actions. It is in this stage that we see the initial symptoms of dissociation.

The flag response occurs if there is still no resolution of the threatening situation. The flag response is the collapse, helplessness, and despair that signals parasympathetic based nervous system shutdown and immobilization. Dissociative reactions dominate this phase. Voluntary movements including speech become more difficult, sounds become distant, vision blurs, and numbness prevails. The heart rate and blood pressure drop, sometimes rapidly, which in some cases leads to the sixth stage, "faint.

The faint or flop response appears to serve several purposes from an evolutionary and survival perspective. When the body succumbs to a horizontal position blood supply increases to the brain. Furthermore, fainting is connected to disgust; an emotional response which rejects toxic or poisonous material. According to Schauer & Elbert, experiencing or even witnessing horrific events such as forced physical or sexual violence can trigger vasovagal syncope (Vagus nerve dysregulation) which promotes nausea, loss of bowel control, vomiting, and fainting.

The fawn response is often associated with trauma that involved a lot of emotional and attachment trauma. The person may be overtly people pleasers, scared to say what they think (overly passive communicator), rarely talks about themselves, may use flattery to avoid conflict, empathic to a point of negative functioning for self, easily manipulated or exploited, and a strong focus on social standing or social acceptance.

Finally, a less severe response that still impacts functioning and occurs as stress or trauma response is known as the fidgeting response. Fidgeting is often associated with boredom. However, whilst there are other causes such as stimulation seeking or sensory seeking, fidgeting can also be a trauma response when used as a distracting or grounding tool. This is often overlooked due to the minimal impact on functioning.

Relating to the fight and flight responses, some people can develop phobias of internal body states, such as the phobia of the upper body feeling "too relaxed". This is because the internal body state can then be associated with previous stress or trauma, and the brain then sees the relaxed state as a potential threat state. This can have obvious repercussions for a person trying to overcome their trauma related difficulties and is something professionals must think about when assisting people.

Adverse Childhood Experiences (ACE) include any negative, often traumatic experiences during the childhood (such as emotional, sexual, physical abuse, neglect) and can include discrimination. As the brain's right hemisphere develops first, any trauma received during young childhood impacts many areas of a person's mental health including increasing or suppressing negative emotions, withdrawal behaviours, difficulty with interpersonal and internal emotional attunement, difficulties regulating prosody (tone of voice), unhealthy neural circuits of attachment, poorer overall awareness of body, poorer self-regulation, difficulties experiencing or demonstrating empathy, and poorer intuition.

The trauma definition that I use for clients is "any event where a person feels helpless, hopeless or powerless may be catalogued by the brain as trauma", even if a person doesn't meet the DSM-V related criteria for a trauma diagnosis. This will often impact a person's biological, psychological and social functioning. There are many variations of health frameworks that are used by professionals and individuals. The fundamental framework I use is known as the Biopsychosocial model. The model includes the biological aspect of our health, the psychological aspect of our health and the social aspect of our health. Its simplicity allows for almost any person to learn it and expand on their understanding of their health. It also has room for added complexities when needed, such as expanding on one of the three areas in more detail such as social health. Many people forget that humans are animals, and we are a social species of animal, that greatly benefits from social interaction and can have poorer health when our own individual social needs are not met (under or over social stimulation). This does mean that everyone needs to be an extrovert, rather it is helpful for people to understand their own social needs and aim to have these needs met. Research has suggested that healthy social engagement and social bonding can lead to internal feelings of emotional safety and emotional bonding and lead to healthy external behaviours of interpersonal contact and healthy proximity.

What we call emotions are neural and chemical states and pathways that are always changing. Emotions influence and are influenced by our perceptions, interpretation of internal and external stimuli, content of our memories, how our memories are encoded and retrieved, are attentional capacity and other executive functioning, our motivations, our gut health and many more. Our perception of reality dictates how we interpret (not see) the world around us. This perception is largely influenced by our life history, then the emotion at the time of the event/thing, then the context of the event of thing, then the event/thing itself, in real time, i.e., watching your favourite sports team or musician with someone who has an opposing view. As well as influence our daily idea of life, perception also influences personal and professional language around health such as blaming women, age, gender identity, etc. This is seen in the history and ongoing use of language when discussing mental illnesses and some physical illnesses. Medical and insurance-based terminology is still in practice across the globe today and often can lead to a negative perception of a person, sometimes even leading to the dehumanising of the person struggling. This may then lead to both the professional and the person struggling to have negative perceptions of self, leading to poorer mental and physical outcomes. By changing our language, we can change perception, and in some cases, this can lead to building or installing hope.

The importance of hope is often understated, but our brains are wired for change, and hope can encourage this neuroplasticity. This means we are all capable of thought and behaviour change, with a lot of work and a bit of good luck. This can be important for many people to know, as often when people are struggling, they can feel that this is the new normal rather than understanding that positive change is possible. Professionals can assist with this by changing language. When a person is dehumanised, hopeless, etc. they can then develop various unhelpful thinking styles. These often arise following trauma and can increase the stress responses in the body. Whilst there are many examples, some include catastrophising, overgeneralising and disqualifying the positive. If the person and or professional can help challenge these unhelpful thinking styles, it can lead a person towards hope, which may improve the outcome for the person struggling.

Regarding stress, there are some useful brain-change related information. Firstly, our hippocampus forms at ages two to three, which is why our earliest memory is rarely before two years of age. The more emotion, the better the memory's accuracy, and negative emotion can be more powerful than positive. However, too much negative/trauma emotion can lead to fuzzy memory. If there is too much emotion during an event, the stored memory can be fuzzy and then the person can inappropriately be triggered or have inappropriate generalisations and associations. I.e., all dogs are dangerous, instead of one specific dog is dangerous. The thalamus sorts incoming sights and sounds and then signals the appropriate parts of the cortex. This raw information is then interpreted by the cortex and an assessment of threat is made. If threat is relevant, the amygdala will then trigger the fear response, and emotional significance is added. Finally, the BNST (Bed Nucleus of the Stria Terminalis) perpetuates the fear response causing longer term unease regarding the stimulus as a safety response. However, this safety response if left on for too long, can turn into anxiety, trauma responses or other health difficulties.

Towards the end of this chapter various tools that people can self-practice, will be discussed. Many of these tools have modernised names and western scientific research as evidence, but most of these tools are still variations of mindfulness and meditation. I feel it is important to remember this, and to also remember that much of the current mindfulness and meditation practices originated from Tibetan, Buddhist and other Eastern practices including Yoga, Tai Chi, Qi Gong and Martial Arts.

Stress and Trauma Brain and Body changes

Stress and the cortisol response is good in small doses, however an excessive release of cortisol due to long-term stress damages our nerves and triggers a worsening stress response. The presence of stress provides an indicator that we are struggling, the feeling of a loss of control which leads to ineffective thinking. Sustained stress is a warning sign that a person needs to change or adjust their thinking or environment. Stress can be helpful for motivation, as it can help improve our focus, speed, and overall output, in small doses. It is the accumulation of unproductive stress that has the greatest negative impact on our functioning. It can remain active when we are constantly thinking and feeling pressure and/or when we feel powerless/hopeless. Positive change is still moving into the unknown, so a level of conflicting emotions is present.

There are many physical and mental health impacts of prolonged cortisol and adrenaline resulting from stress and trauma. The physical, emotional and behavioural impacts of prolonged stress and trauma include: a shutting down of the frontal cortex and associated regions, anxiety, aphantasia (lack of cognitive visual ability), attachment trauma responses (ambivalent and disorganised attachment are most common in people who experienced childhood trauma), autoimmune disorders (rheumatoid arthritis, multiple sclerosis, lupus, thyroid issues, Latent Autoimmune Diabetes of Adulthood/LADA diabetes, fibromyalgia), breathing pattern disorders, bronchial dilation, cardiovascular diseases, chronic inflammatory responses, chronic pain, contracting rectum, darkness on the eyelids, depression, diarrhoea or constipation, digestive disorders (Gastroesophageal Reflux Disease/GERD, microbiome issues), dilated pupils, dissociative disorders (Pain, substance misuse, eating disorders), eating disorders, emotional distress and other physiological response, excess glutamate triggering cell death in the brain, faster more shallow breathing, feelings of whelm, fluid retention, focus difficulties, gastrointestinal issues, gritting of teeth (TMJ), high acidity in the body (which can lead to a general stiffening of the body's fascial system), increase in heart rate and blood pressure, increase in sweating or shivering, increased anger and aggression, increasing heart contractions, inhibition of digestion, inhibition of salivation, insomnia and other sleep disturbances, intermittent explosive disorder, Irritable Bowel Syndrome (IBS), jelly-like legs, loss of hair quantity and health, memory difficulties, mitochondrial illnesses (mitochondrial diabetes, chronic fatigue syndrome, fibromyalgia), nausea, pain, perception/attitude towards food, poorer nail health, poorer self-image, postural issues, premature orgasm ejaculation, puffiness under eyes, relaxing bladder leading to increased risk of peeing, rigid or overly tense muscles, self-harming behaviours and urges (NSSI), stationary hyperventilation (observed as excessive sighing), stimulating epinephrine and norepinephrine release to unhealthy levels, stimulating glucose releases (increasing) by the liver, substance misuse, trembling, type 2 diabetes, and weight changes (loss of muscle, holding of fat).

As a side note here regarding medical illness relating to stress, it has been suggested that up to 66% of people with Fibromyalgia, and 76% of people with Rheumatoid Arthritis have trauma in their history, as well as at least 50% of people with IBS have a complex childhood trauma history.

Complex trauma is also a major risk factor of Central sensitisation. Central sensitisation is a condition of the nervous system that is associated with the development and maintenance of chronic pain. It has two main characteristics that both involve a heightened sensitivity to pain and the sensation of touch, and these are known as allodynia (person experiences pain with things that are normally not painful) and hyperalgesia (when a stimulus that is typically painful is perceived as more painful than it should).

The disordered breathing mentioned above, leads to increased muscular pain, skeletal displacement, hyperventilation syndrome (over breathing), brain hypoxia, depression and headaches, and an overactive SCM (jutting out). This can also lead to jaw tightness, poorer posture and pain in the back and spine.

Grief and loss is another effect that trauma can cause but is rarely discussed. If the trauma has impacted the person's functioning to such a point that they lose the ability to complete their previous level of normal behaviours, they may experience an emotional response known as grief and loss. This can then become a further risk factor for developing other mental illness as well as worsening or developing poorer self-image.

Sensory sensitivities can also arise following trauma. Trauma can trigger or worsen sensory sensitivities such as light, heat, movement etc. This can be a direct response where the nerves are in a constant heightened or stress response level or can be a specific paired association trauma response where the sensory sensitivities is only triggered when specific environmental and internal conditions are met.

Prolonged stress and subsequent prolonged exposure to cortisol in the body, can also become a risk factor for developing psychosis. If a person already has a genetic risk factor such as a family member with hallucinations, then prolonged exposure to stress increases the risk of this genetic factor being expressed. The person may experience a single episode of psychosis and then never again have this experience, or the single episode may change into regular experiences of hallucinations or delusions. Several brain related studies have demonstrated that when a person is experiencing a hallucination, the same area of the brain is firing as if that hallucination is real. For example, a person experiencing a tactile hallucination, will have the same tactile region firing in their brain, therefore making it real to that person. This psychosis related response to prolonged stress can also become confused and intertwined with other physical, sensory and neurological pain and experiences. Trauma can cause this prolonged exposure to cortisol if the person is unable to process the negative event(s) and subsequent impacts, further highlighting the need for sufficient support.

Prolonged stress and trauma can impact our sleep, leading to insomnia and impacting our circadian rhythm. Symptoms of a disrupted circadian rhythm caused by stress include – adrenaline, premenstrual tension, cravings, headaches, SCM and trapezius muscle pain and spasms, alcohol intolerance, indigestion, vertigo, poor memory, palpitations, ligament, laxity, insomnia, less tolerance for environmental changes, more emotionally reactive, poor concentration, fatigue, confusion, depression, physical weakness, food allergies, autoimmune diseases, hives and sensitivity to sunlight. Insomnia also increases the risk of low blood sugar (hypoglycaemia). For those who may experience hypoglycaemia, eating a small snack (55-85gram) before sleep can help break the cycle of middle insomnia. Lastly, Circadian rhythm disruption can turn into a disorder which may then lead to bipolar and bulimia. ADHD people can also be greatly impacted by a disrupted circadian rhythm more than non-ADHD people, and young people with symptoms of ADHD can find their symptoms drastically lessen through correct and healthy chronotype behaviours. Some nutrients that can assist in resetting the circadian rhythm include Melatonin and vitamin B12 (Methylcobalamin or Hydroxocobalamin are good, NOT Cyanocobalamin). Melatonin may help to regulate the if the person is experiencing circadian rhythm difficulties and B12 may assist in regulating the cortisol peak. Other nutrients and behaviours that may assist in lessening the insomnia and circadian rhythm difficulties include a magnesium sulphate bath, Epsom salt bath, oral magnesium dependent on bowel tolerance, sleep hygiene, and balancing hormones through diet/natural supplements.

Self-Image is one aspect of trauma that can be overlooked by professionals. Most people who have experienced trauma, have lower self-image, have poorer interpersonal boundaries and rarely use assertive communication. This low self-image can lead to avoidance behaviours such as passive communication as well as physical avoidance or isolation. These are known as safety behaviours. These help a person to feel emotionally safe but can often lead to further difficulties later in life. They can be very effective and even encouraged in the short term to allow a person to complete tasks, however, when replied upon they can become problematic.

This low self-image can be reinforced by societal expectations and can lead to a person wearing a metaphorical mask. When a person has experienced trauma, and a lower self-image is the response, the mask and need to fit in socially, may often be used as its own type of safety behaviour. Societal ideas and education provided operate bidirectionally. It suppresses every non-conformist tendency through penalties of withdrawal of support and simultaneously encourages the individual to form values that force them to overcome and discard spontaneous desires. This may lead to the mask forming and becoming more entrenched in the person's idea of self. The need for constant support from other people may become so great that most people spend the larger part of their lives fortifying their masks. Often enough the individual becomes so adjusted to their mask, and identifies with it so completely, that they no longer sense any individual drive or satisfaction. This can lead to unhealthy ideas of self, goals, and of others.

As well as safety behaviours, the passive communication may lead to a build-up of unprocessed negative emotions which can cause a person to become more angry and eventually aggressive. Anger is often a symptom emotion triggered by other emotions and may lead to aggression, but doesn't have to, with the right knowledge and skill development.

Finally, pain is a physical and medical difficulty that can be triggered or worsened by prolonged stress or trauma. Stress leads to muscle tension, which leads to pain, which leads to stress. Pain is an inflammation response that can lead to and be caused by substance misuse. Often caused by injury, poor nutrition and trauma. It can be helpful to understand that pain is part physical, part mental. The physical part of pain is the physical damage done to the nerves, muscle, organ etc, and includes the inflammation response that then elicits a pain response. The mental side of pain includes our relationship with pain, how much attention we give the physical pain and our level of stress or calm.

The hippocampus is surrounded by cortisol receptors. Overtime cortisol can cause atrophy and destroy the hippocampus, impacting trauma responses and memory. Some sensory information such as smell can skip the hippocampus and is thought to be the most powerful memory/trigger as it goes straight to the amygdala.

The amygdala is also known as the body's fear brain or smoke alarm, which means when the smell reaches the amygdala, the corresponding memory may be stored inaccurately depending on what emotion was being experienced at the time of the smell. A person with hyperarousal can learn to ignore danger signals in the amygdala in an unhelpful way such as police officers who are used to being in this state can then miss actual danger in their environment or when a car alarm continues to be active for more than three hours, at first, we keep checking it, but eventually we will ignore it.

The Insula and Amygdala communicate perceived negatives and feeds this system of negative thoughts and emotions and can cause an addiction to negative experiences. Smells and touch information bypass the Thalamus and go straight to the amygdala. This is why smells can evoke stronger positive or negative memories or emotions than sights, or sounds, and is important to remember for professionals who assist in trauma management. Paired Association triggers hyper-reactivity through the Insula. Depression and some addictions involve a hypo-activation of Insula often, because of complex trauma. A poorer functioning insula may impact one of senses known as Interoception. Interoception is a person's internal body awareness. Most people will understand when they are hungry, understand roughly what emotion they are feeling etc. When a person has trauma from a young age, it is a common response for the Insula in our brain to shrink thereby lessening or limiting the person's ability to understand their own body and emotions. This can lead to poorer outcomes across most life areas including health, relationships, employment, etc., and can be a strong correlator for many medical conditions. It also can impact our ability to understand pain such as knowing when pain is safe (safe stretching), and when is not safe (being punched). The poor internal awareness of a person's emotion can be a form of poor Interoception and is known as Alexithymia.

The last brain area discussed here is known as the Cingulate Cortex. It is the self-regulation Centre, part of the Cerebral Cortex and Limbic systems and assists behaviour and thought decisions. It is used to assist with cognitive dissonance, and error detection centre but can often be impacted by trauma leading to poorer decision making, more negative or extreme thinking and greater emotional intensity. When the Cingulate Cortex is overactive the error detection centre is overactive, and this may lead to OCD.

Psychology of Sensory Systems

This section will discuss our body's senses mostly from a mental health related angle. It will briefly discuss two alternative models for looking at our senses and then discuss one of the more current scientific models for our body's sensory experiences.

There is one model that breaks down our sensory experiences into 33 different senses. The 33-sense model has some outdated information and doesn't include other sensory inputs but can still be of interest to people when discussing the body's sensory information. This model separates the proposed 33 senses into nine sensory sections. Vision includes light, colour, red, green and blue wave; Hearing its own category; Smell is noted to have more than 2000 receptor types (not detailed); Taste includes sweet, salt, sour, bitter and umami; Touch includes light touch and pressure; Pain includes cutaneous, somatic and visceral; Mechanoreception includes balance, rotational acceleration, linear acceleration, proprioception, kinaesthesis, muscle stretch via Golgi tendon organs and muscle stretch via muscle spindles; Temperature includes heat and old; and Interoceptors include blood pressure, arterial blood pressure, central venous blood pressure, head blood temperature, blood oxygen content, cerebrospinal fluid pH, plasma osmotic pressure (thirst), artery-vein blood glucose difference (hunger), lung inflation, bladder stretch and full stomach.

There is another radical model of the senses that looks at 50 possible senses, although their definition of a sense is different to the traditional model. Again, some of their model may not be accurate, but has a lot of very useful information regarding our body both internally and externally. Their model has four main categories including Radiation Sensitivities, Feeling Sensitivities, Chemical Sensitivities and Mental Sensitivities.

The radiation sensitivities include sense of light and sight (including polarised light), sense of seeing without eyes, sense of colour, sense of moods and identities attached to colour, sense of one's visibility or invisibility, sensitivity to invisible radiation, sense of temperature and temperature change, sense of season and electromagnetic sense and polarity (including the ability to generate current as in brain waves or other energies).

The feeling sensitivities include hearing (including resonance, vibration, sonar, ultrasonic frequencies), awareness of pressure, sensitivity to gravity, sense of excretion, feel (particularly touch) on the skin, sense of weight and balance, space or proximity sense, Coriolis sense (Earth's rotation), and the sense of motion (body movement sensations and sense of mobility).

The chemical sensitivities include smell with and beyond the nose, taste with and beyond the mouth, appetite and hunger for food water and air, food obtaining urges including hunting and killing, humidity sense including thirst, evaporation control, acumen to find water and hormonal sense such as pheromones and other chemical stimuli.

The mental sensitivities include pain (external and external), mental or spiritual distress, sense of fear (dread of injury, death, or attack), procreative urges (sex awareness, courting, love, mating, child rearing), sense of play (sport, humour, pleasure, laughter), sense of physical place (navigation senses, position of celestial bodies), sense of time, sense of electromagnetic fields, sense of weather changes, sense of emotional place, (community, belonging, support, trust, and thankfulness), sense of self, (friendship, companionship, and power), domineering and territorial sense, colonising sense inc. receptive awareness of one's fellow creatures, horticultural sense and ability to cultivate, language and articulation sense, (used to express feelings and convey information), sense of humility, appreciation, and ethics, senses of form and design, reasoning, (including memory, logic and science), sense of mind and consciousness, intuition or subconscious deduction, aesthetic sense (creativity, appreciation of music and beauty), psychic capacity, sense of biological/astral time, (awareness of past-present-future events), capacity to hypnotise other creatures, relaxation and sleep (dreaming, meditation, brain wave awareness), sense of pupation- cocoon building and metamorphosis, sense of excessive stress and capitulation, sense of survival by joining a more established organism and spiritual sense (conscience, sublime love, ecstasy, sin, profound sorrow and sacrifice).

The nine basic senses commonly used in psychology include taste, touch, sight, sound and smell, as well as Interoception, Vestibular, Proprioception and Exteroception. Taste, touch, sight, sound and smell are the five most well-known senses, and it is because of Aristotle that many people still believe that we only have five senses. Three of the five basic senses (sight, sound, and smell) are known as having double organs – two eyes, two ears and two nostrils, which is suggested to have been useful in the wild from an evolutionary perspective. The Vestibular sense is responsible for balance, postural control, eye movements and alertness, but too much vestibular input reaching the brain may make a person feel nauseous. Proprioception is our body's awareness in space and is also involved in balance and the grading of force and pressure. Exteroception is how environmental sensory information impacts our functioning and is often referred to in more detail when discussing sensory quadrants or sensory modulation.

Interoception can be explained as the body's internal body awareness. This internal body awareness can encompass hunger, fullness, thirst, pain, illness, body temperature, sleepiness, toileting needs, anger, anxiety, distractions, focus, calm, boredom, sadness, personal space needs, time perception, and many more. When a person has poor Interoception regarding their internal emotional experiences this can lead to Alexithymia. Alexithymia is when a person struggles to identify their own emotions and as a result will often miss the emotional and physical warning signs when they are stressed, struggling or other. This can then lead to disproportionate responses to smaller stressful events or stimuli. It is very common in people who have experienced childhood trauma (as the brain's safety response) and neurodivergent people. A simple way of explaining this is a person without Alexithymia, experiences warning signs of their emotions, then physiological changes and finally behaviours; whereas people with alexithymia often only understand their emotion based on physical and behaviour change only. Whilst this has the minor benefit of not consciously stressing over smaller stressors, it drastically increases the risk factor for developing stress related mental and physical illnesses.

Another one of body's senses is known as Neuroception. It is the neural detection of safety or threat based on the unconscious bodily awareness. This then triggers reflexive bodily changes in psychological states that serve as neural platforms for specific domains of behaviour. This is very helpful when the threat is shorter-term but becomes an issue (often leading to illness) when a person cannot not return to the rest state.

When discussing our body's senses in a health and mental health setting it is often helpful to look at if a person experiences the senses within the average range of if they have hypo and hyper responses. People who have experienced trauma and neurodivergent people are more likely to have sensory difficulties. One way of investigating sensory experiences is known as the Sensory Quadrants. The sensory quadrants model includes low registration, sensation seeking, sensory sensitivity and sensory avoiding responses. The person will answer questions with a qualified psychologist or mental health OT who then assists the person understanding what their responses mean on a Likert-like scale of one to five ('much less than most people' to 'much more than most people').

Another way of exploring the level of sensory input a person experiences is known as Sensory Modulation. Dr. Ayres' sensory modulation looks at three sensory modulation types (Sensory Sensitive, Sensory Slow and Sensory Seeking). When a person's sense is sensitive it means their brain doesn't block enough of the sensory input and as a result, their brain is hyperresponsive, such as experiencing moderate sounds as intense sounds. When a person's sense is slow it means their brain blocks too much of the sensory input and as a result their brain is hyporesponsive, such as experiencing strong smells as neutral. Finally, when a person's sense leads to seeking behaviours, it means the person is seeking or craving that specific sensory input to relax or stimulate themselves. A person can be sensitive in one sense and slow in another. Organic (from birth) brain difference, medical difficulties, trauma responses, brain injuries and other, may cause a person's senses to be sensitive or slow or seeking. It can be useful for a person to understand their own sensory needs to make their life more comfortable and to lessen the risk of developing a mental or physical illness or having inappropriate behavioural responses to sensory stimuli.

As discussed, impacts of sensory overload or sensitivity occurs when the brain becomes overloaded by sensory information from the environment. This can lead to an increased risk of anxiety, increased risk of social isolation and avoidance as a safety behaviour, poorer focus, poor cognitive ability, poorer emotional understanding and management, larger even inappropriate or disproportionate emotional responses to stimuli, avoidance of specific foods, and can lead to sensory anxiety. Sensory anxiety is when a person experiences the traditional physical, behavioural and emotional difficulties of anxiety, but the cause is sensory related. This can make it difficult for a person to understand why they may be struggling and can make it difficult for them to seek appropriate professional assistance. The person experiences anxiety due to the discussed sensory overload, impacting and metaphorically, shutting down their frontal regions and triggering larger emotional responses.

A person who is sensory slow can also have behavioural difficulties and risks. A person who is sensory slow regarding smell and taste may be less likely to know if a food or chemical that isn't labelled is still okay to use or consume, the person who is sensory slow for sound may play their music too loudly leaving to socially related difficulties, a person who is sensory slow for touch may apply inappropriate levels of force when picking up objects and a person who is sensory slow for sight may damage their eyes from overexposure to artificial light more easily than the average person.

A sensory sensitive and sensory slow experience may lead to sensory seeking behaviours. Sensory seeking is when the person seeks the specific sensory input to help them calm, focus, etc. The behaviours can be small in practice such as smelling own cologne but can lead to social and other difficulties. It may lead to odd or socially unacceptable seeking behaviours such as sniffing people, licking objects, playing music too loudly in quiet areas, etc.

Our emotions also directly influence how we experience our sensory world. When a person is emotionally elevated (including happiness, excitement, stress or trauma reexperiencing), their sensory experience often heightens. This can include heightened external experiences such as taste, touch, sight, sound, smell, or heightened internal experiences such as feeling the heart rate increase. This again demonstrates the multidirectional communication within our body and its many systems.

Enteric Nervous System (nutrition and mental health)

Due to the discussed stress responses in the body, people will often either eat more or eat less when stressed. When the body is chasing a chemical high (comfort eating), the person will often eat more food of a poorer quality. This assists in the person' low mood for a short time, but leads to further low mood, fatigue and increases the risk of developing negative food and eating behaviours. When the body's stress response draws blood away from the digestive system and sends it to the muscles, the person may eat less as their food related stress response. This is because the idea of food, or the chewing of food may trigger nausea, or they may have less appetite due to the slowed digestive system. Furthermore, during this stress response, some people may experience nausea when chewing food due to the salivation response telling the digestive system to get ready, but the digestive system having less available blood to assist in the process.

When the quality of food (based on health) is poorer for an extended period of time, it can lead to a poorer microbiome. A poor microbiome is a risk factor regarding a person's psychological ability to manage and process trauma events. This is because the stomach is our second brain and what we eat impacts our mental health and vice versa. Our stomach communicates to our main brain via our gut-brain axis (enteric nervous system) and via our central nervous system and we have over 100 million nerve cells in the stomach. As well as the quality of food, we need to eat enough calories for our body including our brain. Our front brain requires a lot of calories often gained from glucose being converted from carbs. If we don't consume enough calories for our body, then the front brain doesn't receive enough fuel to perform its higher duties. As well as this, if we don't consume enough calories for our body longer term, we can start to lose muscle which may lead to an increase in joint pain and inflammation in the body.

The Microbiome Revolution: Modbiotics, Prebiotics, and Probiotics for Optimal Health

Brief Microbiome Explanation

Microbiome is still a developing area of science as such there are two primary definitions. Ther first definition states that the Microbiome refers to the entire habitat, including the microorganisms (bacteria, archaea, lower and higher eukaryotes, and viruses), their genomes (i.e., genes), and the surrounding environmental conditions. The second definition states that the metagenome of the human microbiome is the total DNA content of microbes inhabiting our bodies and is variable between individuals. The DNA difference between individuals is minimal, however, individual's microbiome can vary greatly.

Some microorganisms that humans host are commensal, meaning that they co-exist without harming humans and others have a mutualistic relationship with their human hosts. Certain microorganisms perform tasks that are known to be useful to the person, but the role of most of them is not well understood. Those that are expected to be present, and that under normal circumstances do not cause disease, are sometimes deemed normal flora or normal microbiota. The individual's microbiome begins from birth, can improve from breast milk, and continues to interact with the environment. Microbes interact with specific markers that are secreted by cells or found on their surfaces and use these chemical cues to "know" where to develop. This provides evidence that the individual's DNA directly influences what microbes survive after they enter the person. The first two years of life is considered the most important and a process of mutual selection between the baby and the microbe occurs. The microbiome changes after the age of two as a result of diet, antibiotics, new environments, stress, etc. The microbiome includes more than bacteria, and includes viruses, fungi, archaea, and single-celled eukaryotes.

The human genome that each baby inherits from their parents includes approximately twenty thousand genes, whereas the collective genomes of the microbiome is approximately eight million genes. Genes act as a set of instructions to produce a protein that performs tasks. For example, carbohydrates such as sugar and starch are a class of chemical compounds that are synthesised by all living organisms and are extremely diverse. During digestion the carbohydrates are broken down to provide the person with energy. Human genome has less than twenty carbohydrate-digesting enzymes, meaning the individual relies on the gut bacterium genome to digest the carbohydrates.

Bacterial genomes can change quicker that the human genome, leading to bacteria that are distantly related exchanging genetic material, which provides selective advantages in a particular environment. This is helpful but can also lead to unwanted human side effects such as antibiotic resistance being shared across bacterial genomes. Broad-spectrum antibiotics can have a profound and often long-lasting effect on the body's microbiome, with the antibiotic being used to treat the infection or disease, but also having the unwanted human side effect of increasing risk of future infection.

Microbes form "communities" with the three most common being the skin, mouth and gut. Microbes live on all skin surfaces as well as within the skin's pores and sweat glands, and along hair shafts. The skin microbe composition varies with dry areas having fewer and different microbes than moist or oily areas. Approximately one thousand microbial species have been found in the human mouth, with a person hosting between 100-200 species. There are different microhabitats including the tooth surface, tongue, cheek and gums. The line between oral health and diseases seems to depend on maintaining a well-functioning community of microbes that exist in harmony with the immune system.

The gut contains the largest, densest and most diverse microbial community in the human body, with the microbial community in the human large intestine containing one hundred billion to one trillion cells per millimetre. The gut microbiome acts as a bioreactor, helping to extract energy and nutrients from the food we eat, and protects against pathogens, and is in constant communication with the immune system. The gut microbiome has multiple complex effects on the human metabolism. Changes to the composition of the microbiome have been linked to various inflammatory diseases such as Bowel disease, autoimmune disorders, inflammatory bowel disease, Chron's disease, diabetes, asthma, cancer, coeliac disease, heart diseases, anxiety, insomnia and obesity. Some diseases are associated with a disturbance (altered proportions of various normal "members") in the microbial community. Some human gut microorganisms benefit the person by fermenting dietary fibre into short-chain fatty acids (SCFAs), such as acetic acid and butyric acid, which are then absorbed by the person, and Intestinal bacteria also play a role in synthesising vitamin B and vitamin K as well as metabolising bile acids, sterols, and xenobiotics (Prebiotics). Fermented foods such as yoghurt, cheese, and contain sauerkraut microbes that are similar to those found in the Gastrointestinal tract and are known as 'Probiotics'. Consuming a combination of these can assist in the positive change of the microbiome.

The foods we eat directly influence these processes and the flora and microbiota in our gut. Here we will briefly look at Probiotics, Prebiotics, Modbiotics & Synbiotics and Antibiotics.

Modbiotics and Synbiotics

Modbiotics may be beneficial for the body for people who have a poorer gut microbiome. A modbiotic is a type of prebiotic that helps to modify and regulate the gut microbiome. Some research has suggested that the modern diet contains too many overprocessed foods which have an adverse impact on our guts microbiome, leading to various diseases. Natural sources of modbiotics include Acai berry, Apples, Barley sprout, Black Cherry fruit, Broccoli, Cacao fruit powder, Cinnamon bark, Cranberry, Daikon Radish fruit, Ginger root, Kale leaf and sprout, Larch Heartwood, Nutmeg powder, Pomegranate fruit and peel, Rosella flower, Rosemary leaf, Schisandra berry and Turmeric powder.

Synbiotics refers to food ingredients or dietary supplements that combine probiotics and prebiotics in a synergistic form (work better together). Some synergistic food combination examples include Apples with oatmeal, Olives with garlic, Peas and quinoa, Raw cheese and flaxseed bread, and Yogurt, Blueberries, and slightly unripe bananas.

Role of Prebiotics

A simple way to think about Prebiotics is that they help to "grow the garden". Prebiotics are often referred to as soluble indigestible fibre which helps clean the colon, encourages health microbes to be released, improves satiation and assists the microbiome "garden" in the colon by assisting the probiotics and microbiota to flourish and lessen the harmful bacteria to propagate. Examples include raw and cooked onions, garlic, Jerusalem artichokes, leeks, asparagus, wheat, beans, bananas, agave, dandelion root and chicory root. Chia is also a useful prebiotic as it contains soluble and insoluble fibre and is rich in omega three and is best when soaked in water prior to consumption.

Probiotics

Using the garden analogy, Probiotics can be thought of as "adding to the garden". Probiotics are also known as Psycho-biotics and there are 400-500 different kinds of healthy microbiota in our gut. Probiotics can be used to promote a healthy digestive system, prevent infections, prevent diarrhoea, lessen inflammation, improve immune health, assists in the production of Vitamins K, B, Lactic acid and Folate, assists in GABA and Serotonin production and lessen anxiety and stress responses in the stomach. Fermented foods promote intestinal and brain health including yoghurt and cheese with live cultures, kefir products, sauerkraut, kimchi and miso, kombucha, brewer's yeast, Yakult and micro-algae. It is important to note that yoghurt probiotic function is often only active for several days, not weeks as advertised so people buying yoghurt only for health, should speak with the dietician if unsure.

Role of Antibiotics

Antonie van Leeuwenhoek, Joseph Lister, Louis Pasteur, Robert Koch, Bartolomeo Gosio, Paul Ehrlich, Gerhard Domagk, Alexander Fleming and many more, all advanced scientific understanding of microorganisms and eventually these advances led to a basic understanding of antibiotics, with the use of antibiotics beginning in the early and mid-1900's.

Antibiotics are medicines that fight bacterial infections in people and animals and enable vital therapies and procedures. They work by killing the bacteria or by making it hard for the bacteria to grow and multiply. They can be taken Orally/by mouth (pills, capsules, or liquids), Topically (cream, spray, or ointment that you put on your skin, eye ointment, eye drops, or ear drops), and via injections. As antibiotics are easy to administer and easy to measure, they have become a cornerstone of the medical model when treating many infections and diseases. Prior to the understanding and widespread use of antibiotics many people died from infectious diseases such as the plague.

However, research in the last twenty years is showing that some of the unwanted side-effects can outweigh the benefits, with an increasing number of bacterial strains becoming antibiotic resistant. Keeping with the 'garden theme', albeit negative view, allied health and complementary medical practitioners discuss antibiotics as "destroying all or the majority of the garden, to kill the weeds".

Summary

Gut health is very important for overall health and until recently has been overlooked by the medical model. There are still many challenges for the medical model and the maintenance of gut health. The body systems all communicate, and a healthy microbiome directly influences almost all body systems, and nutrition and sleep are still the simplest things we can do to improve our health, including our microbiome health.

With the growing body of research and evidence, it is hoped that gut health can be incorporated into the medical model approach more effectively in the near future. Whole genome sequencing (WGS), Quorum-Quenching (QQ) method, studying Bacteriophages and Humanised monoclonal antibodies, are all areas of current and future study to reduce antibiotic resistance while maintaining the positives of what antibiotic treatment can offer.

There are many supplements available today sold as prebiotics, probiotics, and modbiotics. This has made it helpful and convenient for people to improve their gut, skin, vaginal and hair health. However, people should always ask their medical or allied health professional if they are unsure, as supplements are more likely to cause negative side effects because of their potency and lack of current rules and legislation surrounding the ingredients and efficacy of these supplements.

Key Points & Relevant Personal/Professional Experiences

Very Brief Introduction to Molecular Biology: The Building Blocks of Life

DNA, Genes, and the Blueprint of Life

DNA stands for deoxyribonucleic acid and it is a molecule that consists of two long polynucleotide chains composed of four types of nucleotide subunits. Each of these chains is known as a DNA chain/strand and the hydrogen bonds between the base portions of the nucleotides hold the two chains together. Nucleotides are composed of a five-carbon sugar to which are attached one or more phosphate groups and a nitrogen-containing base. In the case of the nucleotides in DNA, the sugar is deoxyribose attached to a single phosphate group, and the base may be either adenine (A), cytosine (C), guanine (G), or thymine (T). The nucleotides are covalently linked together in a chain through the sugars and phosphates, which form the "backbone" of alternating sugar-phosphate-sugar-phosphate. Each polynucleotide chain in DNA is analogous to a necklace (the backbone) strung with four types of beads. The three-dimensional structure of DNA known as the double helix, arises from the chemical and structural features of its two polynucleotide chains. Because these two chains are held together by hydrogen bonding between the bases on the different strands, all the bases are on the inside of the double helix, and the sugar-phosphate backbones are on the outside.

Genes carry biological information that must be copied accurately for transmission to the next generation each time a cell divides to form two daughter cells. The genes in our body carry instructions for producing proteins, and the properties of a protein, which are responsible for its biological function, are determined by its three-dimensional structure, and its structure is determined in turn by the linear sequence of the amino acids of which it is composed. The genetic information stored in an organism's DNA contains the instructions for all the proteins the organism will ever synthesise; and in eucaryotes, DNA is contained in the cell nucleus.

Most humans are born with twenty-three pairs of chromosomes that consists of a single two-stranded DNA molecule containing between 50 million nucleotide pairs and 250 million nucleotide pairs (building blocks). Human's first chromosome, Chromosome 1 is the largest human chromosome, with approximately two hundred and forty-nine million DNA building blocks (base pairs) representing approximately eight percent of the total DNA in cells. Human's smallest chromosome; whilst chromosome 21, contains approximately 48 million base pairs representing 1.5 to 2 percent of the total DNA in cells. Chromosome twenty-three is different between the biological male and biological female.

The X chromosome is one of the two sex chromosomes in humans, containing approximately 155 million base pairs and representing approximately 5 percent of the total DNA in cells. Each person usually has one pair of sex chromosomes in each cell. Females typically have two X chromosomes, while males typically have one X and one Y chromosome. Early in the embryonic development of people with two X chromosomes, one of the X chromosomes is randomly and permanently inactivated in cells other than egg cells. This phenomenon is called X-inactivation or lyonization. X-inactivation ensures that people with two X chromosomes have only one functional copy of the X chromosome in each cell. Because X-inactivation is random, normally, the X chromosome inherited from one parent is active in some cells, and the X chromosome inherited from the other parent is active in other cells. Some genes on the X chromosome escape X-inactivation. Many of these genes are located at the ends of each arm of the X chromosome in areas known as the pseudo autosomal regions. Although many genes are unique to the X chromosome, genes in the pseudo autosomal regions are present on both sex chromosomes. As a result, males and females each have two functional copies of these genes. Many genes in the pseudo autosomal regions are essential for normal development. The X chromosome contains approximately 900 to 1,400 genes that provide instructions for making proteins.

The Y chromosome is one of the two sex chromosomes in humans containing approximately 59 million base pairs and representing approximately 2 percent of the total DNA in cells. The Y chromosome likely contains 70 to 200 genes that provide instructions for making proteins. Because only males have the Y chromosome, the genes on this chromosome tend to be involved in male sex determination and development. Sex is determined by the SRY (Sex-determining Region Y) gene, which is responsible for the development of a foetus into a male. Other genes on the Y chromosome are important for enabling men to father biological children (male fertility). Many genes are unique to the Y chromosome, but genes in areas known as pseudo autosomal regions are present on both sex chromosomes.

The role of genetics in health and disease is complex, and the more scientists learn about the human body and genetics, the more they learn about its complexity. Presently, genetic testing is helping identify risk factors and protective factors, however, interpretations beyond this are often misunderstandings or purposeful manipulation of scientific data. The primary reason for exploring genetics and disease is to improve the efficacy and effectiveness of treatments.

However, there is also a negative field colloquially known as "pop science" where large companies use genetic data to falsely identify racial and cultural heritage, which is based on people living in a particular country today, and has minimal causation, and a weak correlation to people's genetic geographic history. For example, the global economy, combined with advances in technology now allow whole families to move from one side of the world to the other, which would directly influence the outcome of these claims.

Returning to a positive note about genetics, is an ever-improving field known as epigenetics. Epigenetics is the person's gene expression which is directly influenced by environmental factors including nutrition, age, stress, disease and exercise. Put simply, the DNA epigenetics organise the available genes and the RNA epigenetics dynamically adjust their use. This exciting field promises to improve future medical treatments further once a more thorough understanding of genetics and epigenetics is established.

Extra Information to discuss with a medical or allied health professional

Medication can be beneficial for some people who are struggling with their mental health, whether for shorter-term use or lifelong use. However, like anything we ingest, there are potential side effects the person should discuss with their medical professional. Some side effects often not discussed include mitochondrial dysfunction via inhibiting the mitochondrial respiratory chain, longer term use may increase toxicity in the body and may lead to other mental and physical health side effects, carnitine deficiency leading to lower energy, lower ATP production, impacted sleep and lower nutrition absorption. Some Benzodiazepines are unhelpful and contra-indicated for PTSD as it has been found to increase anxiety, sleep disturbance, nightmare and irritability in most people, they may exacerbate suppression of autonomic nervous system and reduces healing mobilisation through the sympathetic nervous system. Stimulant medications are often helpful for assisting people with ADHD but have also been found to have similar effects when prescribed to a person during the early stages of unresolved trauma.

The use of melatonin in children and teenagers impacts healthy teenage brain development but can be helpful short-term. Prescribed medication including Sedatives, Hypnotics including Benzodiazepines may impact REM sleep and therefore the sleep cycle and may also increase risk of dementia. Nonsteroidal Anti-Inflammatory Drugs (NSAIDs) effectiveness is influenced by the time of day the person takes them for pain; in morning they may work with the circadian rhythm and at night they may work against the circadian rhythm.

There are many helpful tests for people that may require GP, or Dietician referrals, however, these may be forgotten, too expensive or deemed not relevant by the treating professional. These include Pharmacogenomics, Vitamin D panel, Tissue Mineral Analysis, Cortisol Specific Saliva Test APOE Gene test, MTHFR Gene test, COMT Gene test, Neurotransmitter tests, Hormone panels, Mould tests, Food sensitivity tests, Digestive and gut panels, Vitamin Deficiency test, Metabolic Test (fast, slow or mixed oxidiser test), and Mould test.

It is difficult for GPs (General Practitioners) to keep up with all of the latest scientific breakthroughs as GPs have to know information about a lot of different health aspects. As such it is helpful for a person to take information about these tests to their GP so their GP can explore the information to see if they are able to assist. Even in countries such as Australia where scientific and medical understanding is thought to be advanced, some of these tests are still not recognised by medical practitioners due to the tests' infancy in the medical field.

Technology, Artificial Intelligence and Surgical Interventions

Apart from pharmaceutical treatments, the medical model also makes use of technology to assist in improving treatment outcomes. This technology is commonly referred to as medical devices or medical instruments.

These can include instruments, machines, implants, or other articles used for medical purposes in patients. These devices vary in function and complexity. Diagnostic devices include tools used to detect or diagnose diseases, such as X-ray machines, MRI scanners, CT scanners, and ultrasound devices.

Therapeutic devices treat or manage medical conditions, including pacemakers, insulin pumps, dialysis machines, and radiotherapy equipment. Surgical instruments are tools that are used during surgeries, including scalpels, forceps, retractors, and endoscopes.

Implantable devices are placed inside the body to replace or support damaged structures, such as artificial joints, stents, heart valves, and cochlear implants. Smart implants and monitoring devices are devices that can monitor their own performance, track vital signs or other health indicators and send data back to healthcare providers, allowing for more personalised and timely interventions, with examples including diabetes management, blood pressure monitors, glucose meters, and wearable heart rate monitors.

Biodegradable stents and implants are designed to dissolve after fulfilling their purpose, reducing the need for follow-up surgeries. Prosthetics and Orthotics are external devices that replace a missing body part or enhance the function of a limb, such as artificial limbs, braces, and orthopaedic shoes.

Assistive devices are tools that help individuals with disabilities perform activities of daily living, including wheelchairs, hearing aids, and communication devices for those with speech impairments. A new and developing areas is that of 3D Printing, where specialists can create custom-made implants, prosthetics, and even organs, to improve treatment outcomes and reduce costs.

Another new and advancing field slowly being utilised in the medical model is that of Artificial Intelligence (AI). AI is already being integrated into diagnostic devices such as skin cancer cameras, surgical planning, and real-time decision-making during surgeries, as well as being used in skin cancer treatment and early identification. This is a very new sub-field and as machine learning and data sets improve, this area offers medical specialists an extra tool they can utilise to improve treatment outcomes.

Surgical interventions have long been used around the world when treating severe disease or injury such as limb removal. However, modern surgical interventions refer to the medical procedures involving an incision with instruments, typically performed in a sterile environment, to treat disease, injury, or other health conditions.

There are various types of surgical interventions. Elective Surgery includes planned procedures that are not emergencies, such as cosmetic surgery, hernia repairs, or joint replacements. Emergency Surgery includes unplanned surgeries that are often lifesaving, like appendectomies, trauma surgery, or caesarean sections in complicated births. Minimally Invasive Surgery includes procedures performed through tiny incisions using specialised instruments, including laparoscopic surgery and robotic surgery. These methods often result in shorter recovery times and less post-operative pain.

Reconstructive Surgery is focused on repairing damaged tissues or organs, often after trauma, congenital defects, or cancer surgery, and can include skin grafts, breast reconstruction, and cleft palate repair. Transplant Surgery involves replacing a diseased organ or tissue with a healthy one from a donor, such as heart, liver, kidney, or bone marrow transplants. Cardiac Surgery includes procedures like coronary artery bypass grafting (CABG), valve repairs, and heart transplants. Orthopaedic Surgery focuses on the musculoskeletal system, including joint replacements, fracture repairs, and spinal surgeries. Finally, Robotic Surgery is the use of robotic systems to assist in precise, minimally invasive surgeries, often controlled by a surgeon through a computer interface. Robotic surgeries when combined with advances in AI, offer a promising area of medical intervention.

Pharmaceuticals: Role of Drugs in Targeting Specific Symptoms or Pathogens

As discussed in an earlier section, the modern use of medication (pharmaceuticals) began in the early to mid-nineteen hundreds.

Pharmaceuticals (prescribed drugs) are chemical substances used to prevent, diagnose, treat, or manage diseases. They can be categorised based on their therapeutic use, chemical structure, or the biological systems they target. The primary goal of pharmaceuticals is to alleviate symptoms, combat pathogens, or restore normal physiological functions. The terms 'Pharmaceutical Categories' and 'Pharmaceutical Classes' are used interchangeably here for simplicity. However, different countries and different areas of research might use these terms differently.

There are various categories of pharmaceuticals for physical health and mental health, and various medication mechanisms. Pharmacists complete extensive training to understand Pharmacokinetics and Pharmacodynamics which both are very important regarding how medication works. In summary pharmacodynamics and pharmacokinetics are the 2 branches of pharmacology, with pharmacodynamics studying the action of the drug on the organism and pharmacokinetics studying the effect the organism has on the drug.

In practice, medication often fit multiple categories, however for simplicity I have provided a list to assist the lay person in understanding medication. The physical health medication often prescribed under the medical model include:

Analgesics
Medications that relieve pain. There are two main types: non-narcotic analgesics for mild pain, and narcotic analgesics for severe pain.

Antacids
Medications that relieve indigestion and heartburn by neutralising stomach acid.

Antiarrhythmics
Medications used to control irregularities of heartbeat.

Antibacterials
Medications used to treat infections.

Antibiotics
Medications made from naturally occurring and synthetic substances that combat bacterial infection. Some antibiotics are effective only against limited types of bacteria. Others, known as broad spectrum antibiotics, are effective against a wide range of bacteria.

Anticoagulants and Thrombolytics
Anticoagulants prevent blood from clotting. Thrombolytics help dissolve and disperse blood clots and may be prescribed for patients with recent arterial or venous thrombosis.

Anticonvulsants
Medications that prevent epileptic seizures.

Antidiarrheals
Medications used for the relief of diarrhea. Two main types of antidiarrheal preparations are simple adsorbent substances and drugs that slow down the contractions of the bowel muscles so that the contents are propelled more slowly.

Antiemetics
Medications used to treat nausea and vomiting.

Antifungals
Medications used to treat fungal infections, the most common of which affect the hair, skin, nails, or mucous membranes.

Antihistamines
Medications used primarily to counteract the effects of histamine, one of the chemicals involved in allergic reactions.

Antihypertensives
Medications that lower blood pressure. The types of antihypertensives currently marketed include diuretics, beta-blockers, calcium channel blocker, ACE (angiotensin- converting enzyme) inhibitors, centrally acting antihypertensives and sympatholytics.

Anti-Inflammatories
Medications used to reduce inflammation, redness, heat, swelling, and increased blood flow found in infections and in many chronic noninfective diseases such as rheumatoid arthritis and gout.

Antineoplastics
Medications used to treat cancer.

Antipyretics
Medications that reduce fever.

Antivirals
Medications used to treat viral infections or to provide temporary protection against infections such as influenza.

Barbiturates & Benzodiazepines
The two main groups of medications that are used to induce sleep are benzodiazepines and barbiturates. All such medications have a sedative effect in low doses and are effective sleeping medications in higher doses. Benzodiazepines drugs are used more widely than barbiturates because they are safer, the side-effects are less marked, and there is less risk of eventual physical dependence.

Beta-Blockers
Beta-adrenergic blocking agents, or beta-blockers for short, reduce the oxygen needs of the heart by reducing heartbeat rate.

Bronchodilators
Medications that open the bronchial tubes within the lungs when the tubes have become narrowed by muscle spasm. Bronchodilators ease breathing in diseases such as asthma.

Cold Cures
Although there is no medications that can cure a cold, the aches, pains, and fever that accompany a cold can be relieved by aspirin or acetaminophen often accompanied by a decongestant, antihistamine, and sometimes caffeine.

Corticosteroids
These hormonal preparations are used primarily as anti-inflammatories in arthritis or asthma or as immunosuppressives, but they are also useful for treating some malignancies or compensating for a deficiency of natural hormones in disorders such as Addison's disease.

Cough Suppressants
There are two groups of cough suppressants: those that alter the consistency or production of phlegm such as mucolytics and expectorants; and those that suppress the coughing reflex such as codeine (narcotic cough suppressants), antihistamines, dextromethorphan and isoproterenol (non-narcotic cough suppressants).

Cytotoxics
Medications that kill or damage cells. Cytotoxics are used as antineoplastics (drugs used to treat cancer) and as immunosuppressives.

Decongestants
Medications that reduce swelling of the mucous membranes that line the nose by constricting blood vessels, thus relieving nasal stuffiness.

Diuretics
Medications that increase the quantity of urine produced by the kidneys and passed out of the body, thus ridding the body of excess fluid. Diuretics reduce water logging of the tissues caused by fluid retention in disorders of the heart, kidneys, and liver. They are useful in treating mild cases of high blood pressure.

Expectorant
A medication that stimulates the flow of saliva and promotes coughing to eliminate phlegm from the respiratory tract.

Hormones

Chemicals produced naturally by the endocrine glands (thyroid, adrenal, ovary, testis, pancreas, parathyroid). In some disorders, for example, diabetes mellitus, in which too little of a particular hormone is produced, synthetic equivalents or natural hormone extracts are prescribed to restore the deficiency. Such treatment is known as hormone replacement therapy.

Hypoglycemics

Medications that lower the level of glucose in the blood. Oral hypoglycaemic drugs are used in diabetes mellitus if it cannot be controlled by diet alone, but does require treatment with injections of insulin.

Immunosuppressives

Medications that prevent or reduce the body's normal reaction to invasion by disease or by foreign tissues. Immunosuppressives are used to treat autoimmune diseases (in which the body's defences work abnormally and attack its own tissues) and to help prevent rejection of organ transplants.

Laxatives

Medications that increase the frequency and ease of bowel movements, either by stimulating the bowel wall (stimulant laxative), by increasing the bulk of bowel contents (bulk laxative), or by lubricating them (stool-softeners, or bowel movement-softeners). Laxatives may be taken by mouth or directly into the lower bowel as suppositories or enemas. If laxatives are taken regularly, the bowels may ultimately become unable to work properly without them.

Muscle Relaxants

Medications that relieve muscle spasm in disorders such as backache, and can include antianxiety drugs (minor tranquilisers).

Sex Hormones (Female)

There are two groups of these hormones (estrogens and progesterone), which are responsible for development of female secondary sexual characteristics. Small quantities are also produced in males. As drugs, female sex hormones are used to treat menstrual and menopausal disorders and are also used as oral contraceptives. Estrogens may be used to treat cancer of the breast or prostate, progestins (synthetic progesterone to treat endometriosis).

Sex Hormones (Male)

Androgenic hormones, of which the most powerful is testosterone, are responsible for development of male secondary sexual characteristics. Small quantities are also produced in females. As drugs, male sex hormones are given to compensate for hormonal deficiency in hypopituitarism or disorders of the testes. They may be used to treat breast cancer in women, but either synthetic derivatives called anabolic steroids, which have less marked side-effects, or specific anti-estrogens are often preferred. Anabolic steroids also have a "body building" effect that has led to their (usually non-sanctioned) use in competitive sports, for both men and women.

Tranquiliser
This is a term commonly used to describe any medication that has a calming or sedative effect. However, the drugs that are sometimes called minor tranquilisers should be called antianxiety drugs, and the drugs that are sometimes called major tranquilisers should be called antipsychotics.

Vitamins
Chemicals essential in small quantities for good health. Some vitamins are not manufactured by the body, but adequate quantities are present in a normal diet. People whose diets are inadequate or who have digestive tract or liver disorders may need to take supplementary vitamins.

Medication use in mental health is always evolving as understanding of the brain and body improve. The mental health medication often prescribed under the medical model include:

Antianxiety
Medications that suppress anxiety and relax muscles (sometimes called anxiolytics, sedatives, or minor tranquilisers).

Antidepressants
Antidepressants are used to relieve psychological and physical symptoms of depression, with the benefit of treatment increasing with severity. There are several main groups of mood-lifting antidepressants including Monoamine oxidase inhibitor (MAOI), mood stabilisers, Serotonin-Norepinephrine Reuptake Inhibitor (SNRI) Tricyclics, and Selective Serotonin Reuptake Inhibitors (SSRIs).

Antipsychotics (including Atypical)
Drugs used to treat symptoms of severe psychiatric disorders and relieve symptoms such as hallucinations, delusions or disordered thought. These drugs are sometimes called major tranquilisers. Atypical antipsychotics have largely replaced traditional agents as first-line therapy in the treatment of schizophrenia. Toxicologic exposures and fatalities associated with atypical agents pose a persistent problem in the United States and elsewhere.

Lithium Carbonate
Lithium carbonate is given to prevent manic or depressive episodes in bipolar disorder. Due to potential toxicity, regular blood tests are important during treatment.

Stimulants
These include medications that are used to treat Attention Deficit Hyperactivity Disorder (ADHD), narcolepsy, and occasionally early treatment of Post Traumatic Stress Disorder (PTSD).

Revisiting role of diet, exercise, and lifestyle changes in preventing chronic diseases

This section will revisit how nutrition directly and indirectly impacts our health. Nutrition is a very large and open-ended area of research and understanding. As such, the majority of information presented here, will be focusing on its impacts on mental health whether directly or indirectly.

There are many different types of diets/food plans that people around the world follow, and often what is generalised advice won't work for everyone. Each person has their own dietary needs, and some practiced diets include Ancestral, Atkin's Carnivore, Paleo, Modified Carnivore, Ketogenic, Anti-Inflammatory, Gut and Psychology Syndrome (GAPS), Mediterranean, Raw, Vegetarian, Ayurvedic, Chinese Five Element, Macrobiotic, Vegan, Fasting and Detoxification. The individual's genetic difference means that our biochemistry is the main determinant about what foods/fuel is better for a person, and the rate of glucose oxidation is the rate at which our body burns fuels. This means that some nutrition plans may be harmful or counterproductive. Our cultural-genetic heritage is a strong determinant regarding if the individual will do better with higher percentages of fats and proteins, or better with less fats and higher percentages of carbohydrates.

The main role of carbohydrates is to provide the body and all its cells with energy. Carbohydrates can be divided into at least five different categories including monosaccharides, disaccharides, oligosaccharides, polysaccharides, and sugar alcohols. The brain and red blood cells rely heavily on carbohydrates being converted into glucose for energy. Fibre is important and can come as either Dietary Fibre or Functional Fibre, although these terms are often used as the same in the general population under the label Fibre. Dietary fibre is the carbohydrates and lignin that are found in plants and are not digested and absorbed in the small intestine. Functional fibre consists of isolated or purified carbohydrates that are not digested and absorbed in the small intestine and have beneficial physiological effects in humans. The main purposes of fibre include laxation, attenuation of blood glucose levels and normalisation of serum cholesterol levels. Proteins form the major structural components of all the cells of the body and function as enzymes in membranes, as transport carriers and as hormones. Amino acids are elements of protein and act as precursors for nucleic acids, hormones, vitamins and other important molecules needed in the body. Consuming fats aid in the absorption of fat-soluble vitamins and carotenoids.

People who benefit more from fats and proteins are known as 'Fast Oxidisers'. Fast oxidisers burn glucose too rapidly and require more protein and fats (such as the traditional Inuit peoples). Fast oxidisers often benefit more from carnivorous diets, animal proteins, fats, purine food, organ meats, sardines, anchovies, fruits, vegetables and few grains (approximately 30% protein, 20% carbohydrates, 50% fats). Fast oxidisers will still often meet their body's glucose needs as they will metabolise glucose from the amino acids found in dietary proteins. People who don't burn glucose rapidly enough and require a higher glucose percentage (such as Indian peoples and people living in Tropical countries) are known as 'Slow Oxidisers'. Slow oxidisers often benefit more from vegetarian and pescatarian nutrition plans, plant proteins, nuts, legumes, fish, eggs and low fats (approximately 25% protein, 60%

carbohydrates, 15% fats). The majority of the modern-day population fall under the 'Mixed Oxidisers' heading. Mixed oxidisers are people who, as the name suggests, benefit from a mixed protein-fat-carbohydrate diet to balance the rate of oxidisation (approximately 30% protein, 40% carbohydrates, 30% fats). This information is helpful and can be used to help a person direct their efforts such as eating to their type.

Many health difficulties arise following extended periods of poor sleep and poor nutrition. This statement is simple, but important to reiterate. In the modern world where life can often be faster, more stressful, and require more from a person, many people look for a quick fix to their difficulties. However, most of a person's individual health difficulties can be managed or assisted through the correct nutrition.

Nutrition Information

Preparing fresh food where possible may have mental health benefits and can be used as a relaxation or family building tool. It also allows a person to have more control over what they are consuming. Healthy foods to prepare in kitchen for overall mental health and mood improvement include Organic meats (beef, lamb, chicken), pinto beans, eggs, wild caught or wild canned salmon or tuna, olive oil, coconut fat, sweet potatoes, blueberries, raspberries, lemons, oats, green tea, beets, basil, figs, and bitter green vegetables. Dark Leafy greens and Cruciferous vegetables are best when lightly cooked/steamed (still green and slightly crunchy).

When cooking, it is useful to know that oils have different smoke points (when the oil starts to burn and lose nutrients) so if nutrition is important to a person's cooking process, they can adapt the temperature at which they prepare food. Where possible it is advisable to eliminate additives, preservatives, hormone additives, toxic pesticides and fertilisers on food, consume healthy fats, eliminate refined sugars (including carbohydrates) and eliminate refined fats.

Eating antioxidants should form part of the daily or at least weekly practice as they are the body's protection against free radicals that age us and impact many areas of our physical and mental health. Eating the colours of the rainbow (fruit and vegetables) can help to ensure the body is getting the required fuel as different colours in natural foods mean different pigments. Anthocyanins (blues and purples), Betalains (reds and violets), Carotenoids (deep yellow, reds and orange) and Chlorophylls (greens), means different chemical compounds are found in the different coloured foods. Anthocyanins are represented as red and are found in blue berries and cherries; Carotenoids are represented as Beta-Cryptoxanthin, Beta-Carotene and Lycopene, Beta, Cryptoxanthin which are all precursors for vitamin A, are highly bioavailable, and are essential for eyesight, growth and immune response and can be found in orange rind, egg yolk, apple skin, and mandarins. It is suggested that Carotenoids are useful for digestion, especially after large fatty meals. Chlorophylls are represented in leafy green vegetables, green herbs and other foods and can assist with wound healing, assist with iron, and lessen inflammation in the body. Eating a spectrum of food proteins (meats, nuts, eggs, dairy), and a spectrum of Carbohydrates (root vegetables, soluble fibres such as psyllium seeds, fruits and vegetables, fresh greens, fermented foods, fruits, and grains) are recommended. Healthy fats and other supporting foods are also beneficial.

When cooking with oil there are several ideas and options to think about. Is the oil stored in a dark green bottle to lessen light exposure damage, if not can you afford to buy an alternative that is. Some research has suggested when oil receives too much light exposure damage, it can lose nutrient quality. Ghee is an optimal cooking oil and butter replacement, and it may assist with absorption of positive effects from herbs and spices. Coconut fats can be an alternative for cooking as it can help with internal and external health difficulties. Sesame oil (raw) in small amounts can be useful as it helps with lessening gum health difficulties which can also assist the body in lessening heart disease and dementia risk.

As well adding or being a base for flavour, "cooking" herbs can assist in overall health with basil, oregano, cardamon, cinnamon, curcumin, turmeric, ginger and garlic being examples. Sea Salt is often used to naturally enhance flavours, but it is also rich in minerals, supports adrenal function and may help to lessen stress (pink and grey sea salts are recommended). Different vinegars can also assist in flavour and health in cooking with fruit vinegars being the most recommended (such as apple cider vinegar). The health benefits of fruit vinegars can include better management of blood glucose control, increasing levels of vitamin C, antimicrobial, antifungal, boost energy and reduce mild anxiety.

Everyone has been told that eating vegetables are good for you, and there are different types with different benefits. Cruciferous vegetables such as Broccoli, Kale, Brussel Sprouts, Broccoli Sprouts, and Parsley have many health benefits. These include Anti-carcinogenic, Antioxidant, Anti-inflammatory, reversing oxidative stress and improving mitochondrial function, helping to detox body, balancing oestrogen metabolism and helping to release it and assisting the Glutathione production in the body. Nightshade vegetables such as eggplant have many health benefits including fibre, antioxidant and anti-inflammatory. However, they may also cause intestinal permeability and inflammation which may lead to more reflux and pain. For people who have a negative response to nightshade vegetables alternatives such as plantain can be beneficial. Seaweed has been called the vegetable of the sea and has many health benefits. These can include being rich in calcium, phosphorus, magnesium, iron, iodine, sodium, Vitamin C, Vitamin A, Folacin, Vitamin B complex, protein, helping thyroid function, assisting in constipation management and losing weight; and some variations such as brown seaweeds (such as Royal Kombu) help to detoxify heavy metals (such as from air pollution) in the body by binding with the excess metal and radioactive isotypes. Mushrooms can also be beneficial and are sometimes used as meat replacements. Reishi mushrooms are thought to be good for the immune system, Shiitake mushrooms for Vitamin B, Niacin, Choline, Folate, Selenium, Copper, Zinc and Manganese, and Lion's Mane mushrooms for brain and nervous system support, PTSD support, and for improving mild cognitive impairment.

As discussed throughout this book, eating fat can be a good thing if we are consuming healthy fats. Healthy Fats provides the body with energy and lubrication for the brain and insulation for body organs and are essential for the absorption of fat-soluble nutrients (vitamins A, D, E and K). The three main types of healthy fats are saturated, monounsaturated, and polyunsaturated. Monounsaturated fats from olives and avocado assists with digestive and gallbladder health due to the chlorophyll and can also be consumed as lamb, beef, and wildlife animals. Polyunsaturated fats can become toxic when used as cooking oil for frying, etc. and can increase inflammation, pain and depression risk; as a result, these should be eaten through nuts, seeds, leafy greens and fatty fish. Fats from animals, vegetables, nuts, and seeds that are extracted via a "cold process" should be integrated into daily schedule if possible. Eggs are rich in Choline and should be consumed daily for brain and memory health. Males often require more EPA, and females often require more DHA in their diets, but it is important to remember that DHA and EPA needs change through the life stages. DHA is often required at younger ages (for structural support) and EPA in later ages. DHA supplementation may assist younger people with managing learning and behavioural difficulties, and it is useful to know that the adult brain is approximately 60% DHA fat. Saturated fats have various benefits including anti-bacterial, anti-fungal and anti-inflammatory, and can be consumed through butter, coconut, tallow, suet (from cows and lambs), ducks, geese, chickens, turkey, and pig lard. The different types of saturated fats include Butyric Acid (found in butter), Lauric Acid (found in coconut oil and palm oil), Myristic Acid (found in dairy products), Palmitic Acid (found in meat and palm oil) and Stearic Acid (found in meat and cocoa butter).

Trans-fatty acids are known as unhealthy fats and should be avoided where possible. Remove Trans-fatty acids such as Hydrogenated Vegetable oils found in margarine, etc as they increase the risk for – Liver damage, reproductive health, respiratory health, digestive disorders, neurological damage, unhealthy weight gain and impaired immune function.

Essential Fatty Acids (EFA) are essential and can only by obtained from foods with three types including Omega 3, 6 and Arachidonic Acid (AA). As discussed throughout, our genetic history/bio-individuality determines how a person metabolises DHA and EPA. DHA and EPA are important as they improve communication between synapses, improve dendritic spines on postsynaptic neurons, improve brain volume, assist with treatment of brain injury, assist in management of depression, are anti-inflammatory and may assist with eyesight. The fatty acid Omega 6 is known as Gamma Linoleic Acid (GLA) and can be consumed from Borage seed, Evening primrose seeds, Black currant seed, Hemp and Spirulina. It may assist with dermatological issues, menopause, PMS, Uterine cramps, PCOS and endometriosis.

Saturated fats such as Medium Chain Fatty Acids may improve cognition and memory and promotes neuronal communication by increasing dendrites and can be consumed in coconut and palm oils. There is also a special type of fat called Phospholipids which comprise neuron membranes and support communication between neurons, such as Spinach and Krill oil. A lack of phospholipids reportedly increases the risk of depression and schizophrenia.

One of the reasons we should eat the aforementioned foods is for the essential vitamins and minerals our body needs. Essential vitamins can be water soluble or fat soluble. Water soluble vitamins are not stored in body, so risk of overdosing is low; whereas fat soluble vitamins are stored in body, so the risk of overdosing is higher. Fat soluble vitamins include vitamins A, D, E and K and are absorbed into fats but also need fats for the body to absorbs these.

Vitamin A helps immune system to protect against viruses, assists the eyes, skin and lungs, assists in helpful gene expression and can assist in reproduction. There are at least four forms of Vitamin A including retinol, retinal, retinoic acid and retinyl esters. One of the side effects of insufficient Vitamin A is corneal and other eye related difficulties and degeneration. Vitamin A is mostly stored in the liver, and when there is an insufficient level of Vitamin A ingestion, it will be slowly released from the liver.

Vitamin E contain eight different fat-soluble antioxidants that help the respiratory system and mitochondria and lowers risk of cognitive decline and Alzheimer's disease. Vitamin E also assists by preventing the spread of free-radical reactions in the body. One of the eight forms of Vitamin E (a-tocopherol) is contained is the body's plasma. Insufficient Vitamin E longer term may lead to poorer pain management, and neurological, muscular and skeletal health.

Vitamin K assists the body by functioning as a coenzyme for biological reactions involved in blood coagulation and bone metabolism. There are two different types K1 and K2. Vitamin K1 assists with cognitive function in older adults and vitamin K2 is essential for nerve health in the brain.

Vitamin D Is not really a vitamin but a Neurohormone which helps the body to absorb calcium, magnesium, phosphate, iron, and zinc. The Vitamin D receptors in brain also increase serotonin production and improves mitochondrial functioning and can assist people with Depression, pain and immune problems. Vitamin D also assists in bone health by assisting the bones in their absorption of calcium. Vitamin D is high in foods such as fatty fish and eggs.

Vitamin C is a water-soluble nutrient that acts as antioxidant. It may help the immune system, improve mood and cognition, and assists in the biosynthesis of carnitine, neurotransmitters, collagen, and other connective tissue components, and modulates the absorption, transport and storage of iron. It can be found in banana pulp, citrus, pulp, and many other food sources.

Vitamin B has many types which generally supports the management of blood glucose, support serotonin, and improves cognition and neurological health. Vitamin B1 (Thiamine) assists in the metabolism of carbohydrates and branched-chain amino acids. Vitamin B2 (Riboflavin) assists with various oxidation–reduction reactions in several metabolic pathways and in energy production. Vitamin B3 (Niacin and Niacinamide) may help as a mood stabiliser and sedative, assists with fatty acid synthesis, assist with arthritic pain, and sometimes is used in natural treatments and management of schizophrenia and alcohol misuse. Vitamin B5 (Pantothenic Acid) is a water-soluble vitamin that is essential for fatty acid synthesis and degradation, transfer of acetyl and acyl groups, and a multitude of other anabolic and catabolic processes. Vitamin B6 is comprised of six related compounds and supports Neurotransmitter function, assists with insomnia, hypertension, poorer cognitive functioning, PMS, and irritability, and may assist with the symptoms of depression and anxiety. It is rare, but insufficient levels of Vitamin B6 may worsen depression and increase cognitive confusion. Vitamin B7 (Biotin) promotes appropriate function of the nervous system and is essential for liver metabolism.

Vitamin B8 (Inositol) may be effective for depression, panic attacks, agoraphobia, obsessive compulsive behaviour, bulimia, and binge eating and may also be effective for SSRI resistant people. Vitamin B9 can be from folate (natural form and healthier option) or from folic acid (synthetic form and less healthy). Some of the difficulties with folate arise from needing levels of the enzyme 5-MTHF to convert folate, and approximately 40% of western populations have difficulties converting folate as a result. Some research has suggested that people with bipolar, depression, schizophrenia, Autism and ADHD are more likely to have a deficiency of the 5-MTHF enzyme. Vitamin B12 may assist with the symptoms of depression, fatigue, anxiety, cognition and psychosis, and sufficient levels are essential for healthy blood and neurological function.

Choline is required by the body for the structural integrity of cell membranes and is involved in methyl metabolism, cholinergic neurotransmission, transmembrane signalling and lipid and cholesterol transport and metabolism. Choline (Cytidine-5-Diphosphate Choline) is an essential nutrient that breaks down into Phosphatidylcholine, then into Alpha-GPC. Alpha-GPC, allows the choline to assist in memory and cognitive functioning, may assist in recovery for people with TBI, may assist with treatment of some addictions such as Cocaine cravings and may reduce manic symptoms in bipolar. Choline can be consumed through beef, liver, eggs, fish, chicken, and milk. Insufficient levels of choline may lead to liver damage.

Essential minerals help the body "get stuff done" and helps various body systems. It includes macro-minerals and trace minerals. As the name suggests, macro-minerals are needed in larger amounts and include calcium, phosphorus, magnesium, sodium, potassium, chloride, and sulphur. There are many different forms of magnesium and different benefits. In general, magnesium assists with stress, anxiety, cognitive function, and mood regulation, improves serotonin synthesis, and reduces inflammation and oxidative stress. Magnesium Citrate is best for digestive health, bowel health, leg cramps, sleep; Magnesium Malate is crucial for ATP production and may assist with fibromyalgia; Magnesium Glycinate is great for calming, and back pain relief; Magnesium Aspartate may assist rapid cycling bipolar management; Magnesium cream may assist in management of muscle cramps; and Magnesium L-threonate was developed to cross blood-brain barrier to improve short-term memory and overall cognitive functioning, assist depression management and may dampen traumatic memories (such as nightmares). Potassium is the main intracellular cation in the body and is required for normal cellular function and has two types Orotate and Citrate. Potassium is often lower in people with PTSD, heart problems, bulimia, and anorexia. Calcium plays a key role in bone health and is also involved in vascular, neuromuscular, and glandular functions. Phosphorus helps maintain a normal pH in the body and is involved in metabolic processes. Sodium and Chloride are often found together in food and are necessary to maintain extracellular fluid volume and plasma health.

Trace minerals are required but only in smaller amounts an include iron, manganese, copper, iodine, zinc, cobalt, fluoride, selenium, chromium, lithium orotate and rubidium. Chromium helps in glucose regulation, may assist with depression and mood regulation and may decreases carbohydrate cravings and binge eating. Manganese is involved in the formation of bone and in specific reactions related to amino acid, cholesterol, and carbohydrate metabolism. Iron is an essential component of several proteins in the body including enzymes, cytochromes, myoglobin and haemoglobin. Fluoride protects against dental cavities, can stimulate new bone formation and is essential for the health of teeth and bones. Lithium Orotate is often used for cognitive and mood disorders, memory loss, alcohol recovery and relapse prevention, and may also assist thorough its neuroprotective and anti-inflammatory properties. It has also been found to help hippocampal volume and Brain Derived Neurotrophic Factor (BDNF), lessens risk of Alzheimer's and dementia, and assist in sleep quality.

Selenium is an antioxidant nutrient involved in the defence against oxidative stress and regulates thyroid hormone actions. Selenium may also elevate mood, reduce inflammation, and enhance immunity. Zinc is crucial for growth and development as it facilitates several enzyme related processes related to the metabolism of protein, carbohydrates, and fats. Zinc also helps form the structure of proteins and enzymes and is involved in the regulation of gene expression. Zinc may also assist in depression management, bulimia and purging and anorexia disorders and may also assist the immune system. Copper regulates cellular energy, assists in production and neurotransmission, may assist in prostate health, and assists with depression management. However, some research has found that copper can be negatively impacted by antacid medications. Iodine assists with fatigue management and may assists in thyroid health. Rubidium may assist with depression management, stimulate the dopamine, norepinephrine and epinephrine pathways may assist in nervous and stress symptoms and is synergistic with potassium. It primarily comes from red meat, but can also be found in Brazil nuts, pecans, sesame and sunflower seeds, potato skins, eggplant, mushrooms, cucumber and avocado.

Coenzyme Q10 is a vitamin-like substance that acts like a vitamin is fat soluble and is found in mitochondria. There are two types Ubiquinol and Ubiquinone. Ubiquinol accounts for 90% of coenzyme Q10 and is the most absorbable form. It may assist in treatment of bipolar, depression, fatigue, fibromyalgia and schizophrenia and supports the mitochondria.

Phosphatidylserine is a phospholipid which is a key component of the cell membrane and is essential for the transfer of biochemical messages into cells within the brain and CNS. It also assists in regulating cortisol levels, increasing acetylcholine in brain, may be used in management of chronic stress, depression, ADHD, PTSD and brain injury and is found in egg yolks and liver.

Bromelain is a proteolytic that inhibits the cyclooxygenase enzyme, reduce swelling and can be the foundation of anti-inflammatory treatment including for pain and fibromyalgia.

Acetyl-L-Carnitine (ALCAR) is made from L-Carnitine in the body and is often used as it may assist with cognitive improvement, and it increases acetylcholine, increases nerve growth factor in brain, increases metabolism and cellular energy and decreases insulin resistance. It crosses the blood brain barrier and is extra important for vegetarians.

Chocolate (no added sugar or sugar alternatives) such as cacao nibs. Natural, sugar free chocolate has anti-inflammatory compounds including Flavanols and antioxidants (epicatechin highest in chocolate), may assist the liver and gallbladder as a bitter herb/food, may support mitochondria, may be used as a prebiotic via the flavanols, increases endorphins such as Dopamine, may increase focus, is high in magnesium and may assist the respiratory system.

Amino acids are the precursors to neurotransmitters, and are affected by our diet (low protein, poor fats). Some professionals use Amino Acid Therapy as substitutions for psychotropics and prescribed psychotropics. The top seven neurotransmitter essential nutrients include Free Amino Acids, Probiotics, B-Complex, Magnesium, Theanine, Curcumin with black pepper and Tyrosine.

Mental Health and Nutrition revisited

We know now that the brain and stomach are connected via what is known as the enteric nervous system and the Gut Brain Axis. What we eat directly impacts our mental health for better or worse and directly influences our main brain centres including the Hypothalamus-Pituitary-Adrenal axis (HPA), Hippocampus, Cerebral Cortex, Amygdala and Brain Stem. The prebiotics, probiotics and mod-biotics were discussed earlier and are very relevant to mental health.

One aspect of nutrition and mental health that has received more attention in recent years is over-nutrition. In the modern world where there are vitamin pills for almost anything, it is easier for people to have too much of a particular nutrient. This overloading of a particular nutrient can cause many health side effects including a worsening of mental health. Some research found that people with an overload of copper, methionine, folic acid, or iron are likely to deteriorate if they take supplements containing these nutrients. Whilst it is true that good food is a primary need for a healthy self, a person may benefit from seeking professional assistance before self-medicating with vitamins. The professional such as dietician can assist a person in carefully identifying the specific nutrient overloads and deficiencies possessed by the person. Some studies found that people living in countries such as Australia waste close to two billion dollars annually on over-nutrition.

Chronic low-grade inflammation is caused by poor nutrition, stress and leads to further stress, early ageing, proinflammatory cytokines that suppress natural serotonin and neurotransmitter function, cardiovascular disease, metabolic disease, neurodegenerative disorders, shortening of the telomeres gene, cancers and poor mental health such as depression. Neurotoxins may impact mood stability that may present as a mood disorder such as depression. Neurotoxins may be ingested by eating foods that contain dough conditioners, artificial seasonings, yeast extract, synthetic carrageenan, maltodextrin, hydrolysed vegetable protein, WPC (Whey Protein Concentrate), aspartate and aspartame. Aspartame has been suggested to worsen depression and irritability and may increase risk and severity of migraines, oxidative stress, diabetes, seizures, blindness, obesity, neurological disorders, and is considered a carcinogen. Sugar has also been theorised as a risk factor for maintaining depression. To help manage mood disorders such as mild to moderate depression various foods, herbs, minerals, fats and other should be ingested. Some of these include turmeric (with added black pepper to increase bioavailability), curcumin, ginger, black or green tea, berries, vitamin D, vitamin E, omegas, Kimchee and other fermented foods (increase Brain Derived Neurotropic Factor to lessen depression and dementia risk), vitamins and minerals with L-Methylfolate, Omega 3 Oil (Green Lipped Mussel or Krill oil), Gamma Linoleic Acid (GLA) (borage or evening primrose oil), Free amino acids, Probiotics, Vitamin D, Vitamin B6, Niacinamide, Methylcobalamin, Lithium Orotate, Magnesium, Tryptophan (precursor for 5-HTP), L-tyrosine, and glandular foods (Adrenal Glandular and Hypothalamus Glandular).

Nutrition can influence and be used to improve other areas of mental health other than depression. If a person is anxious carbohydrates and health fats combined may help to lower their anxiety and lessen the need for comfort or craving related eating behaviours. Foods that are rich in Vitamins and Minerals with L-Methylfolate, Omega 3 Oil, Gamma Linoleic Acid (GLA), Free amino acids, Probiotics, Vitamin D, Vitamin B6 and B12, Niacinamide, Magnesium L-threonate or glycinate, Choline foods (Alpha GP-Choline precursor), Tryptophan (precursor for 5-HTP), Lithium Orotate and Taurine can be helpful. Some examples of these foods may include bananas, figs, fruit vinegars, walnuts, and almonds. Support the production of GABA through food has also been suggested to lessen the severity of anxiety. Glandular foods have also been used in some cultures to manage mental health difficulties. Glandular animal meats can include Brain, Hypothalamus, Pituitary, Adrenal, Thymus, Liver, Pancreas, Heart, Thyroid, Lung. They can be used to assist treating or managing stress, supporting immune function, metabolism, fatigue recovery and weight loss, managing depression and substance misuse recovery, supporting digestion, sugar metabolism and fat digestion, managing immune function and some research suggests it may improve cognitive functioning. Glandular meats have been traditionally prepared as Tripe, Lung, Thymus Sweetbread, Heart, Liver, Tongue, Testicles, Kidney.

Tracking our food can be difficult, especially when we live busy lives. There are many apps and methods that a person can use to track their food, however, most of the ways people track their food, don't consider their mental health. A 'Food Mood Diary' such as the one developed by Dr. Leslie Korn, can help develop insight including identifying patterns of food and mood and highlighting any possible addictive and mental health patterns. Ideas such as the food mood diary can also help a person manage disordered eating by identifying patterns and possible triggers. In the modern world overeating and still being micronutrient deficient is a commonly found issue with many clients who have high stress lives such as trauma, event stress, relationship issues, and other stressors.

The overlapping and also competing ideas of overeating, rigidity in calorie counting and other behaviours have, in some cases, increased the risk of developing eating disordered behaviours in westernised countries. Disordered eating includes diagnosed eating disorders but also includes the behaviours that impact a person's function, even if they don't have a formal diagnosis. Regarding nutrition and disordered eating, there may be foods and food profiles that can assist in managing these behaviours. Foods that are rich in Tryptophan (healthy fats and complex carbohydrates) help to metabolise serotonin, and help a person feel full, which can be helpful in managing disordered eating behaviours. Some examples of these foods may include Whey protein (as it can help satiate a person and lessen purging related behaviours, whilst also containing the nine essential amino acids), oats and nuts and seeds. Another disordered eating behaviour that isn't officially recognised by the DSM-5 is Orthorexia. I and many other well trained fitness professionals have seen first-hand when the fine line between healthy calorie/macro counting turns into disordered eating. Orthorexia is thought to include – fixated, rigid, or righteous eating (Veganism, Keto, Raw Food only diets, etc.) being extrapolated to other people if it works for the one person and may also include the person becoming addicted to the claims of recovery. It is thought it normally starts with positive intent such as wanting to be healthier, or because of chemical/allergic responses to foods, but then leads to the unhealth expression of these behaviours.

Circadian rhythm has been discussed elsewhere, but I will briefly revisit it here in the context of mental health and nutrition. The term Chrono-nutrition can be defined as the time of day and meal frequency and refers to how nutrition and other foods are used to regulate the body's circadian and metabolic rhythms. A large amount of research has found that the disruption of circadian rhythm is correlated and sometimes causated with, insomnia, mood disorders, PTSD and other complex trauma. A metabolically healthy person has the physiological ability to switch between macronutrient sources for energy needs and to not substantially lose physical and cognitive performance in the short-term (24hours or less) in the absence of food. The body's circadian and metabolic rhythm are affected by factors such as sleep, physical activity (or sometimes lack of) and nutrients in the blood stream (including blood sugar and fatty acids). Difficulties here can contribute to Sleep/Wake disorders. Sleep/Wake disorders can be defined as longer term difficulties with sleep patterns and can include Dyssomnias, Parasomnias, Insomnia, and Circadian rhythm disruption. Eating foods rich in Vitamins and Minerals with L-Methylfolate, Omega 3 Oil, Gamma Linoleic Acid (GLA), Free amino acids, Probiotics, Vitamin D, B12, Magnesium Threonate, Lithium Orotate, Choline foods (Alpha GP-Choline precursor), Melatonin and Tryptophan (precursor for 5-HTP) can assist in the management of sleep/wake disorders.

Another area of mental health that can be impacted by poor nutrition includes alcohol and other substance recovery. Alcohol and other substance use has many causes and serves a variety of purposes. One of the causes for maintaining high levels of alcohol use includes the pleasure and or focus a person may temporarily feel from the dopamine rush from alcohol. Again, nutrition can be one of the tools a person can implement to lessen the need for the alcohol. Eating foods rich in L-Tyrosine (to increase the amount of dopamine secretion), Vitamin C (ensuring enough water is consumed), L-Glutamine (increase to lessen the physiological cravings for alcohol), Lecithin (increase to assist with Inositol, Choline and B Vitamins, and metabolise fats out of the liver), Chromium (increase to manage mis-metabolism of carbohydrates and help control blood sugar levels), Magnesium, Antioxidants, L-Methylfolate, Omega 3 Oil, Gamma Linoleic Acid (GLA), free amino acids, Probiotics, Vitamin D, Thiamine, Choline, Liver Glandular, Adrenal Glandular, Hypothalamus Glandular, Niacinamide, Potassium, Lithium Orotate, Tryptophan (precursor for 5-HTP), Melatonin foods and Thiamine can improve this.

Micronutrients are the elements required in small quantities to sustain life, and these have also been linked to mental health. Some examples include Magnesium and Vitamin B that have been demonstrated to reduce symptoms of depression, and anxiety, dietary fibre, probiotics, and prebiotics directly influence the gut health which is where approximately 90% of the body's serotonin is produced. When people are lacking in micronutrients it can be tempting to use multivitamins as the first and quickest way to fix this deficit. However, more recent research has found that using multivitamins as the primary or only tool of increasing a person's micronutrient intake can be detrimental and, in some cases, harmful to the person's health. The phrase "eating a rainbow" is still the best advice for many people to follow, as most people will benefit from this approach. Micronutrients and hormones that assist in the body's circadian rhythm include vitamin B12, lithium and melatonin. Novak and colleagues reviewed two of the most important micronutrients – Vitamin D and Omega Fatty Acids.

Vitamin D is used in over 1000 different biological processes in the body. This means that there are many opportunities for a deficiency, such as people living in the northern hemisphere or extreme southern hemisphere. Some of the Vitamin D receptors can be found in the cortex, hippocampus and cerebellum, and are used to help regulate movement, memory and cognition. Vitamin D also helps to transport serotonin to the brain and improves calcium absorption (alongside vitamin K). Vitamin D is also associated with an increase in Brain Derived Neurotrophic Factor (BDNF) which is thought to be important for neuronal health and growth, Glial cell Derived Neurotrophic Factor (GDNF), and nerve growth factor which is thought to help maintain and improve the structures of the brain. As discussed earlier, individual needs vary, but some research suggests that 10-25mcg of Vitamin D per day is beneficial.

Omega Fatty Acids including Docosahexaenoic Acid (DHA) and Eicosatetraenoic Acid (EPA) are considered healthy fats, while trans fats are known as unhealthy fats. Low DHA and EPA has been correlated with many mental health conditions including Schizophrenia, Attention Deficit Hyperactivity Disorder (ADHD), Depression and Bipolar. The main benefits of sufficient DHA and EPA include the inhibition of cytokine synthesis (which can cause inflammation when there is too much), assist in the dopaminergic and serotoninergic systems (which most mental health medications target), assist with receptor functioning, assist in the manufacturing of more synapses, assist in the maintenance of cell and neuron structure integrity and assist with neuroplasticity. The recommended source for DHA and EPA includes seafood related oils such as fish, krill and green lipped mussels, and nuts and seeds. Recommended dosages range from one to ten grams daily.

Macronutrients include protein, carbohydrates, and fats. They are the basic building blocks for energy and also provide important nutrition to the brain for emotional, cognitive and relational functioning. Hydration is also important here. Protein provides the brain with amino acids that are crucial for cellular integrity and the form the basis of neurotransmitters (such as Tryptophan and Serotonin) that regulate mood. When a person doesn't consume enough protein, it can lead to brain fog and a depressed mood. Carbohydrates include simple carbohydrates (fruits, vegetables and sugars) and complex carbohydrates (whole grains, starchy vegetables and beans) and provide the brain and body with fuel. When a person consumes simple carbohydrates, they receive a temporary boost in mood, but this can then cause a crashing effect in the body. When a person consumes complex carbohydrates, there is a slow release of glucose into the bloodstream. When a person doesn't consume enough complex carbohydrates their front brain functioning can be negatively impacted (thinking, problem solving) as can their other brain centres relating to mood and stress management. Fats can be naturally occurring (saturated, monosaturated and polysaturated) and engineered (hydrogenated/trans-fats). The natural fats help to lubricate the brain and body organs, help with memory, and transport vital minerals and vitamins to the brain. Whilst, engineered fats may impair learning and memory, lead to weight gain and damage the body's essential processes. Hydration is very important for a healthy body. Dehydration has been found to alter the function and structure of the brain resulting in problems in cognition, attention, focus, emotional control and irritability. A person needs to drink at least 1.8-3ltrs a day depending on weight, activity level, temperature, etc., to avoid hyponatremia (low blood sodium levels) and to avoid hyperhydration. Despite the various "optimal ratios" that are taught to us in the fitness world, told to us by nutritionists, etc., there is no one rule fits all to this ratio. Genetic heritage is a large determining factor regarding what ratio is best suited to an individual. The individual's needs are determined by their genetic heritage, current location, activity level, medication conditions, emotional state and current physical health. Groups such as the National Academies of Science have reference tables with the minimum amounts of macronutrients a person needs based on age.

Hypoglycaemia is also known as Low Blood Glucose. It occurs when the level of glucose in the blood drops below what is a healthy normal level for that person. Some research has suggested that by stabilising our glucose levels, we can directly impact or influence our mood. There are reportedly two types of hypoglycaemia, known as Primary Hypoglycaemia and Reactive Hypoglycaemia. Primary Hypoglycaemia occurs from the inadequate supply of carbohydrates, whereas Reactive Hypoglycaemia is the excessive release of insulin following a meal with high amounts of refined carbohydrates. Hypoglycaemia can be a risk factor for people withdrawing from addictions such as tobacco, nicotine, and other stimulant related addictions, as the refined carbohydrates often release a shorter-term chemical high that the person may be looking for. The healthiest way to manage Hypoglycaemia is through consuming protein, healthy fats, starchy and non-starchy vegetables, complex carbohydrates and eating regular smaller meals. Hypoglycaemia can cause irritability, anxiety, nervousness, craving refined sugars, panic, crying, fainting, motor weakness or poorer functioning, personality changes, headaches, visual disturbances, confusion and shakiness. It may also be misdiagnosed and mistreated (but also comorbid with) – anxiety, bipolar, irritability, insomnia, tantrums, hyperactivity and depression.

Food allergies, sensitivities and subsequent need for adapted or special diets are varied with some people having minor sensitivities to one food, while other people can have life threatening responses to specific food compounds. Food allergies often occur immediately after ingesting food but can take up to several hours later. Risk factors for food allergies include genetics, chronic infections, poor quality or pro-inflammatory foods, nutritional deficits and chronic stress. Food sensitivities and intolerances are the most common diet induced inflammatory response, and symptoms can include skin changes, digestive issues, respiratory issues, fibromyalgia, GERD, IBS, obesity, migraines, depression, insomnia and chronic fatigue syndrome. In the westernised countries, one the most common food sensitivity or intolerance is lactose, with up to 70% of the westernised population being lactose intolerant.

If your pulse raises more than normal after eating a specific food, it may be a sign of a food sensitivity. One of the other most common food sensitivities or intolerances is gluten. Gliadin and Glutenin are two proteins in grains that may trigger an immune system response. Type one sensitivity is known as Coeliac and is an autoimmune response in the small intestines. Gluten intolerance may trigger Gluteomorphins to be released in the brain which may then trigger an opioid-like effect on the brain. Type two gluten sensitivity is known as Non-Coeliac Gluten Sensitivity (GS) and is an immune response that leads to digestive and neurological difficulty and often goes undiagnosed. Approximately 1 in 250 people in the USA have Coeliac disease and approximately 1 in 10 people in the USA have gluten sensitivity. Alternative foods to gluten rich foods include Basmati rice, potato, coconut, almond, buckwheat, sorghum, sweet potato, legumes and tapioca. If a person is sensitive to gluten, there is approximately a 50% chance of the person also being sensitive to casein (found in milk). Some studies completed in USA have found that despite individual difference there are some geographic cultural averages regarding lactose intolerance. Cultures where dairy animals are not native and therefore people didn't genetically be exposed to dairy historically leads to intolerances (80-100% of African and Asian peoples are Lactose or dairy intolerant, 70-80% of African Americans and Mexican native peoples are Lactose or dairy intolerant, 60-90% of Mediterranean and Jewish descended peoples are Lactose or dairy intolerant, and 1-5% of Northern Europeans are Lactose or dairy intolerant).

A common medical disorder known as Alzheimer's is now being investigated as type three diabetes. This is because the conditions that lead to type two diabetes are almost the same as the conditions that lead to Alzheimer's disease and dementia. As well as lifestyle and nutritional changes such as managing the amount of grains and refined sugars ingested, there are other supplementary behaviours that may assist in lowering the risk factor for Alzheimer's disease. These include the use of Hyperbaric Oxygen Therapy, and by lessening inflammation in the body by consuming more turmeric, hops, rosemary, gingko, vinpocetine and vitamin E. Childhood trauma, toxic accumulations (such as from mould spores), brain injury, and the APOE gene are other risk factors.

Nutrition can directly influence the health of our Mitochondria. Mitochondria are known as the cells power plants and are essential for mental health. Viruses, stress, immune issues, poor nutrition and poor mental health can cause mitochondria dysfunction. To assist the body in its absorption of nutrients, improve gas, bloating and GERD, consuming digestive enzymes are important. The key Digestive Enzymes – Proteolytic Enzymes (digests proteins and inflammation), Amylase (digests Carbohydrates), Lipase (digests fats), Cellulase (digests fibre), Maltase (converts complex sugars into glucose), Lactase (digests milk sugars such as lactose), Phytase (helps to produce B Vitamins) and Sucrase (digests most sugars).

This section has focused on nutrition rather than weight goals or an individual's fat percentage. This is because a person's weight is only one indicator of their overall self and health and in our modern world is often used in a negative context. A person's weight and weight fluctuation can be influenced by bone density, water retention, genetic response to stress, and other factors that may not be considered in a medical or sales environment. The Body Mass Index (BMI) is still used today in a medical setting for a base line only and should not be used as a true indicator of a person's health. Focusing on weight also increases the risk of poorer mental health, which can then create a cycle of weight related difficulties and poor mental health. A person with an average BMI may be unhealthier than a person with a larger BMI due to fats being stored around the organs. This highlights the importance of speaking with your GP (General Practitioner) as a starting point and then speaking with a dietician regarding specific nutrition advice if weight and food related health difficulties are a concern. The GP can be a great place to start, however, as GP's know a lot about many areas of the human body, they can't be expected to have a full understanding of human nutrition as well.

Key Points & Relevant Personal/Professional Experiences

Brief Dip into Physics, Psychology and Physiology

Physics provides a foundation for understanding the principles that govern biological systems, and it can be used to explain the energy transformations and interactions at a cellular level, which Western and Eastern physiology describe as biochemical and energy flows, respectively. Physics focuses on the structure of matter and its interactions between fundamental parts of the observable universe including the physiology of plants and animals, whereas psychology focuses on the mental processes and behaviour in animals. At the macro level these can be seen as very different areas of study however, at the micro and social levels these two areas of study and learning share many similarities.

Biochemical reactions, energy metabolism, and thermodynamics are all areas stemming from physics that are used in the medical model to examine physical health, and some of this language has entered psychology and social language use such as feeling warmth towards someone or feeling drawn to an activity or person.

The relationship between an established theory of physics known as supersymmetry and a less recognised theory known as asymmetry-induced symmetry is relevant to health and psychology. In non-physics language, there are instances in which the observed behaviour of the system can be symmetric only when the system itself is not. This can also be explained as the microlevel being asymmetrical which then leads to the observable (macrolevel) becoming symmetrical. In psychology there is a similar idea where the individual is always different to everyone else, but at the macro level (society, town, culture, etc.) the differences or "chaos" averages out to behaviours known as socially acceptable or common behaviours.

At the microscopic level, quantum mechanics explains phenomena such as molecular bonding and electron behaviour, which are essential for understanding biochemical processes. Quantum mechanics discusses how everything is connected by energy and this idea is again relevant to feelings of social connection, and even interoception of emotions often referred to as "gut instinct".

The observer effect and the role of consciousness in quantum mechanics is another physics area that states that the process of observing a particle changes the way the particle behaves. The same has been found to be true when examining a person's physical health through scans or physical fitness assessments, as well as through social observation and the resulting change of a person's behaviour.

Physics concepts such as JND (Just Noticeable Difference) are relevant in counselling settings when discussing goal setting, motivation and stages of change models, but physics can also inform how a person learns. When taking a more wholistic health approach in psychology, physics concepts such as Wolff's law can be relevant to arthritis, nutrition and exercise discussions. Finally, when discussing social connection to people who are either very scientific or to people who are very spiritual in their life approach, the physics idea of quantum entanglement theory can be used to discuss connection. Quantum entanglement theory briefly discusses that "things" are connected by energy, and many spiritual beliefs discuss that people are connected by energy.

Brief Dip into Physics, Psychology and Physiology

The psychology, health and physics overlaps are also useful in a learning environment. Every person has a different way of learning and retaining information (microlevel). However, despite schools and teachers trying their best to individualise education, they still have to use macrolevel education standards and tools.

Psychology and learning

Defining learning

Learning is defined by most dictionaries as "the acquisition of knowledge or skills through study, experience, or being taught". This starting definition helps to illuminate the idea of learning as being more than only remembering definitions. The word 'skills' is included, as a skill is something that can be taught theoretically, but also requires practice, leading to an improvement in that behaviour or task. The skills need to be tested and practiced allow the learning to be improved and embedded, leading to even deeper learning and more accurate memory.

Learning is also discussed as an increase, often through experience, of problem-solving ability. Researcher and author Washburne developed a formula they used to attempt to measure learning in a quantifiable way. Washburne's formula of m/r meant that 'm' represented the memories which aided in the extension of experience towards the goal, and the 'r' represented the resistance to the attainment of the goal (such as habits, conflicting goals, etc.). Their research suggested that when the ratio m/r increases, learning is proportional to cue reduction.

Neurologically speaking, for those who do not experience blindness, to learn we must see the stimulus. This stimulus is then transmitted into our Visual Cortex, which then transmits this information to our Visual Association Cortex, and finally to our various association parts of the brain. For example, when a person reads, the words are seen by the eyes, transmitted to the Visual Cortes, then to the Visual Association Cortex and then to the Language Association Cortex. People who are considered more creative (in arts, dance, business, science, etc.) have been shown via imaging, to have more powerful association cortices (more pathways, more neuronal firing and more interconnection).

Another important aspect of learning that is often overlooked is motivation, also known as 'the why'. This will be discussed later in the book, but it is important to raise this point here. When a person or team understands why they want to learn something or improve, they are more likely to work towards this. Alongside an individual's motivation is their perception. No one sees the world exactly as it is. Every person has their own perception based on their life experiences, their emotions and the context of the event or "thing" which influence how they understand and therefore how they respond to their reality.

Many of the learning theories discussed in this book will be rooted in a Western cultural viewpoint, informed by both my personal experiences, research and professional insights.

To assist in any form of learning, healthy eating, sleep and other positive life practices are beneficial, but will not be discussed in this book due to the focus being specifically on learning. However, this is an important side note, as we don't learn in isolation, and our ability to learn is directly influenced by our health.

We learn every day, often known as informal or implicit learning. We learn when we speak to other people, we learn by reading, participating in activities, repeating the same task, attempting a new task, we even learn when watching a cartoon or movie. Our brain is always adapting and as a result we are always learning even if we are not aware of this fact. Even when asleep, we are still learning as our dreams act as thought and experience consolidation, as well as assisting in emotional processing and reorganising of the day's events.

This book will focus more on formal learning also known as *structured learning or learning with intent*.

When thinking of formal learning one of the first ideas people may remember is that of formal schooling. For many people daycare is their first example of formal learning, often taught to children through play or in primary school often taught in classrooms. This semi-structured and later structured learning environment is used to help teach many people the basics that their state or country has legislated as required learning. The modern-day school helps many people learn basic mathematics, language, science, and health concepts often through wrote learning and visual learning. The modern school is also a common place where young people learn social skills and emotional skills from their teachers as well as from other peers.

Understanding how we learn is useful as this knowledge can be used to improve our efficiency at learning. Motivation, memory, learning styles and sensory barriers are all areas relating to learning.

Memory Summary

Memory can be defined as the mental capacity of retaining and reviving information including facts, events, emotional impressions, etc. Memory forms part of a person's perception of their reality but is not 100 percent accurate. When memories are being encoded, they can be impacted by various internal and external influences such as our own emotion, any relevant life history prior to the event or information, the context of the event or information, the event or information itself as well as various other sensory inputs. Memories can be encoded as various types, most of which have a strong overlap with each other including interpersonal (between people), intrapersonal (understanding of self) memory, fact or information-based memory, emotional memory, and somatic memory.

Somatic memory is when the person's body remembers the event or information physically such as a muscle tension response when the person sees an animal they fear, or a release of tension through a relaxing sigh when a person remembers a positive event from the past.

As well as somatic memory there are other types of memory known as Short-term memory, Long-term memory and Working memory. Short-term memory is a term used to describe the information a person can remember for a short period of time, often 15-30 seconds. Traditionally this often includes seven items of information plus or minus two, such as writing a short list or writing a person's phone number. Working memory often lasts up to 15 seconds and is the information the person is receiving. The level of focus and investment from the person during this time can greatly impact the accuracy and manipulation of information that is transferred to short or long-term memory. Long-term memory happens when the short-term memory is stored for longer term use and can include information that is older than 30 seconds. As will be seen throughout this book there are various ideas and frameworks in which academics and researchers have theorised, we learn, store and retrieve memories.

There are various areas of the brain responsible for memory and the type of memory can influence what part of the brain is activated. The most common brain areas used in memory activation include the – Prefrontal Cortex, Neocortex, Basal Ganglia, Amygdala, Hippocampus and Cerebellum.

Different types of memories often require an activation from different brain areas. Explicit memories that can include direct experience and facts, often activate the Hippocampus, Neocortex and the Amygdala. Implicit memories such as motor memories often activate the Basal Ganglia and the Cerebellum. Working memory relies heavily on the Prefrontal Cortex and is therefore vulnerable when a person is under intense stress, or their environment provides a sensory information overload (which can also trigger a stress response).

To improve the chance of memory recall in the future several ideas are useful. Firstly, paying mindful attention to the event/idea/person/behaviour improves the amount of neural firing (pathways) attached to the memory. Next trying to acknowledge the emotions relevant to the memory improves encoding pathways. Lastly, consciously storing the memory with all relevant information including sensory information can greatly improve the ability of future memory recall.

The idea that the brain has memory types is a practice that we have developed to understand and compartmentalise our new and old understandings. The brain regions don't stick to their "type of memory" but instead there is often communication across the brain regions. Memory has been broken into the three types to assist in learning the basics only.

Learning Across the Lifespan

There are many metaphors used to explain the human brain. Combining two metaphors, the human brain works somewhere between a supercomputer and a sponge. The early childhood brain is absorbing lots of information from their environment which is forming the base for their future learning and perception of reality. This base combined with their inherited genetics forms the basis of their coding, with which they will use and adapt for the rest of their lives. The way the individual child learns best is dependent on this combination, which is why the mass education movement from the industrial revolution has seen drastic changes in recent years.

The healthy newborn baby has approximately 100 billion neurons, which make at least 100 trillion interconnections. First the connections begin to change from undifferentiated brain cells, to migrating toward a predetermined location in the brain, and then differentiates into specific types of cells appropriate to that location. Next the aggregation of similar types of cells changes into distinct brain regions, forming connections among the neurons within and across the regions. Next the competition for energy among these connections results in the selective elimination of many of the neurons resulting in the 100 trillion plus interconnections.

This process doesn't occur in a rigid sequence, instead overlapping in time, from about 5 weeks after conception onward. After about 18 months of age, no more neurons are added, and the collection of cell types into distinct regions is roughly complete. Next comes the synaptic pruning.

During the first year of life, the number of synapses in the brain of an infant grows tenfold. By the age of 2 to 3, an infant has about 15,000 synapses per neuron. During the second year of life, the number of synapses being to drop dramatically. Synaptic pruning happens very quickly between ages 2 and 10. During this time, about 50 percent of the extra synapses are eliminated. In the visual cortex, pruning continues until about 6 years of age. These years are vital for a young child's development in the areas of motor movement patterns, basic emotional understandings, basic reading and writing skills and the exploration of interests. The young child's environment will strongly influence how they manage their own emotions and interact with others' emotions for the rest of their lives. Children often learn best when interacting with people they know and trust, or when learning material from their favourite characters or influences. Fun is the key to learning in this age range. The first seven years are also known as the core attachment years.

During adolescence the synaptic pruning continues through adolescence, but not as fast as before. The total number of synapses begins to stabilise, even though the pathways developing are beginning to utilise these synapses very differently to young childhood.

Adolescence is a vital time for learning and exploration and is a larger risk reward time. Adolescent brains don't have much access to their frontal lobes and as such, they are much more likely to be adventurous in their exploration leading to great feats such as in gymnastics and motorcross, but also greater risks such as speeding and drug taking. It is also a very important time in social learning. During Adolescence the core identity is beginning to form, separate from the parents, and it is this combined with the greater risk taking that leads to the adolescent brain listening more to their peers. This combination can lead to a healthy self-identity base, but also means the adolescent is vulnerable to social and emotional manipulation and bullying from peers. Future thinking is minimal during early adolescence despite efforts from the environment (parents, teachers, organisations, etc.).

The synaptic pruning continues into early adulthood stopping in the late 20s. During this time the pruning occurs mostly in the brain's prefrontal cortex, which is the part of the brain heavily involved in the decision-making processes, personality development, and critical thinking. The pruning is taking place because of our brain's brilliant neuroplasticity, and it is this ability to adapt that can either assist or hinder our development. Even our IQ (Intelligence Quotient), once thought to be set in stone changes during our teenage years, with one third of people's IQ going up, one third staying close to the same, and one third going downwards. The brain's pruning and adaptation has been found to be different between the male and female biological sex with females having greater volume in the prefrontal cortex, orbitofrontal cortex, superior temporal cortex, lateral parietal cortex, and insula. While males, on average, had greater volume in the ventral temporal and occipital regions. Each of these regions is responsible for processing different types of information. This difference in the brain development focus and synaptic change is thought to be highly influenced by the reproductive hormones, again highlighting the importance of understanding the body's systems as an interacting network.

Adult learners are more goal-oriented, activity-oriented, or learning-oriented than children. Four principles that can be applied to adult learning include – Involving Adult Learners as adults need to be involved in the planning and evaluation of their instruction; Taking into account the Adult Learners' Experience which can inform and provide the basis for learning activities; understanding the Relevance & Impact to Learners' Lives as most adults are most interested in learning subjects that have immediate relevance and impact to their job or personal life; and, using a Problem-Centred approach as adult learning is problem-centred rather than content orientated.

Research has also identified learning phases adults often go through. Dissonance is identified as the primary learning phase when the learner's existing knowledge is incomplete and is influenced by resources, motivation, stage of development, learning style, age, etc. Elaboration and Refinement involves the new learning concepts being facilitated through task completion, research, reflection, and discussion. Organisation allows reflection in action for the integration of the new learning into schemata which fits the learner's new understanding. Feedback stage is an essential phase for the learner to articulate and refine their knowledge and is influenced by the quality of feedback provided by the environment (including those in responsible for the teaching). Consolidation is the final phase involving reflection on action, for learners to better understand the learning process and content.

The saying use or lose it applies heavily in the context of the brain. Our conscious, subconscious and unconscious thoughts (such as dreaming) and actions all heavily influence the synaptic pruning, especially as we enter adulthood. When we stop thinking or using a particular behaviour, that pathway is slowly pruned, and experienced as a loss of skill or knowledge. Our overall health also directly influences this process, as all body systems interact, and influence outcomes on each other, including our brain. Some researchers have suggested that over pruning is a risk factor for developing various motor and mental health difficulties such as Epilepsy, Alzheimer's Disease or Schizophrenia.

As we age, more and more pathways continue to be pruned. This is a basic survival response helpful in the wild (by allowing for efficient use of brain resources) but leads to various difficulties in today's complex modern world. The older aged adults can often be observed to experience a sudden cognitive decline however, this decline was happening in the background. A common example includes the older male who in their youth knew how to complete basic banking activities, but as they aged alongside their partner, they stopped using these brain pathways and instead relied on their partner. When the partner leaves them or dies, the older male has lost many of the pathways (knowledge, skill and confidence) relating to performing the basic banking.

Various examples have demonstrated an older adult entering a nursing home after recovering from a fall or being placed in a nursing home after dementia related behaviours have begun. The older adult is then hopefully in a supported living arrangement, which improves their safety. However, this supported living arrangement comes at the cost of reduced activation requirements for the adult including toileting, cooking, basic hygiene, exercise, etc.

A more serious example was an older female who injured in her hip. Prior to the hip, she was able to communicate, play chess, and perform basic home tasks. However, once in hospital, her basic medical needs were met, but her other needs were neglected (physio, social interaction, etc.), and she passed away after two weeks. This last example demonstrates how quickly the synaptic pruning can occur and how the other body systems influence each other.

Any healthy person at any age has the ability to learn new skills or change unwanted behaviours. However, as we age, learning a new skill or changing an unwanted behaviour becomes increasingly difficult because we have less synaptic pathways to utilise.

Pre-learn, learn and drill Theory

Young and colleagues found that learning efficiency benefited from three core aspects he defined as Pre-learning, Learning and Drilling. His research found that Pre-learning was a helpful tool to assist a person in mapping or planning their learning journey. Pre-learning consists of identifying what the person wants to learn, planning what the most efficient and effective way to achieve the goal might be, the best order in which to learn (considering any prior learning that might need to be done) and identifying the most important things to learn with the relevant context. Other research has supported this and suggested that Pre-learning is a useful tool, but no more than 10 percent of the entire allocated learning time should be allocated to Pre-learning. This is theorised to avoid the possible procrastination that might occur during the Pre-learning phase.

Young identified the most important aspect of Learning that needs to be remembered was hard work. A person must spend the time and put in the effort to improve their learning. This can be made more efficient by removing external distractions (noise, other sporadic wants, etc.) and by removing internal distractions (what was for dinner, stress, anxiety, etc.). As discussed in other areas in this book, understanding the value and motivation behind the learning goal can assist in removing the distractions.

Finally Young discussed the term 'Drilling'. Drilling includes understanding what current weaknesses the person has that is relevant to the main goal but needs to be strengthened prior to the official learning taking place. It is thought that by strengthening the weaknesses, the rest of the learning journey and memory retention of the topic would be improved.

Using Young's structure can assist in improving how efficiently a person learns, even if it feels like it might take longer due to the Pre-learning process. Another important aspect is understanding how any other prior learning can assist in the learning process. Some researchers have used the term 'Lateral thinking' or 'Lateral learning' which can be loosely defined as the ability to use other information from topics that might not seem relevant to improve the outcome of the current goal or behaviour. One example in psychology might include using a physics example of 'Just Noticeable Difference' and instead applying it to goal setting and behaviour change.

Kolb's Experiential Learning Model

The model was first published in 1984 by David Kolb, an American psychologist, professor and education theorist. Kolb was born in 1939 and earned his undergraduate degree from Knox College in 1961. He then earned a PhD in social psychology from Harvard University. Kolb's experiential learning theory was influenced by the work of other education theorists, including Jean Piaget, John Dewey, and Kurt Lewin.

Kolb's learning style model contains two continuums in the centre – a Perception Continuum (How we think about things) and a Processing Continuum (How we do things). There are four learning stages on the outside of the model – Concrete Experience and Learning (Feeling), Reflective Observation (Watching), Abstract Conceptualisation (Thinking) and Active Experimentation (Doing). The four stages of Kolb's model are portrayed as an experiential learning cycle where learners can enter the cycle at any time. Kolb reported that learners have natural preferences for how they enter the experiential learning cycle based on their hereditary equipment (genes), past life experiences, and the demands of the individual's environment.

Kolb's learning model has five levels of preference (Very Strong, Strong, Moderate, Low and Very Low Preference) given to the person based on how much they scored for each of the four main types of learning. The four learning styles are Activist, Reflector, Theorist and Pragmatist. After completing the required assessment, the person's results are scored, and they are then combined into a profile known as Kolb's learning styles.

Kolb's Reflector learning style contained two significant features – Observation and Consideration. The reflector prefers to gather a lot of information and gain experiences, before making their conclusion. Cooperation is vital to the reflector, because they gain a lot of ideas from listening to others. A reflector is process oriented before they act but is not very good at working towards a final result, on short deadlines or by prioritizing tasks.

Kolb's Theorist learning style benefits from qualified knowledge in a system, as they gather theory, they store all of it into a system / model / scheme / structure, etc. In opposition to the reflector, the theorist prefers to work alone to ensure that the work is done properly. On the other hand, the theorist is good in concluding, they don't keep in the background, and they would like to participate in discussions with their knowledge.

Kolb's Pragmatist learning style prefers to have the opportunity to experiment and would like to tear everything apart and repair it once again, to see how it works. A learning path must be manageable with a clear purpose, and the processes must not come on hold, or else the pragmatist will get impatient very quickly. In opposition to the theorist, the pragmatist doesn't read a manual from cover to cover but prefers to try things out for themselves.

Kolb's Activist learning style benefits from being given space to explore the content on their own right away. They are often very impulsive and become bored quickly. The activist is good at working with deadlines under a lot of pressure and is often only involved in several activities in any one moment. Furthermore, they are good at finding alternative solutions and often discovers something new and exciting but often say yes to too many tasks at once.

Kolb's model has many more layers that explore the depth of learning including Behavioural Complexity, Symbolic Complexity, Perceptual Complexity, Affective Complexity, Acquisition, Specialisation and Integration.

Transformational Leadership and Learning

The term was first coined in 1973 by Downton. Later Burns linked the roles of leadership and followership in 1978 identifying two types of leadership (Transactional and Transformational). They reported that Transactional leadership focuses on exchanges between leaders and followers (politicians winning office from public, teachers giving students grades for work), whereas, Transformational leadership is when the person engages with others, creates connection, raises level of motivation and morality in both leader and follower. In 1976 House published a similar theory known as charismatic leadership.

The goal for healthy leadership is to be a Transformational leader that motivates followers to do more than expected. This type of leader focuses on improving performance of followers and developing them to their fullest potential, Empowers followers, nurtures them, raises consciousness, helps them transcend their own self-interests for the sake of others, are strong role models, have highly developed set of moral values & self-determined sense of identity, are confident, competent, articulate, express strong ideals, listen to followers, develop spirit of cooperation with followers, create a vision, are social Architects and are effective at working with people.

The strengths of this model include – it is widely researched, has intuitive appeal (advocates change for others), broader view of leadership that augments other models, emphasis on followers' needs, values and morals, and evidence that transformational leadership is effective. The weaknesses of the model include – it lacks conceptual clarity, difficult to define exact parametres, the validity is challenged and difficult to measure, it treats leadership as a personality trait rather than a learned behaviour and has been accused of being elitist and antidemocratic. However, some practical uses include – recruitment, selection and promotion, training and development, and improving team development, decision making groups, quality initiatives.

Learning Styles

There is some debate among academic circles regarding the efficacy of learning styles. The term 'Learning Styles' was made popular during the 1960s following the theory of Multiple Intelligences from Howard Gardner. Since then, there was a strong focus, almost to the extreme about learning specific ways. Some research has suggested that learning styles are irrelevant, and it is the person's determination and passion that determine if they will learn the desired goal. However, I strongly suggest that learning styles are relevant but should be incorporated alongside passion and determination when learning. Understanding a person's motivation will assist in directing their passion and determination alongside their learning styles.

Many people don't learn with only one learning style, and often have multiple areas of strength when learning. For example, a person who studies for an exam by reading the content aloud while audio recording their own voice is implementing visual learning, auditory learning, and elements of kinetic and wrote learning. The learning styles a person uses, may also change based on the context of the learning, i.e., from a book in a library or in the middle of a busy workplace. There are many different learning styles that will be discussed with different academics using different terms for similar interpretations, which may lead to overlap across the learning styles.

Informational learning

Informational learning can include linguistic and mathematical subsets. The linguistic learning subset will often involve learning through words and can have a strong overlap with the verbal and auditory learning styles. A Linguistic learner utilises language as their foundation for most learning.

Mathematical learners often learn better with numbers, structure, and reasoning. The Mathematical learning style has a strong overlap with the Sequential and Aural learning styles. People who utilise the Mathematical learning style often have a strength in Informational Learning, and often work in engineering or similar fields. Some people who have this strength may also use this alongside their music learning or career.

Visual/Spatial learning

Visual learning refers to when a person learns by watching, reading, or seeing information or behaviours. The term 'Visual Learning' refers to the learner using their sense of sight to encode information or employ their internal ability to visualise the information. Today's technology allows visual learners to excel in many areas with an enormous amount of video content and electronic books available to the average person. Other examples include diagrams, flow charts, colour, and images.

This visual strength often translates to a better spatial awareness when performing physical tasks such as building.

Auditory learning

Auditory learning refers to when a person learns by hearing and listening to the discussed information and can include listening to the instructions of what is required for behaviours or outcomes. The term 'Auditory Learning' refers to the learner's ability to use their sense of hearing to process information by listening. This can include listening to a recording, debate, podcast, etc.

Verbal learning

Verbal learning involves using sound. Often this can involve a person reading text aloud, having group discussion, and interactive questioning of information. There is a strong overlap here with the Interactive and Aural learning styles.

Aural/Musical/ Rhythmic/Melodic learning

Aural or Music learning involves the use of rhythm and sound to assist in the learning process. The person may sing information or use musical melodies or rhythm while reading or speaking to assist in memory retention. A common example of this is the alphabet song, nursery rhymes and other learning songs. Aural learning also utilises subtle mathematic patterns or structure. Unfortunately, many westernised schools and workplaces often teach people that this style of learning is only for young children, leading to less effective learning when people move from primary school to high school and then to the workforce.

However, there has recently been improvements made in some schools, with some schools having entire music programs that utilise and encourage this learning strength as part of their core curriculum.

Kinaesthetic learning

Kinaesthetic learning refers to when a person learns by doing. This may involve physically attempting the behaviour or task or attempting to add a practical behaviour to a theoretical concept, such as building a solar system diorama when learning about space. It can also involve field trips, interactive experiments, and role-playing. Kinaesthetic learning helps activate the person's brain pathways and utilises the Proprioceptive and Vestibular senses which may be beneficial for some people.

Tactile learning

Tactile learning involves touch. This often involves the learner touching and manipulating objects to assist in learning. Examples of this can include the use of playdough to roll and make letters, shapes, numbers, etc. Science experiments in the classroom are a common Tactile learning tool. There is a strong overlap between Tactile and Kinaesthetic learning.

Sequential learning

Some people learn best when information is presented in specific orders. This can include alphabetical order, progress order, timelining and can also include flow charts. A common example is seen in public and school libraries where the Dewey Decimal system is used to display books, utilising a form of sequential learning.

Wrote learning

Wrote learning refers to the physical practice of writing information or completing a task enough times that the person can remember it effectively. This can still be seen today in formal education and is also used in sports, martial arts, and some trades. There is a strong overlap with Wrote learning, Tactile and Kinaesthetic learning, although some academics may disagree.

Reflective/Intrapersonal Learning

Reflective or Intrapersonal learning involves the person using their reasoning skills to solve problems and interpret complex information. This can involve brainstorming possible solutions to dilemmas, analysing material, and having discussions that explore deeper interpretations. Intrapersonal learners often find psychology, philosophy and other fields that require self-reflection easier and more interesting. The intrapersonal learner will also often be more aware of their own internal emotions and needs.

Interpersonal/Interactive learning

The Interpersonal or Interactive learning style often involves group type learning. Debates, group activities and any activity that involves another person can be beneficial. This doesn't have to involve face-face learning and can also be done through question-answer scenarios or through open-source coding examples. This type of learning has a strong overlap with many of the other learning styles and is considered by some people, a practical example of combining different learning styles.

Implicit/Indirect learning

As discussed earlier, implicit learning often happens without our full conscious awareness, and is known as a "nonintentional automatic learning mechanism". Implicit learning may occur when a person fails an attempt, through social conversation, or from watching fictional movies. Implicit learning includes indirect (reading, etc.) and direct (life experience). Field trips, and apprentice programs can also be examples of this learning style. This implicit learning often happens slowly and can assist a person in developing what they may refer as "common sense". Some researchers also suggested that "muscle memory" is an example of implicit learning.

As a side note, the term "Implicit learning" can be helpful, however, terming it "common sense" may become unhelpful. Common sense as a term is often used in negative connotations but can be explained as 'assumed knowledge'. If a person can frame their previous implicit learning as 'assumed knowledge', it can allow them to appreciate their own life experiences without negatively impacting another person's.

Learning Styles Summary

As can be seen there are many different learning styles that with different academics using different terms for similar interpretations. Despite differences in terminology and opinion, advocates for the learning styles agree that a multisensory approach is best and where possible the learner, teacher, facilitator, etc., should implement a combination of learning styles. Understanding that the learning styles are useful frameworks rather than strict boxes can also be beneficial. Examples of multisensory learning includes group presentations utilising movement, PowerPoint, etc., drawing images and flow charts, and writing and performing songs, skits, etc.

Sensory Impacts/Barriers for Learning

Sensory and Senses Introduction

As discussed in a previous section, there are many senses that we use to experience our environment. There are also various 'Sensory Models', including Dr. Winnie Dunn's model, and Dr. Ayre's Sensory Integration model. However, due to my own professional training, I will be utilising the model from Dr. Miller's, 'Sensory Modulation Model'. This model separates a person's sensory difficulties into 'Sensory Sensitive', 'Sensory Slow' and 'Sensory Seeking'. A person can be 'Sensory Sensitive' to a type of stimuli but also use a variation as a seeking behaviour, however, it is most common that a person who is 'Sensory Slow' will also be 'Sensory Seeking' with that same sense.

Sensory Sensitive

'Sensory Sensitive' is defined as a sensitivity to a particular sense, often causing discomfort or distress. It can include – Only eating familiar foods, disliking strong tasting lollies, gag reflex when presented with new foods, disliking most fragrances from perfume or bath products, distress at smells that other children do not notice, disliking bright lights, greater than normal distress in unusual visual environments (e.g. bright colourful room, wall decorations), discomfort with fast moving images on television or movies, preferring the blinds/curtains closed, easily distracted visually, disliking loud, unexpected sounds (sirens, school bells), might cover ears or cry when presented with loud noises, larger than average startle response to unexpected sounds, easily distracted by background noises such as television or music, difficulty with higher pitched sounds such as hand driers, disliking having messy hands, disliking haircuts, disliking specific food textures, disliking specific fabrics, disliking teeth brushing more than other people, avoiding swings or trampolines, fear of heights and disliking feet off the ground and/or travel sickness or motion sickness. Ideas that can help with 'Sensory Sensitive' related difficulties include packing meals that are blander and serve sauces on side, using fragrance free washing detergent, having dark spaces for relaxing zones, using specific music or sound frequencies played through headphones, using vibration or heavier touch contact, using slow linear and rhythmic movements, and many more.

Sensory Slow

'Sensory Slow' is defined as being under responsive to sensory stimuli, often leading to seeking behaviours. It can include – Not noticing or care if food is spicy or bland, being unable to distinguish between different smells, not noticing noxious/ dangerous/ offensive smells, seeming oblivious to details of an object and the surrounding environment, not noticing when others walk into or leave a room, walking into objects or people as if they were not there, not responding when his or her name is called, not hearing sounds in the environment, appearing as if in their own world, making their own noises for fun (can also be related to stimming), not noticing if hands or face are messy or dirty, being unaware of temperature changes, not noticing if bumped or pushed, bumping into things or falling over objects, losing balance unexpectedly when walking on an uneven surface, having poor muscle tone or appearing more floppy than people of similar age, having poor endurance, becoming tired easily especially when standing or holding the body in one position, leaning on walls or slumping on furniture and/or walking loudly as if feet are heavy. Ideas that can help with 'Sensory Slow' related difficulties include cooking with sour or sweet flavours, using specific fragrances or fragranced washing detergents, using movement combined with visual cues or activities, having uneven or faster beats or visuals, buying different textured clothing, using higher intensity exercise or circuit training, encouraging team sports with lots of movement use environmental reminders for basic tasks such as eating enough or sleep routines.

Sensory Seeking

'Sensory Seeking' is defined as behaviours that involve the person wanting more of that specific sensory input and spending energy in meeting this sensory need. It can include – Adding salt & spice to their food, preferring spicy food, putting objects into their mouth prior to playing with them, enjoying music and television at extremely loud volumes, making noise in the background while doing other tasks, smelling people, animals and objects, touching people to the point of irritating them, seeking vibration, jumping/crashing/spinning/swinging/rolling, rocking in chair, jumping on bed or sofa excessively, loving fast movement input and/or grinding teeth. The ideas that can help with 'Sensory Seeking' related difficulties often have a very strong overlap with the ideas that help with the 'Sensory Slow' ideas.

Sensory Summary

All people have different levels of sensory input needs. Some people's brains filter close to the right amount of sensory information, and this leads to the person experiencing minimal sensory related stress. However, many people have at least one of their senses that either are sensitive leading to a sensory related stress (also known as sensory anxiety) or are sensory slow requiring seeking behaviours to help find the sensory homeostasis. Understanding our own sensory needs can assist in our own learning journey but also help with communicating with people we might be assisting in understanding their own sensory needs. When a person's sensory needs are met, they are much more likely to want to learn and be able to retain the learnt information.

5E Model of Instruction

The 5E model was developed as an approach to science teaching and learning. It was developed by the Biological Sciences Curriculum Study in 1987 with the goal to improve the experience of learners and the effectiveness of teachers. The 5E model was strongly influenced by a previous model for learning by Atkin and colleagues known as the Atkin and Karplus Learning Cycle. The 5E Model of Instruction consists of five teaching phases – Engagement, Exploration, Explanation, Elaboration and Evaluation. Each phase serves a specific function and overall, they aim to help the teacher provide a more coherent instruction, as well as assisting the learner to engage in the learning to better understand and retain the scientific knowledge. Research conducted in schools from different socioeconomic backgrounds, over the last several decades have supported the efficacy of the 5E model. Other studies have suggested that the model assisted in developing a better conceptual understanding of scientific ideas and models, had positive effects on general achievement in science, improved the level of learner's wanting to pursue further scientific study after school and led to a more positive attitude towards science.

The first of the five areas in the 5E model is known as 'Engage'. 'Engage' involves the teacher introducing a problem or event in a familiar context that the learners cannot yet explain with their current knowledge, because their current knowledge does not yet fit in with the new challenge or experience. As a result of this a cognitive conflict arises for the learner. This conflict plays an important motivational role and provides an opportunity to activate and elicit the learners' prior knowledge. From the cognitive learning perspective, this stage of the 5E model, is important because it addresses several processes which have been proven to be critical for enhancing meaningful, durable, and transferable learning.

Research from various academic, psychology, neuroscience and learning experts has shown that encouraging learners to recall relevant knowledge from previous courses or their own life experiences can facilitate the integration of the new material. Strategies such as asking learners questions specifically designed to trigger recall or providing learners with a relevant context can help them use prior knowledge to aid the integration and retention of new information. The research has stated time and again that prior knowledge plays an essential role in the processing and retention of new information. Information that learners need to learn, depends on what they already know because learning is a constructive process, building foundations of prior knowledge in their long-term memory. This foundational knowledge and memory then must be activated via prompting to become useful during the learning episode. This means that it must be activated in the long-term memory and enter the working memory when needed so that the learner can hold and manipulate the information.

When this manipulation happens, the new learning is generated with some pieces of the new information being connected to semantically related pieces of knowledge that the learner had retrieved from long-term memory. Following this, when the learner wants to retrieve what has been learned, they will be able to reconstruct the memories using the related knowledge from different learning episodes. Research has suggested that human memory does not store redundant information, instead using information that is already consolidated in long-term memory to build on new memories that share those features. However, many learners were found to have difficulty accessing their prior knowledge and required explicit opportunities to do so, often in the form of guidance from the teacher. This guidance also helps to protect against inappropriate use of prior knowledge or context.

Learning involves an assimilation process but also requires an accommodation process, where the prior knowledge and conceptual structures of the learner need to be fundamentally restructured to allow an understanding of the intended knowledge. Activation of prior knowledge with assimilation leads to memory updating, also known as learning. It is thought to be essential to activate prior knowledge because only memories that become activated are prone to change according to the cognitive neuroscience research. Once the assimilation, accommodation and activation processes have been used, a reconsolidation needs to happen, often guided by the teacher. This reconsolidation of learning combined with the appreciation of the real-life implications of the knowledge assists in long-term memory retention and more accessible knowledge for the future.

This 'Engage' stage of learning is hugely important for the cognitive and emotional/motivational dimensions involved in the learning process. It also allows for group discussions and cooperative learning, which are also important for socio-cognitive learning, which has been suggested to be more beneficial for both the teachers and the learners.

The second of the five areas in the 5E model is known as 'Explore'. The 'Explore' stage is about the guided inquiry activity that provides opportunities for students to address alternative conceptions and build new explanations that make sense to them. The 'Explore' stage is where the learner investigates phenomena, share their observations, suggest explanations, and discuss their interpretations. During this stage the teacher will facilitate, guide and scaffold the learners' thinking, which is what most effective teachers do anyway. This stage focuses on the promotion of connections between the learners' prior knowledge and the new information. To help the learner with the exploration of information, a guided inquiry-based approach is used, to assist in fostering thinking and sensemaking during the learning task. This is because people are thought to learn and remember better when they think about what they are learning in in terms of meaning, when they are prompted to connect information in ways meaningful to them.

The 'Explore' stage provides the learner with opportunities to reformulate their explanations by inferring them from new experiences and observations. According to the classical model of conceptual change by Posner and colleagues, after recognising conceptions are inconsistent in a new given situation, the learner needs to find an adequate new conception that successfully explains it. The new explanation must be able to be grasped by the learner and the learner needs to understand how it is consistent with prior knowledge. This can be completed with small groups, where the role of the teacher is to once again make sure the learner can help others to solve problems by building on each other's knowledge, ask questions to clarify explanations and suggest avenues that assist in moving the group towards the goal. Learning in the group setting also allows for cooperation in problem solving activities as well as debate/argumentation which has been suggested to enhance the learner' cognitive development in areas of learning, thinking, and reasoning. The teacher's role also requires careful guidance and extensive scaffolding to facilitate learning and may also include learning through investigation to assist in sensemaking, developing evidence-based explanations, collaborating and communicating ideas. Lastly, this stage provides the learner with opportunities to explore specific information, thereby creating a "time for telling", setting up the next stage known as the 'Explain' stage.

The 'Explain' stage is where the new concepts that had been grasped during the 'Explore' stage are formalised. This allows the teacher to formally introduce the concepts and help the learner to organise their new knowledge in a way that facilitates encoding and later retrieval of the information. Lots of learning related research has suggested that when the learner is provided with an organisational structure to fit new knowledge, they learn more effectively, when compared to being left alone to deduce this conceptual structure for themselves. In this stage the formalised definitions and explanations of the intended models and concepts are cooperatively built by the learner with the close guidance of the teacher.

The fourth stage of the 5E leaning model is known as 'Elaborate'. Activities in this stage require the learner to apply the concepts and procedures they have learned to solve new problems in new contexts. The new concepts offer the opportunity to prove they resolve the previous anomalies whilst also leading to new insights and discoveries for the learner. Activities in this stage also provide opportunities for the learner to transfer their new knowledge to a wide diversity of contexts. This is often done via exposing the learner to multiple contexts to promote deeper understanding and assist in abstracting the relevant features of the concepts and develop a flexible representation of the knowledge. By providing multiple contexts of applicability for the same overall concepts, it assists in creating several retrieval routes to access the learned information, which in turn increases the probability of the learner being able to find a match between the cues given in the transfer task and the stored memory. Extended practice is essential if something new is to be learned, especially if the goal is for the new knowledge to be retained over time and transferred to new situations.

The final stage of this learning model is known as the 'Evaluate' stage. The knowledge and abilities acquired by the learner are assessed through an activity that challenges their understanding. This has often been more subtly completed throughout the other stages, often informally through feedback and discussions, and is another form of learning. During the 'Evaluate' stage, the learner is often provided with tests or other forms of formal evaluation to determine the learners' level of understanding and abilities, whilst also serving as a tool for the learner to self-evaluate. Testing also provides another opportunity for the learner to retrieve information from their memory which in turn changes the memory and may increase the probability of successful retrieval in the future, through active repetition. Whilst testing has many benefits to the learners' memory and knowledge retrieval, it can cause some learners' distress which may negatively impact their ability to access the learnt information and negatively affect future memory and knowledge retrieval.

The '5E Model of Instruction' was designed in the late 1980's and then later adapted with the goal of improving a person's ability to learn more effectively and efficiently. The research that is used throughout the model believes that when the pattern of neural connections that represent a memory in the brain is reactivated, the brain experiences a new round of consolidations which works to strengthen and adapt the original memory with the newly learnt information through an active reconsolidation process. The model can be used in one-on-one settings but was designed for group use such as in classrooms.

Illusion of learning

Illusion of learning is when a person is physically attempting to learn information or a behaviour, but their mind is no longer paying conscious awareness. It also refers to a person who believes they understand a topic or task, but the person only recognises it. An example would be when a person studies for an exam for six hours without breaks and later only remembers the first or last hour of their study. A practical example might be a person who is fixing a car engine, finishes their task and finds a small piece left over. This suggests that at some point in their fixing, their mind stopped paying conscious attention and they relied on their muscle memory to finish the task. A personal example of the illusion of learning is when I was attempting to study a psychology topic. After two hours of study, I noticed I was now paying attention to the physics behind how bees fly. It is important for a person to understand the difference between learning and retaining information (learning and therefor knowing it) versus being with the information or task but not retaining it (illusion of learning).

Understanding the term 'illusion of learning' can be helpful and can be utilised to improve a person's study behaviours and memory retention. A person can use structured and semi-structured rests to help their learning retention and focus. A structured example may include setting an alarm for 2 hours and having a timed break such as 20 minutes. When the 20 minutes is finished, the person then returns to the study or task knowing they only must attempt to focus for 2 hours. A semi-structured approach would be when a person is studying or attempting a task, as soon as they notice their thoughts are on any other task or information such as food, they have a timed break such as 20 minutes, and when the break finishes, they return to their task or study.

This can improve a person's efficiency with learning, which is especially important when there are pressures such as due dates, fast-paced online workshops, etc.

Key Points & Relevant Personal/Professional Experiences

Psychology Specific Learning Frameworks and Ideas

There is a long history of psychology investigating how people learn including behavioural learning theories, cognitive learning theories, conditioning, and various others. This section will discuss the most common ideas including Journey vs Destination, Motivational Interviewing, Positive Thinking, Neuroplasticity, Conditioning, Observational/Social Learning, Stages of Change, FAIL, Proficiency and Becoming Great and the Time to Change.

Journey vs Destination

The Journey vs Destination argument is relevant to learning and the answer or outcome is individual and often context based. In some psychological frameworks such as Acceptance Therapy, they encourage people to identify what their destination is, but then try to redirect the person's attention back to their journey to assist in enjoying or appreciating their journey. It is important to acknowledge the destination as this allows the person to understand what their efforts are working towards. The destination can be 10 years away, or it can be within a month. The many concepts discussed in this book outline how and why the destination is important. Another more common word used in place of 'destination' is 'goal'.

One aspect often overlooked in modern societies around the world is the journey. Most people who are considered successful discuss that they learnt more from their failures along the way to their success and that their destination changed several times. Despite this, modern societies often place a strong societal and often peer-peer pressure on achieving, and less focus on appreciating and sometimes even enjoying the journey. Enjoying the journey is about being present in the now, mindful of the experiences and appreciating the positive and acknowledging the negative. When a person is solely destination focused, they might miss opportunities to adapt, might miss opportunities to enjoy, and might miss opportunities to improve. This last point can be summarised with the song lyrics "life is what happens when we are busy making plans".

Motivational Interviewing

Motivational interviewing is a client-centred counselling style used by professionals to encourage and guide behaviour change. It was originally developed by clinical psychologists William R. Miller and Stephen Rollnick and has had various updates to the framework. Most health professionals use the core principles of Motivational Interviewing, even if they don't use the formal structure of it. Motivational Interviewing can also be used by people in management positions to help understand and guide their staff towards a common goal.

The core principles of Motivational Interviewing include Expressing Empathy, Developing Discrepancy, Rolling with Resistance and Supporting Self-Efficacy. Expressing Empathy often involves conveying that as the listener, you understand some of their emotional experience even if you may not fully understand their individual experience. Often this involves listening for key thoughts, feelings, and statements of facts, normalising the person's responses to a difficult situation, reflective paraphrasing and phrases with genuine emotion.

Developing Discrepancy can include discussions regarding their future goals, barriers to improving, and discussions about what happens if nothing changes. Rolling with Resistance can include reframing towards more goal directed or positive language without arguing with the person who is seeking assistance. Finally, the listener or professional should try to encourage as much Self-Efficacy as possible to enhance a person's belief in their ability to begin, maintain or complete a task or behaviour. The four processes of Engaging, Focusing, Evoking and Planning are the practical steps the professional might use to assist the person.

One suggested structure within Motivational Interviewing that is used to improve the outcome is known as OARS. OARS stands for – Open-ended questions, Affirmations, Reflective listening, and Summaries.

Other tools used in Motivational Interviewing that won't be explored here can include Agenda Mapping (also known in other frameworks as mind mapping), Brief Action Plan, Elicit-Provide-Elicit model, Patient Dilemma focus (focusing on the concern and barriers to change), Evoking (exploring the Pros and Cons), Readiness Rulers (such as a 1-10 Likert scale) and various other goal frameworks, discussed elsewhere in this book.

Positive Thinking

The idea of thinking positively has been discussed for thousands of years through various spiritual practices, each with their own interpretation and causal explanations. There was a scientific movement investigating the idea of positive thinking as a tool to improve health in approximately the 1940s and 50s. More recently there have been a plethora of books and self-help guides using the idea of Positive thinking. Positive thinking can be loosely defined as looking at the brighter side of situations and is related to positive emotions and other constructs such as optimism, hope, joy, and wellbeing. Positive thinking is a mental attitude that admits into the mind; thoughts, words and images that are conducive to growth, expansion, and success. The idea is that if a person can change the words they use, they not only influence their perception, but can directly influence their overall health including physical and mental health.

As mentioned in the book 'My Eclectic Human Body', a field of science known as 'Psychoneuroimmunology' has been investigating the idea of positive thinking through a scientific and slightly spiritual lens. They believe that the interaction of our conscious thoughts and emotions can directly influence our neurology, mental health, and immune system. An emotionally induced illness is physical (felt in the body) and not imaginary due to the mind-body connection. Research was demonstrated in 1975 and is now known as Biochemical Perception. Biochemical perception highlights what a person can do to change the negative biochemical responses to stress. How a person perceives an event, directly impacts our immune system, thereby affecting our emotional and physical health. This provides an understanding of the importance of managing internal and external emotional conflict. The biochemical perception is also about how our internal environment is affected by stress, and that our perception of this can influence whether the stress increases or decreases. Emotions have a direct impact on our immune system as the body communicates with the brain via bidirectional communication. This suggests that changing our language use from negative to positive or to goal directed language can improve our stress management.

Psychoneuroimmunology research has found that almost every cell within the body responds to the way we think. The emotional aspects of a person influence their physical manifestation as evidenced by how stress modulates the activities of the nervous, endocrine, and immune systems.

The physiology of hopefulness can help the body to fight disease, whereas longer term emotional stress quietly harms the immune system and other systems in the body. Nerve proteins known as neuropeptides affect our emotions as well as our physiology. A feeling in the mind will translate as a peptide being released somewhere in the body, as peptides regulate every aspect of the body including digestion and immune system responses. Neuropeptides' neuronal signalling of molecules influence the activity of the brain in specific ways.

Different neuropeptides are involved in a wide range of brain functions, including analgesia, reward, food intake, metabolism, reproduction, social behaviours, learning and memory. When we change the way we think, we can change the way we feel and this creates a perceptual change, which in turn allows for a deeper level of self-governance around our thinking. Every emotion has connection with a physical counterpart, and every ailment has an emotional attachment.

A researcher and author Candance Pert discussed that the body and mind are one and that what a person thinks and how they speak, directly impacts the state of the body's cells. The spleen, every lymph node, and all floating immune cells are in close communication with the brain. Emotions live and run every system of the body, and are in bidirectional communication with the nervous, endocrine, and immune systems. Our emotional state is directly affected by perception, suggesting that a negative mind will lead to an unhealthier body.

Our perception changes, life changes, etc. trigger an epigenetic response, meaning they change our genetic memory and gene expression. Genetic memory can be altered through the process of positive thinking and visualization (for those without Aphantasia), which stimulates a positive emotional state and adjusts to a negative one. Generating pleasant feelings helps a person to gain a sense of control, build hope, and increase the ability to generate and experience love, laughter, empathy, joy, confidence etc. The body's goal is homeostasis; however, the responses are not always accurate, and a stress response may be activated when there is nothing to fear, dependent on the emotions and thoughts a person is experiencing in the moments prior, during and following. Whilst the goal is to generate positive emotions and thoughts, to assist the body's health and recovery, we also don't want to suppress the negative emotions and emotional awareness. If we ignore our needs and suppress our emotions, our subconscious mind will alert us to the fact that something is wrong, which may result in a physical manifestation of emotional strain and medical illnesses. This highlights the ever-increasing importance of self-interventions.

As discussed, thinking positively can directly improve our overall health and mental health. Thinking positively is not about dismissing the negative impacts of an event, emotion, or thing, rather about helping a person gain some control over their health and responses. Changing our language towards positive or goal-directed does not mean ignoring or dismissing negative experiences. Rather, it means encouraging a person to acknowledge and learn from their negative experiences, and then find ways to change their language use, in order to improve their health.

Neuroplasticity

Neuroplasticity involves the brain's ability to change by internal and external stimulus. It can be defined as brain's ability to change, remodel, and reorganise for purpose of better ability to adapt to new situations. Prior to 1890 it was commonly thought in many westernised cultures that the brain stopped developing after the first few years of life. It was commonly thought that only during the early "critical period" as a young child, that connections formed between the brains nerve cells which then remained fixed in place as we age.

As such it was considered that only young brains were able to change and thus able to form new connections. Because of this belief, scientists also thought that if a particular area of the adult brain was damaged, the nerve cells could not form new connections or regenerate, and the functions controlled by that area of the brain would be permanently lost.

However, in 1890 a psychologist William James, released his work known as the 'Principle of Psychology'. His work suggested that human brain including the adult brain was able to adapt and change, however his work was not widely accepted until 1948 when a neuroscientist Jerzy Konorski coined the term 'Neuroplasticity' and suggested that over time neurons that had 'coincidental activation due to the vicinity to the firing neuron would after time create plastic changes in the brain', meaning the brain can and will change. Again, it took time for this idea to be accepted by the scientific and psychological societies, taking until the late twentieth century. There is now a lot of resources discussing this importance.

Today, almost any educator, health worker, and most parents understand to various degrees, that the brain is capable of change. The brain is wired for survival and efficiency. The brain doesn't "care" about our long-term health, it "cares" about keeping us alive and being as efficient as possible. This is very useful as it allows people to learn about potential dangers increasing survivability and learn more efficient ways of performing tasks.

However, there are some negatives to neuroplasticity, with the first one being we are unable to directly choose how the brain adapts. As discussed in other sections of this book, we can influence our thoughts and our behaviours which has the side effect of changing our brain, but we do not have direct control. What we do, feel, and experience during the day is often consolidated and reorganised while we sleep.

We are all capable of change, so instead of letting the brain decide, it is useful to instead make positive life choices where we can, so that when the brain does its job of being efficient, we at least are having some positive input. This is also helpful to know for some people as it can provide hope that change is possible.

Conditioning

One area of psychology that focuses heavily on learning is known as 'Conditioning'. There are two major types – Classical Conditioning and Operant Conditioning. Classical Conditioning often involves an involuntary response and stimulus where Operant Conditioning involves a voluntary behaviour and consequence. Operant Conditioning is focused primarily on behaviours under our conscious control and leaves the automatic and reflexive behaviours to the Classical Conditioning framework.

Classical Conditioning

Classical Conditioning is also known as Pavlovian or Respondent Conditioning because of the experiment first published by Russian physiologist Ivan Pavlov in 1897. Classical conditioning is a type of automatic learning that is created through associations between an unconditioned stimulus and a neutral stimulus. The most famous example involves Pavlov's dog food experiment. Pavlov conditioned his dogs through a process of associating sound (neutral stimulus) and food (uncontrolled stimulus). The original sound of the tone did not produce any greater amount of salivation from his dogs. However, after enough pairings of the sound with the food, when the dogs heard the sound, their brains associated the sound with food and created a greater amount of salivation in anticipation of the food.

In psychology a field known as 'Behaviourism' developed from this idea of classical conditioning and psychologists such as Watson and Rayner strongly led the way using research and experiments. There is some overlap between behaviourism and social learning, the latter of which will be discussed elsewhere.

The underlying principles in Classical Conditioning include – Neutral Stimulus (a stimulus that initially does not trigger a response until it is paired with the unconditioned stimulus), Unconditioned Stimulus (the feature of the environment that causes a natural and automatic unconditioned response such as dog food with Pavlov's dogs), Unconditioned Response (an unlearned response that occurs automatically when the unconditioned stimulus is presented), Conditioned Stimulus (a substitute stimulus that triggers the same response in an individual as an unconditioned stimulus), Conditioned Response (learned response to the previously neutral stimulus), Acquisition (an individual learns to connect a neutral stimulus and an unconditioned stimulus), Extinction (the gradual weakening of a conditioned response by breaking the association between the conditioned and the unconditioned stimuli/unlearning, such as the bell ringing without food being presented), Spontaneous Recovery (return of a conditioned response in a weaker form after a period of time post-extinction), Generalisation (tendency to respond in the same way to stimuli that are similar but not identical to the conditioned stimuli) and Discrimination (process through which individuals learn to differentiate among similar stimuli and respond appropriately to each one).

Classical Conditioning involves three stages – Before, During and After conditioning. The first stage involves the unconditioned stimulus eliciting an unconditioned response. This means that the stimulus in the environment has produced a behavioural response which is unlearned and therefore natural. The neutral stimulus in classical conditioning does not produce a response until it is paired with the unconditioned stimuli.

The second stage involves the originally neutral stimulus being associated with the originally unconditioned stimulus leading to relationship whereby the stimulus is known as a 'Conditioned Stimulus'. The third stage involves the conditioned stimulus now being associated with the unconditioned stimulus to create a new conditioned response.

Classical conditioning can often be evident in stress or trauma responses and in psychology is sometimes known as paired association. An example could include a person who eats chocolate often with no conditioned response, becoming ill, and then having a conditioned response such as nausea whenever they think of eating chocolate again. A trauma response might include a person is hit by a red car, and then has a fear response only to other red cars. Classical conditioning is also relevant, in part, with addiction, fear responses, taste aversions, organisational behaviour and classroom learning where a person learns a response that they previously did not have in relation to a stimulus that was previously neutral.

There were several flaws in Classical Conditioning, however, it formed a strong base in which many other areas of psychology were able to develop and further our understanding of the brain, mental health and learning.

Operant Conditioning

Operant Conditioning involves an association being made between a behaviour and a consequence (positive or negative). Operant Conditioning was first described by Skinner who was an avid and early proponent of behaviourism psychology. Skinner strongly believed that internal thoughts and motivations were not required knowledge and that we only needed to understand the external, observable causes of human behaviour. Skinner used the term 'Operant' and defined it as "an active behaviour that operates upon the environment to generate consequences", which was heavily influenced by the work of Edward Thorndike's 'Law of Effect'. Outside of experimental laboratory conditions, Operant Conditioning often occurs where reinforcement and punishment take place, such as classrooms, therapy sessions or team sports.

In a classroom setting, if a student who raises their hand is rewarded with helpful information or praise regarding their behaviour, they are more likely to raise their hand in the future. This is because their initial behaviour of raising their hand was followed by a reinforcement or desirable outcome leading to the original behaviour being strengthened. The opposite occurs when the original behaviour is followed by an undesirable outcome such as punishment or lack of response. Such as if a student tells the same joke and receives no laughter from their peers. This leads to the original behaviour being weakened/less likely to occur again in the future.

The key concepts in Operant Conditioning include Reinforcement and Punishment, with a third, less spoken about concept known as Neutral Operants. Reinforcement includes positive and negative reinforcers. Positive reinforcers are favourable events or outcomes that occur following the behaviour. A response or behaviour is strengthened by the addition of praise or a direct reward. Negative reinforcers involve the removal of an unfavourable event or outcome after the original behaviour. A response is strengthened by the removal of something considered unpleasant. An example of where both can happen involves a screaming child in a public setting. A child screams as they want a biscuit, when the parent gives them the biscuit under the condition of the child being quiet, the child's screaming behaviour is strengthened (screaming equals biscuit) and the parent's behaviour of providing the treat is also strengthened as the parent is rewarded with silence. When using Positive Reinforcement there is a concept known as the Premack Principle which states that any positive reinforcement should make use of a preferred activity (high-probability behaviour) as the reward for completing a less preferred behaviour (low-probability).

Operant Conditioning has two types of punishment – Positive Punishment and Negative Punishment. Punishment is a tool used to weaken or eliminate a response. Positive Punishment is the addition of an unfavourable event or outcome such as spanking. Negative punishment is a punishment through the removal of a favourable event or outcome such as a removal of a toy or opportunity. Ineffective Punishment may occur when the punishment being used is no longer decreasing the undesired behaviour. One example might include a parent that says no desert if the vegetables are not eaten, but the child forgoes the desert and still does not eat the vegetables. Whilst punishment is often easier to implement than reinforcement there have been several weaknesses found regarding its use including – the behaviour may not be forgotten only suppressed until the punishment is no longer present or effective, there might be an increase in aggression in an attempt to negate the use of the punishment, it might create fear regarding the undesirable behaviour but also anything connected to the behaviour, and it might not guide towards the desired behaviour as it may only teach what not to do instead of the desirable behaviour is.

Neutral Operants are often not discussed when exploring Operant Conditioning but are important to understand as they are variables that may subtly improve or hinder focus. Neutral Operants are the responses from the environment that do not increase or decrease the probability of a behaviour being repeated.

In Operant Conditioning the application of reinforcement has several different types known as different Reinforcement Schedules. The five schedules are known as Continuous Reinforcement, Fixed-Ratio Schedules, Fixed-Interval Schedules, Variable-Ratio Schedules and Variable-Interval Schedules. Continuous Reinforcement is defined as delivering a reinforcement every time a response occurs. This allows for the learning to occur quickly, however, also allows for the extinction (loss of conditioning relationship) to occur quickly once reinforcement stops. Fixed-Ratio Scheduling involves a type of partial reinforcement. Responses are reinforced only after several responses have occurred. Fixed-Interval Schedules involves a partial reinforcement, but the reinforcement occurs only after a certain time interval has elapsed. Responses here remain steady and begin to increase as the reinforcement time draws nearer but may slow immediately after the reinforcement has been delivered. Variable-Ratio Schedules involves a type of partial reinforcement that strengthens a behaviour after a varied number of responses, which can lead to a high response rate and a slower extinction rate. Variable-Interval Schedules involve delivering reinforcements after variable times elapse, which can lead to a fast response rate and a slower extinction rate.

Two examples of Operant Conditioning leading to behaviour modification include Token Economy and Behaviour Shaping. A Token Economy is a reward system where desirable behaviours are reinforced with tokens (that form a secondary reinforcer) and are later exchanged for rewards (a primary reinforcer). This is often used in a classroom setting where teachers reward students who have demonstrated the desirable behaviour, with tokens or a tally that the student can exchange at the end of a term or semester. Behaviour Shaping involves the existing response gradually changing across successive trials towards the desired target behaviour through rewarding exact segments of behaviour. This requires the conditions to receive the reward to gradually shift closer towards the desired behaviour, and Skinner believed that human behaviour such as language learning was an example of Behaviour Shaping.

Conditioning Summary

Classical Conditioning formed an integral base for most of the subsequent behaviourism ideas and led to improvements in various areas such as animal training and factory work efficiency. However, when working with groups and individuals, Operant Conditioning has been found to be more effective at eliciting behaviour change compared to Classical Conditioning and when paired with more modern ideas that include motivation and values it can be used in almost all areas of human behaviour change.

Operant Conditioning had several weaknesses of its own including the dismissal of internal processes and the lack of social learning investigation. However, it still contributed a strong base of ideas that are still used in many modern learning programs.

Observational/Social Learning

Observational Learning, also known as Social Learning, occurs through observing and imitating others. The most famous Social Learning theory came from Albert Bandura, who suggested that people learn through conditioning, but they also learn through observing and imitating the actions of people in their environment. One way of framing Observational Learning is "learning from others' experiences". If a younger sibling observes their older sibling receive a speeding ticket, the theory suggests the younger sibling would be less likely to speed when they drive.

Bandura's most famous experiment is known as the 'Bobo Doll' experiments. This involved people imitating the actions of other people without any direct reinforcement. Young people observed aggressive behaviours towards the inflatable doll and then imitated the aggressive actions of the adult. The children were not directed to act aggressively but were left alone with the doll after watching the behaviour. Bandura's experiments also then added an aspect of Operant Conditioning as they found that young people were more likely to copy the aggressive behaviours when the adult received no punishment or when the adult received a reward, versus being less likely to act aggressively when they saw the adult receive a punishment.

Observational Learning plays an important role in the socialisation process as it indirectly and directly teaches the young person which behaviours are recommended or not recommended. As humans are a social species, the socialisation process is one of the most important learnings that people learn to live a healthier life when they are adults.

There are four stages of Observational Learning – Attention, Retention, Reproduction and Motivation. For a person to learn something from an observation they must be paying enough cognitive attention and remain focused long enough for the learning from the model to be absorbed. Once absorbed, the learning from the model must then be understood enough otherwise the next stage of Retention is unable to happen. Retention happens when the person can recall what was observed, and if they can attach the reasoning behind the behaviour, their retention can be improved. Reproduction occurs when the person can replicate the observed learnings of the original model in a relevant context, even if the reproduction is not exactly the same as the original behaviour or learning. Finally, Motivation is important because even if the person meets the first three stages, if they are not motivated to continue the learnt behaviour or if they are motivated to discontinue the behaviour (such as observing punishment), the learnt behaviour will lessen or cease.

Neurologically speaking, Observational Learning makes use of a basic brain function known as mirror neurons. Mirror neurons are neurons which fire not only when an individual exhibits a behaviour, but also when observing a behaviour. Mirror neurons play a functional role in theory of mind, emotional recognition, empathy, acquisition of language, predicting intention, and imitation. Research has supported the idea that when a person looks into the eyes of another person and discuss difficult topics, over a short period of time, both people's brain waves become very similar, activated by mirror neurons which, in this context can impact a person's emotions and empathy. It has also been suggested that the emotion mirror neurons are stronger than motor mirror neurons. When a person's motor mirror neurons are activated our skin cells and pathways help us understand it is not happening to us. Emotion mirror neurons don't have a skin barrier or defence, meaning greater emotional brain-brain influence, often called empathy.

Whilst the Observational Learning model has been useful for many individuals and professionals regarding improving learning outcomes, there have been some areas of concern regarding its long-term impacts and real-world replication and validation. For example, some studies found that children who played violent video games were more violent. However, more recent studies have found that the children were not necessarily violent because of the video game but did have poorer emotional regulation and greater stimulation seeking which could increase the risk of aggression. Another real-life complication of Observational Learning is the "cyclic argument". Simply put the "cyclic argument" suggests that if a person observed their core parental figure to be an alcoholic, they would learn that this is the normal behaviour. On the surface this sounds accurate, however, it is specious thinking. The observed alcoholic behaviours become a risk factor for becoming a learnt behaviour and therefore becoming an alcoholic but do not then lead to alcoholic behaviours on their own. This is an important distinction often forgotten by many academics and Hollywood movies.

Observational/Social Learning is very useful, but like most learning frameworks discussed in this book, benefits from a combination of other information and learning ideas.

Dunning Kruger Effect & Johari Window

The Dunning Kruger Effect refers to a cognitive bias in which people with less ability and or knowledge suffer from illusory superiority, mistakenly assessing their ability as much higher than it really is. Dunning-Kruger Effect has an inverse corollary that applies to high-ability individuals. Talented people tend to underestimate their relative competence and may erroneously assume that tasks which are easy for them are similarly easy for others. A common example in today's world is "social media experts" where the term refers to people who read one article and then use this as evidence to attempt to disprove real scientific evidence. A common example of the social media expert is people who still believe that vaccinations cause Autism, because they read social media articles and then pursued conspiracy theories to support this idea, even though the original scientists who made the claim, have since debunked their own claim.

The Johari Window is a visual framework used to improve interpersonal communication and relationships while promoting personal development. This can help some people reduce their cognitive bias regarding their ability. It can be used as a tool with multiple people, as an internal tool, or a combination known as the 'New Johari Window'.

When used with multiple people, it consists of a matrix/grid containing four cells (quadrants). Open, or Arena – Adjectives that both the subject and peers select go in this cell of the grid. These are traits that subject and peers perceive. Blind Spot – Adjectives not selected by subjects, but only by their peers go here. These represent what others perceive but the subject does not. Hidden, or Façade – Adjectives selected by the subject, but not by any of their peers, go in this quadrant. These are things the peers are either unaware of, or that are untrue but for the subject's claim. Unknown – Adjectives that neither subject nor peers selected go here. They represent subject's behaviours or motives that no one participating recognizes—either because they do not apply or because of collective ignorance of these traits.

When used internally the Johari window consists of four different quadrants and is built on the meaning of trust. Trust has 3 meanings in this context – the first meaning associated with the English word, "trust," concerning competence, the second meaning concerns intentions, and the third meaning concerns perspective. Open – the person understands the different meanings of Trust; we Know what we Know. Opaque Self – we are usually not "blind" to how other people see us rather, we can see the faint outline or shadow but not the clear detail. At some level we "know" what we don't "know." Our knowledge is opaque, in part, because we view ourselves from a state or contextual point of view, whereas others tend to view us from a trait or personality perspective. We Don't Know what we Know. Protected – we make assumptions and try to "hide" these assumptions but these assumptions become "self-fulfilling prophecies, we can't talk about any of this with other people and are even unlikely to reflect on these dynamics in our own minds; we Know what we Don't Know. Unknown: We Don't Know what we Don't Know.

In the 'New Johari Window' also known as the 'Three-Dimensional Johari Window Model', there are two panes each with four quadrants. Known to Self and Known to Others External Pane – Inadvertent Self; Internal Pane – Presentational Self. Unknown to Self and Known to Others External Pane – Ignorant Self; Internal Pane – Blocked Self. Known to Self and Unknown to Others External Pane – Obtuse Self; Internal Pane – Withheld Self. Unknown to Self and Unknown to Others External Pane – Discounted Self; Internal Pane – Unexplored Self. To the extent that the gap between these two panes is small, there is substantial congruence between our internal and external worlds. To the extent that the gap is large, there is an incongruent state, and the dynamics involved in coping with this gap can be profound. When the gap is large it is because the 'Trust' has been violated. This interpersonal model suggests that there are many ways to view interpersonal relationships. We can focus on the external panes or look deeply into the dynamics of the interior life of each participant in an interpersonal relationship. The double-paned window also points to the importance of interpersonal needs and to ways in which we express and fulfill these needs. Interpersonal needs are not simply shown to the external world. We don't simply ask or demand that these needs be met. Rather, these needs may remain "at home" (the internal panes) and may rarely or very subtly be made known outside our home (the external panes) to specific people in specific settings.

Stages of Change

The Stages of Change was first developed to assist people with addictions to understand and improve their behaviours. The Stages of Change is also known as the Transtheoretical Model and developed by Prochaska and DiClemente in the late 1970s. Today we use the Stages of Change regarding most behaviour change related difficulties including addiction, fitness, health, finance, etc. The model is very useful for people to understand and explore their motivation to change and understand that change can be a lifelong challenge or practice. Often this model is used in professional settings such as psychological counselling, coaching, and in support groups.

The Stages of Change have six stages - Precontemplation, Contemplation, Preparation (Determination), Action, Maintenance and Lapse/Relapse. Precontemplation is that stage when a person does not understand or is not aware that their behaviour is negatively impacting their function. Often people in this stage can feel they and their behaviours are fine, and that if any issues arise, the issues are then externalised onto other people or environmental factors. Often support people can only provide emotional or other support and information but cannot provide direct guidance during this stage of change.

The Contemplation stage is when a person understands there might be an issue with their current behaviour. Often pros and cons regarding their behaviour begin, but change is not yet made as they may not yet have the motivation or still be ambivalent regarding making the change required. For many people going from this stage to the Preparation stage can be the most difficult due to the responsibility of previous behaviours that might be acknowledged.

The Preparation stage involves preparing to change. Often people are ready to make change within the next 30 days, and the person might begin to make small steps towards changing their behaviour. Often motivation and determination can be at its peak.

The Action stage involves people who have recently begun changing their behaviours and intend to keep moving in the forward direction with these changes. This can often look like a person modifying their previous unhealthy behaviours and/or beginning new healthier behaviours.

The Maintenance stage is when the person has sustained their behaviour change for a while, often more than six months, and they intend to maintain the new behaviour(s). For many people the Maintenance stage can become the hardest stage due to its long-term nature. This is even truer for many people with neurodivergence or trauma, as the Maintenance stage can represent a lack of stimulation and boredom. This can then lead to a lapse or a relapse into the previous unhealthy behaviour.

The final stage that can occur at any point between the first five stages is known as Lapse/Relapse. Often these terms are used interchangeably, however, understanding the differences can assist with future recovery and improvement. A Lapse can loosely be understood as when a person drops back a stage or two. The person might have made it to the Maintenance stage then a life stressor occurs, which might then lead to the person returning to the Preparation stage. A Lapse is common and natural and should not be seen as a failure, rather it should be seen as a response to a negative situation and hopefully lead to better responses in the future. A Relapse is when a person might restart the entire cycle again. Often this occurs as a large response to a large stressor or life event. For example, a person who has not used alcohol for two years and is maintaining healthy behaviours might lose a loved one or a job or a limb. This massive loss can lead to previous unhealthy short-term behaviours such as alcohol use. This person is capable of change and can go through the stages again, and if they are fortunate, they might be able to go through the stages more efficiently with the life lessons learnt from their previous experiences. Often this person might require extra supports from professionals and support people to get from the Precontemplation to the Contemplation and Preparation stages.

There have been ten processes of change that have been found to occur and assist when a person is going through the Stages of Change. Different processes can have greater or lesser effect on a person's change depending on where they are on their journey. The ten processes are Consciousness Raising, Dramatic Relief, Self-Re-evaluation, Environmental Re-evaluation, Social Liberation, Self-Liberation, Helping Relationships, Counterconditioning, Reinforcement Management and Stimulus Control.

Consciousness Raising involves increasing the awareness about the healthy behavioural alternatives, Dramatic Relief involves the emotional arousal about the healthy behavioural alternative (can be positive or negative), Self-Re-evaluation is the self-reappraisal to realise the healthy behaviour is part of who they want to be, Environmental Re-evaluation is the social reappraisal to realise how their unhealthy behaviour affects other people, Social Liberation is the environmental opportunities that exist to show society is supportive of the healthy behaviour, Self-Liberation is the commitment to change a behaviour, based on the belief that achievement of the healthy behaviour is possible, Helping Relationships involves finding supportive relationships that encourage the desired change (these can be professionals, family, friends or support groups), Counter-Conditioning involves substituting healthy behaviours and thoughts for unhealthy behaviours and thoughts (and can lead to a lapse or relapse), Reinforcement Management is when the positive behaviours are rewarded whilst the negative behaviours receive less and less reward, and finally, Stimulus Control is the re-engineering of the environment to have reminders and cues that support and encourage the healthy behaviour and remove those that encourage the unhealthy behaviour.

There are several limitations to the model including – it can be ignorant of the social context in which changes occur such as Socioeconomic status; the lines between the stages can be vague with no concrete criteria to determine the person's stage of change; there is no concrete information about how much time is needed to reach and remain in a stage; and the model assumes that the person will make coherent and logical plans in their decision making process, which is often not the case as people are inherently emotional beings, more so when they are struggling. The Stages of Change model can be used as a very structured framework of behaviour change but can also be used more loosely as framework of ideas. Despite the limitations, the Stages of Change model has been found to be very helpful in changing unhealthy behaviours into healthier alternatives.

In the formal learning environment, the Stages of Change model can assist students and educators to identify if there are any less helpful behaviours or routines the person uses regarding learning. Once this is identified then the person (often with assistance from other people) is able to problem solve and work towards a new healthier alternative behaviour that will improve their learning efficiency and reduce their risk of a lapse or relapse.

FAIL, FAILURE & SUCCESS

FAIL

Most people don't like failing and can be impacted by the possibility of failing. For some people it is helpful to see the word 'fail' as an acronym to help change the person relationship with the idea. The acronym FAIL stands for First Attempt In Learning. Some of the greatest human achievements were achieved after many failures such as the light bulb, flight, ACDC electricity and even children's entertainment such as 'Captain Underpants'.

Continuous failure with learning often leads to a person achieving something better than they originally set out to achieve. Failure is an important teacher for those who are willing to learn. When a person can change their internal dialogue and therefore relationship with the idea of failing, a failure changes from a long-term negative to an opportunity to improve.

If a person has sufficient support from their environment, it can greatly improve how quickly the person is able to recover and can also influence what information the person learns from the failure experience.

FAILURE

FAILURE as an acronym stands for Frustration/hopelessness/futility, Aggressiveness (misdirected), Insecurity, Loneliness (lack of "oneness"), Uncertainty, Resentment and Emptiness.

Frustration here, arises when we have set goals that are unrealistic either environmentally or internally (such as an inadequate self-assessment of self or ability). Misdirected aggressiveness occurs when our frustration in achieving the goal blocks our ability to release or direct our anger in healthy ways leading to a buildup. This buildup eventually is expressed as aggression either towards ourselves, those closest to us, or an easy target (known as a scapegoat). The failure and aggression can reinforce any previous insecurities or encourage new insecurities. This occurs when a concept or belief of self and goal are not met and the person feels stuck, leading to various negative emotional interpretations.

Being alone is okay, here loneliness refers to the person alienating themselves or their behaviours alienating them from their peers. Combined with various other aspects of the FAILURE acronym, it can create a self-perpetuating negative cycle. This negative cycle can lead to greater uncertainty and lead to less attempts or avoidance of attempts further reinforcing the cycle. Resentment occurs when the negative cycle begins to form a core part of the person's identity. This can lead to externalisation of behaviours and outcomes, blaming "the system" and others instead of understanding the cause and problem solving. All of this can lead to a sense of emptiness. Once a person gets to this point change becomes more difficult as person might feel they have lost the capacity to enjoy or attempt.

However, everyone is capable of change. Reframing (and being okay with mistakes), connection, goal frameworks, healthy lifestyle and many other factors can contribute to a person achieving success.

SUCCESS

The acronym SUCCESS stands for Sense of direction, Understanding, Courage, Compassion, Esteem, Self-Confidence and Self-Acceptance. A clear sense of direction can help a person understand their purpose which allows them to direct their emotions, energy and effort in a direction they want. The clarity of the direction is our understanding. When a person has clear communication regarding what their direction looks like, they develop a clearer understanding of what they want. Once this is established, the person needs to have the courage to act, even if it involves trying something new, taking a slight risk or doing something they are normally afraid of (without fear there can be courage). Most people can encourage or "bet" on their friends to succeed" but have difficulty doing this for themselves. Compassion here refers to the respect a person has for another human being and is worth striving for. In an ideal world successful people have compassion for themselves, those closest to them and other people, however, this is often the least common attribute seen in people society deems as "successful".

Esteem refers to the opinion we have of ourselves. If our life history, emotions and context influence our perception of reality, why not influence the context ourselves by reframing the challenges and focusing on the positives. This will allow our esteem to improve or flourish. By improving our esteem, it allows us to be confident not just in ourselves, but in the decisions we make, even in the failures. It also makes reframing challenges easier can lead to improvements in our understanding of our direction. With work, and a bit of luck the above attributes can assist in achieving a level of self-acceptance. This allows a person to experience happiness with their core internal self, as well as allow them to appreciate the wins and achievements.

Proficiency and Becoming Great

Proficiency

What is the difference between being proficient and being great? Proficiency is the ability to perform a task or understand and communicate information in a way that is accurate and efficient. Many people reach a level of skill where they become proficient and for some people this is enough. It is okay to be proficient in more than one area and never be great at it. The pursuit of becoming great is an individual want but is also encouraged by many cultures and subcultures around the world.

10 000 Greatness Hours?

There are many assumptions about what it takes a person to become great at something. Apart from the myriad of difficulties trying to define this, there are also individual differences that are discussed throughout this book. One idea of what it takes to achieve 'Greatness' is "thousands of hours of intensely focused practice and work, with the guidance of experienced people". That is probably the most well-rounded definition, however, one idea that is often used as an unofficial rule is the "10 000 hours" rule. This number was first used by Malcom Gladwell in his book 'Outliers: The Story of Success' in 2008. It has been used as a motivational number and a marketable number and can be considered an average at best. The general idea is that if a person practices for approximately 10 000 hours, they will be proficient enough at the skill that they could be considered great.

Quantity of practice is important as it helps the brain pattern the required knowledge and skills so that they may become useable without too much conscious effort. Often known as "blueprinting" or "mechanical repetition", quantity of practice has been a helpful tool for many people in academic settings, sporting settings and trade related skills. However, relying on quantity of practice alone may be detrimental in improving. A person may practice for 10 000 hours, but if they are practicing the wrong technique or practicing the skill with errors, they are becoming more proficient at the wrong thing or in the wrong way.

Quality of practice is very important. Regular assistance and receiving feedback are important. When a person can learn a skill with the assistance of an expert, or at least a very good teacher, it allows their quality of practice to improve. The expert or teacher can assist the person in improving in specific areas relevant to their goal, whilst also allowing for the individual's differences. Differences in a person's learning needs and strengths, their ability starting point regarding their learning goal, and their motivation are all relevant areas that once understood, can be used to improve a person's quality. The next aspect of quality practice is "deliberate practice". Deliberate practice can be defined as – practicing with the intent to be better. This often includes following advice from experts and intentionally pushing oneself out of their comfort zone towards the desired goal. Some research including a meta-analysis from Brooke Macnamara and colleagues, found that deliberate practice can account for up to 26percent of skill variation. This suggests there are many other factors in a person becoming great.

One factor is the age at which a person begins the skill or technique. Research from Burgoyone and colleagues found that people who began practicing chess at a younger age, reached higher levels of skill then those who started in adulthood, even when accounting for deliberate practice.

As well as age, genetics has been found to be an important aspect when working towards greatness. However, as genetics is difficult to accurately use as a defining variable, most research uses twin studies. One such study used 15 000 twins (maternal and fraternal) in a drawing related experiment. The study found that there was a high correlation in skill level with the identical (maternal) twins compared to the fraternal twins. This makes sense as maternal twins often share 99percent of their genetics. Another study found that over 50percent of the variation between skilled readers and unskilled readers were found to be due to genetics. A study in Sweden tested more than 10 000 twins on their basic music abilities in relation to how much they had practiced. Their study found genes influenced approximately 38percent of the musical abilities measured with minimal evidence being found that the amount of practice in the young people influenced the difference in ability (compared to the identical twin that hadn't practiced). Regarding chess ability, there was a large variance in the time it took to reach a 'Chess Master' level of up to 22 times difference.

Other factors that influence the ability to become great at a skill include emotions, mental practice, and value behind the goal, which are discussed elsewhere in this book.

Quality combined with quantity may lead to a person becoming "great" at the chosen skill or technique, should their effort and motivation hold for the duration of their journey. A person may require approximately 728 hours of efficient quality practice, or they may require up to 16 120 hours of efficient quality practice. Not everyone wants to or needs to be great at something, and many people are happy practicing a skill or technique for fun or are happy understanding the basics.

Greene's Mastery

Greene discussed core aspects most people who had obtained greatness in their respective fields had in common – 'Primal Curiosity', 'Learning above all else' and 'Gathering Skills and Combining Skills in a Unique Way'. Primal Curiosity is the innate and individual curiosity that drives a person to want to improve and learn regarding a particular topic or field. Primal Curiosity includes "discovering your life's task", meaning what were the things that meant the most to you as a child and how can you pursue this as an adult. Greene suggests that regular journaling about what the person naturally found interesting when they were young, before they felt the external pressure to conform, can assist an adult in rediscovering their 'Primal Curiosity'.

Greene discussed that 'Learning above all else' is an important and often difficult step that many people who achieved greatness in their field took in their journey. Placing learning first can sometimes include accepting lower pay or reimbursement, receiving no recognition for efforts, facing harsh criticism, or implementing many hours of tedious practice and work. Placing learning first is also known as 'Prime Learning Opportunities', and this can sometimes include having to change most other aspects of your life to learn from the best people or organisations.

Some examples can include early career comedians or actors who often have to move to geographic locations they can't financially afford through to Muay Thai fighters who sleep on concrete for many years so that they can learn from the best coaches in Thailand. It can also include taking on unpaid or unofficial apprenticeships in the area you want to improve in and then working with a mentor that can assist your growth. Finally, this aspect also includes developing or honing your social intelligence. For some people this comes more naturally, whilst for others it is a skill that needs to be practiced. For your learning to assist in your longer-term financial future, a person needs to be able to communicate their knowledge in a way that is understood and eventually appreciated by other people. 'Learning above all else' is about the transformation of the person's mind and character, above all other ideas or rewards.

'Gathering Skills and Combining Skills in a Unique Way' is as the name implies, the act of gathering all relevant information and skills learnt and combining them in a way that is unique to the individual. When a person can combine their higher levels of skills and knowledge in a unique way, it often leads to a new idea, product or in some cases, unique fields of work and study. The combination of a person unlocking their own unique creative way of thinking allows the person to be able to combine the knowledge and their intuition in a way that allows for even better communication and understanding of your knowledge or skill.

Greatness Summarised

Becoming proficient in any task or knowledge is often enough. However, if a person strives for greatness in a chosen field or skill, hard work will always be a key component. Whether a person must practice or study for 700 hours or for 10 000 hours, their quality of study, and the relevant sacrifices they make to achieve their goal of greatness will strongly influence the outcome.

Change is a Direction & Not a Destination

According to the research from various sources, behavioural change can occur from 15-250 days. This is a large number variance and is the culmination of various sources being combined. Change involves a lot of hard work, time and consistency, and these elements lead to brain pathway changes, that then allow for future change. The key for many people is to improve their life a small amount on a regular basis, therefore assisting the person to make a change. Hence the title of this section – "Change is a Direction and not a Destination".

Whenever we have a thought, or practice a behaviour, the relevant neurological pathway in the brain is strengthened. Since the brain's main jobs are to keep us alive and be efficient, the brain will utilise the largest pathways possible for any thought or behaviour. The strengthening of the pathways often happens without us choosing as an adaptive efficiency response. This efficiency response is often a good thing as it allows a person to learn new behaviours or skills and can free up conscious thought for other tasks. The downside of these pathways happening autonomously is that if a person is practicing an unhealthy behaviour the pathways continue to increase and become more efficient with that specific behaviour. This is a neurological reason why behaviour change is difficult for many people. One way of being able to influence the brain's natural pathway response is to form healthy habits by choice.

Some research has reported that building habits can be separated into two phases – Defining and Designing Future Outcomes and Leveraging Your Subconscious. Defining and Designing Future Outcomes includes Defining the Objective and then Designing the Routine. Defining the Objective is used to understand what the overall goal is, such as "being fit" or "learning Spanish". During this part, the person needs to clearly understand why the overall goal is important and it often helps to write both the goal and the reason why it is important down. Designing the Routine involves breaking down the large goal into smaller and manageable steps (many of the goal frameworks discussed in this book can be helpful for this step).

The second phase known as Leveraging Your Subconscious has three aspects – The Start Button, Revisiting the Context & Repeating Actions and Enjoyable by Association. The Start Button is where the person defines a clear trigger mechanism for the routine. This can include a visual pointer such as seeing a specific object, the time of day, workout clothing only being used for working out, etc., and is used to help create the context for your brain to do the behaviour. Revisiting the Context & Repeating Actions is where the person tries to change the brain pathway in their favour. The person uses the Start Button in the Context as regularly as possible. Lastly, associating the habit behaviour with other desirable activities can utilise the Enjoyable by Association idea. This can include listening to your favourite music while working out or using your favourite scent while cleaning.

Change is a direction and not a destination. Making small steps every day towards the larger goal can help form healthy habits and behaviours. Also, aiming for an 80percent compliance with the habit and behaviour in the correct direction allows for natural life events to happen without any negative self-judgement being associated with a perceived failure.

Other Learning & Achieving Frameworks

There are various models and frameworks of learning discussed in psychology and in other fields such as education, sports coaching, teaching, etc. Different coaching frameworks such as AMN Academy and White Tiger Qigong have developed their own tools regarding how to learn a behaviour, both of which I use in my psychological practice. This section will discuss various learning frameworks often not directly focused on in psychology, but which can still benefit people individually and professionally.

Aboriginal 8 Pedagogy Framework

Here I will provide a brief overview of a learning style developed by First Nations People of Australia in collaboration with various education centres. During the process of writing this section, I requested assistance from one of my previous psychology supervisors that identifies as an Indigenous Australian. This was done to check for cultural appropriateness, as I wanted to include this learning framework as it provided a slightly different perspective and has aspects that many people could benefit from.

Aboriginal and non-Aboriginal teachers continue to contribute to the framework in an ongoing cross-cultural dialogue. It is managed by the Aboriginal Education Team at the Bangamalanha Centre (in New South Wales) and is a culturally safe point of entry for teachers to begin engaging with Aboriginal knowledge and cross-cultural dialogue in the community. Research from Louth and colleagues found that four dimensions of empowerment relating to embedding the Aboriginal and Torres Strait Islander perspectives of knowledge, understanding, perceptions and attitudes all increased for the teachers who completed training in the 8 Ways Aboriginal Pedagogical Framework. The Framework allows teachers to include Aboriginal perspectives by using Aboriginal learning techniques. In this way, focus can remain on core curriculum content while embedding Aboriginal perspectives in every lesson. It came from a research project involving DET staff, James Cook University's School of Indigenous Studies, and the Western New South Wales Regional Aboriginal Education Team between 2007 and 2009.

The Aboriginal Pedagogy Framework consists of eight interconnected pedagogies involving Narrative-Driven Learning (Story Sharing), Visualised Learning Processes (Learning Maps), Hands-on/Reflective techniques (Non-verbal), use of Symbols/Metaphors, Land-based Learning (Land Links), Indirect/Synergistic Logic (Non-Linear learning), Modelled/Scaffolded Genre Mastery (Deconstruct/Reconstruct), and Connectedness to Community. However, it is noted that these can adapt to the changing setting and are considered fluid and dynamic, resulting in a strong overlap across the eight areas. The 8 simple pedagogies are merely a starting point for dialogue and should not be considered a framework in the same way as the other frameworks discussed in this book.

Narrative-Driven Learning also known as Story Sharing is assisting the teacher and student to learn through story telling (yarning) instead of the concrete structure often taught in westernised education centres. The story sharing allows lessons to be taught whilst also allowing for the Indigenous Australian language experience to be demonstrated and shared. The story sharing also allows for the ethics, values, storied experiences, cultural meaning-making, place-based significance to be used to improve memory and cognition. Teachers and students are encouraged to share relevant personal stories with each other to help enrich the education material taught to the students whilst also building rapport and trust.

Visualised Learning Processes also known as Learning Maps is used to explicitly map and visualise ideas. The framework suggests that this allows for the Aboriginal intellectual processes to be visualised with the assistance of metaphors grounded in culture and country. Land-based Learning including the relevant Land Links are the dynamic set of relationships that contain vast schematics, knowledge system and intellectual processes that can be used to guide and enrich school systems and curricula. Hands-on/Reflective techniques also known as Non-verbal learning allows for the Aboriginal ways of relating and connecting to knowledge reflectively, critically, ancestrally, and physically. This is also known as seeing, thinking, acting, making, and sharing without words.

Symbols and Metaphors based learning is now becoming understood as a type of visual metalanguage which can be considered the building blocks for memory and the making of meaning, which is cross-cultural and dynamic. Visual images and metaphors can be created orally allowing for a deeper learning experience. Indirect/Synergistic Logic also known as Non-Linear learning is the cultural innovation through the interaction of cultural systems. This can be considered a way of approaching higher order thinking by laterally incorporating seemingly unrelated domains to create complex, real-life problems to be solved by learners using holistic thinking and innovative processes. Modelled/Scaffolded Genre Mastery also known as Deconstruct/Reconstruct learning engages with whole processes and texts, modelling and building upon a person's basic skills and identities and then transferring these successfully from familiar to unfamiliar contexts. This idea can also be thought as the ability to transfer knowledge and skills across forms and contexts.

Connectedness to Community is an important aspect of learning for many Indigenous Australians. The Community Link is the centrality of these relationships to the development and acquisition of all knowledge and highlights the importance of not just knowledge but rapport and cultural relationship. This also highlights the cultural importance of having the right people deliver the information, which is often not considered in the western education system.

It is strongly recommended that anyone wanting to implement this framework after completing the official training, follow some of the following ideas – work with community to identify the local Aboriginal systems in country and culture, explore the values inherent in the local culture, respect any local enduring protocols and, follow any reported processes that are locally used to inform the ways of interacting with changing social and ecological landscapes.

Goal related frameworks

In modern times, goal frameworks often arise from corporate or group learning principles. The frameworks are often used to help a team or business to work towards a shared understanding or target. Many ideas discussed in these frameworks are beneficial for individuals as they may assist the individual in structuring their own personal or professional goals. When employees don't know one another's goals, they are more likely to make unrealistic demands, focus on activities that don't support their colleagues, or duplicate effort.

The ideas of recorded formalised goal setting dates to the ancient Greek philosopher Aristotle who developed his own version of goal setting known as the 'Four Causes'. When assessing today's modern goal theories, there are four common moderators - Ability, Task Complexity, Performance Feedback and Goal Commitment – which all affect us and our outcomes very differently. Goal setting is a theory of motivation that helps to explain what drives us all to perform better and achieve more than others. In more modern times formalised goal setting was formerly introduced by Bloom and colleagues in 1956 in their now famous work 'Taxonomy of Educational Objectives'. Many attribute the various goal frameworks to this work. As well as Bloom, there have been various other influential people such as Peter Druker in the 1950's, Edward Locke in the 1960's, Marcell Telles in the 1980's, as well as various other educators and even spiritual leaders. Finding the correct fit for an individual or team can be difficult, and often elements of goal templates are adapted into work and school settings.

For many the idea of a goal is simultaneously attractive and daunting, and in 2014 a study completed by Shafique, and colleagues found that of the people surveyed, 74 percent had failed in reaching their new year's resolution goals. In a psychology setting similar numbers are seen at the individual level, where people set goals and then fail to achieve them. One of the more common reasons for a person failing to achieve their goal, is a lack of clarity around what their goal means in real practical terms, and a lack of measurability regarding their progress. Whilst there are many variations of goal frameworks the ones discussed in this book include – the Bloom Taxonomy and the acronym frameworks – SMART, FAST, PACT, CLEAR, WOOP, WISE, and CLARITY.

Bloom Taxonomy

Bloom's Taxonomy is recommended as a teaching guide, more than an individual's goal setting tool. According to Forehand and colleagues there are several benefits to using Bloom's Taxonomy or the more recent revised Taxonomy. Firstly, it assists with establishing effective learning objectives so that teachers and students have a similar understanding of the purpose they are trying to achieve. Next it can assist in organising objectives and help clarify objectives for the teachers and students. And finally, it can assist in establishing an organised set of objectives to help teachers plan and deliver appropriate instruction, design valid assessment tasks and strategies, and ensure that instruction and assessment are aligned with the objectives.

The original Taxonomy included six different categories – Knowledge, Comprehension, Application, Analysis, Synthesis and Evaluation. Knowledge involved the recall of specific information and universally known information, the recall of methods and processes, or the recall of a pattern, structure or setting. Comprehension involved the understanding or apprehension of what is being communicated and the ability to make use of the material or idea being communicated without necessarily relating it to other material or seeing its fullest implications. Application involved the use of abstractions in specific and concrete situations. Analysis involved the breakdown of a communication into its constituent elements or parts, so that the usual hierarchy of ideas is made clear and the relations between ideas expressed is made explicit. Synthesis involved the combining of elements and parts so that they formed a whole. Finally, Evaluation involved the judgement about the value of material and methods for the given purposes.

This original Taxonomy had a massive influence in business and education and in 2001 the Taxonomy was revised following a lot of work from cognitive psychologists, curriculum theorists, instructional researchers and testing and assessment specialists. This new Taxonomy was more fluid and dynamic, as the experts believed that the original was too static for current use. The new Taxonomy made use of six aspects and could be explained using a pyramid structure with the first aspect 'Remember' being at the bottom, and 'Create' at the top of the pyramid. The six aspects are – Remember, Understand, Apply, Analyse, Evaluate and Create. 'Remember' sits at the base of the Taxonomy pyramid and involves the ability to retrieve, recall, or recognise relevant knowledge from the long-term memory (such as recalling dates). 'Understand' is the second from the base of the Taxonomy pyramid and involves the ability to demonstrate the comprehension through one or more forms of explanation including comparison and definition. 'Apply' is the third from the base of the Taxonomy pyramid and involves the use of information or a skill in new situations. 'Analyse' is the third from the top of the Taxonomy pyramid and involves the ability to separate and breakdown information into its constituent parts and determine how the parts relate to each other or to an overall structure. 'Evaluate' is the second from the top of the Taxonomy pyramid and involves the ability to make judgements based on criteria and standards. Finally, 'Create' is the top of the Taxonomy pyramid and involves the ability to put elements together to form a new coherent or functional whole or reorganise elements into a new pattern or structure.

Following the success of the revised Taxonomy, some professionals wrote a version with a heavier focus on the types of knowledge used in cognition. The four knowledge types included Factual Knowledge, Conceptual Knowledge, Procedural Knowledge, and Metacognitive Knowledge. Factual Knowledge focused on terminology knowledge and the specific details and elements. Conceptual Knowledge focused on knowledge of classifications and categories, principles and generalisations, and theories, models, and structures. Procedural Knowledge focused on the knowledge of subject-specific skills and algorithms, subject-specific techniques and methods and the knowledge of criteria for determining when to use the most appropriate procedures. Finally Metacognitive Knowledge focused on strategic knowledge, knowledge about cognitive tasks including appropriate contextual and conditional knowledge and self-knowledge.

Another idea that was strongly influenced by the revised Taxonomy is Anderson's '25 Alternatives'. This version can also be seen as a supplementary framework to the revised Taxonomy. Here Anderson and colleague broke down thinking and goal setting into three levels of thinking order, with the Lower Order being for remembering, The Middle Order for Analysing, Applying and Understanding and the Higher Order thinking for Creating and Evaluating. In the Lower Order, Anderson included the following – Silence, Speed/Tone/Volume changes, Signposting, Rhetorical Questions, Questions to Students, Redundances, Class Structure Repetition, Lying, Music relating to content, Videos relating to content, Theatre explanations and the listening to the Invited Speaker. In the Middle Order thinking, Anderson included – Moodle/Academic Tests, Online Contests, Incomplete Presentations and Interactive Activities. In the High Order level, Anderson included – Practical Group Exercises, Practical Individual Exercises, Class Debates, Thinking/Pairing/Sharing, Projecting Basic Learning, Challenge Based Learning, Inverted Classes and Improvised Classes.

The various versions of the Taxonomy were found to be useful in academic settings and for occupational psychology work, and less useful for the individual's goal setting. The following goal frameworks have various purposes, with some being better suited for individual and some better suited for groups.

SMART (Specific Measurable/Meaningful Achievable/Actionable Realistic Timely)

The idea of SMART goals arose in 1981 from Doran and his colleagues who suggested that there was a better way to write goals and they developed the groundwork for today's SMART goals. SMART goals are a basic and structured template that can assist people in understanding how to achieve an end goal. Another interpretation is that SMART goals allow a person to understand their first step in a way that provides a clear understanding and responsibility of the outcome, on their way to achieving their desired result. As people are not robots, aiming for 100 percent compliance with a SMART goal can be unrealistic, and some research suggests aiming for 80 percent compliance.

The S in SMART stands for 'Specific' and SMART goal practitioners believe that goals should be specific enough that the individual and other people can understand what is trying to be achieved. Several prompts can be helpful in this section including – What the individual or team wants to achieve, Who needs to be involved to accomplish the goal, When does the goal need to be completed by and why should the goal be achieved in this exact way.

The M in SMART stands for 'Measurable' or 'Meaningful' and SMART goal practitioners believe that goals should be able to be measured in a clear and precise manner. Understanding how to measure progress and success are important in achieving the goal but also for people as motivation and responsibility. Even if a goal is unsuccessful, if it was measured clearly, the individual or team can understand how and why they failed, which can lead to future improvement. Some people also include the addition/interpretation of 'Meaningful', which to ensure the goal is measured in a way that is meaningful to the overall outcome and reason behind the need for the goal.

The A in SMART stands for 'Achievable' or 'Actionable' and SMART goal practitioners believe that goals should be achievable so that people understand their efforts. Prompts can be helpful such as – is the individual or team capable of achieving the goal, does everyone involved have the needed skills, and if they don't how can these skills be learnt or developed.

The R in SMART stands for 'Relevant' and SMART goal practitioners believe that goals should be understood clearly that any redundancy can be removed earlier in the process. Understanding the 'why' can help people understand why they want to achieve a goal and what the impact of their efforts leads to.

The T in SMART stands for 'Timely' and SMART goal practitioners believe that goals should have an end date. The end date allows for people to measure their progress, provides motivation and can help in assessing the other four aspects of the SMART goal regarding achievement.

A learning example of a SMART goal is – to read five pages, every day, for sixty days. If the goal is to read one 120-page book, then breaking the book down into a number of pages would be the simplest way to demonstrate the smart goal. The page number is Specific, Measurable, Achievable and Relevant, and the number of days is Timed.

SMART goals are best suited for helping a person identify specifics within their large goal and providing the person with steps to direct them and help them start.

In approximately 2010 a variation, sometimes used as a replacement, known as 'SMARTER' was developed. There are variations on was the additional 'E' and 'R' mean with some interpretations including – Evaluative/Ethical and Rewarding or Evolving and Relationship-centred.

FAST (Frequent Ambitious Specific Transparent)

The idea of FAST goals arose because business leaders such as Peter Druker felt that the previous approach to business goals were having a negative impact. One of the barriers to organisations using FAST goals is the fear of transparency. However, an analysis completed by Sull & Sull, found that of the companies that opted for this approach, almost 90percent of employees supported transparency for majority of their work-related goals. They also found that the structure allowed for teams and individuals to improve their performance up to the 80th percentile. The process and outcome of linking goals to measurable results, can often lead to greater value for the people involved in the task once it is completed.

The F in FAST stands for 'Frequently discussed' and FAST goal practitioners believe that goals should be embedded in ongoing discussions to allow for progress, resources, initiatives, and feedback to be assessed and improved. This approach can be helpful as it provides guidance for important decision making, assists in keeping teams focused on what matters most to the group, can link performance feedback to help concrete goals and can be used to evaluate progress and provide correction as needed.

The A stands for Ambitions and FAST goal practitioners believe that goals should be difficult but not impossible to achieve. This is thought to boost performance of the individual and the team, minimise the risk of plateauing and can assist in encouraging innovation.

The S stands for Specific and FAST goal practitioners believe that goals should be translated into measurable concrete metrics that encourage clarity, how the goal will be achieved, and progress measured. The benefits of this are that team members know what is expected of them, it helps to identify what is not working so it can be corrected and may encourage better performance from individuals and the team.

The T stands for Transparent and FAST goal practitioners believe that goals should be made public for all the team to see. This may allow peer pressure to become a motivator, helps individuals to understand the difference they are making, understand other team members' agendas and efforts and highlight redundant or unaligned strategies.

A learning example of a FAST goal is – finish a group project, one week prior to its due date, and edit using a group accessible cloud drive, with all members completing one section each. The group project would require Frequent Discussion regarding information, direction, etc. Finishing it early would be Ambitious as deadlines in formal learning environments and workplaces are often already difficult to meet. The dividing of the project into sections allows for the Specific aspect of FAST to be met. And the use of a cloud drive allows for Transparency.

FAST goals are best suited for tasks or projects that involve multiple people.

PACT (Purposeful Actionable Continuous Trackable)

The history of PACT goals is unclear; however, some business professionals believe the focus of PACT is more conducive to achieving company goals than SMART goals. The PACT approach focuses on the output instead of a specific outcome. It's about continuous growth rather than the pursuit of a well-defined achievement. PACT goals are also thought to work well for neurodivergent people such as ADHD instead of the traditional SMART goal approach.

The P in Pact stands for 'Purposeful' and PACT goal practitioners believe that goals should be meaningful to a longer-term purpose in life. This approach can be helpful because when a goal has value or purpose it assists with internal motivation, motivation to improve, and or achieve.

The A in Pact stands for 'Actionable' and PACT goal practitioners believe that goals should be controllable and actionable. This approach can be helpful as it assists in shifting a person's mindset from longer-term outcomes in the future to present outputs the person can control. It also helps in making the person feel their desired learning outcome is within reach, acting today rather than overplanning for tomorrow.

The C in Pact stands for 'Continuous' and PACT goal practitioners believe that goals should be simple, flexible and repeatable. This approach can be helpful as it can lessen the choice paralysis that many people experience from having too many possibilities or choices. Once the person starts, they begin to learn more, which allows for adaptation as they work towards their learning goal. The idea is that continuous improvement may be less daunting to people compared to a specific outcome.

The T in Pact stands for 'Trackable' and PACT goal practitioners believe that goals should be trackable instead of measurable. This approach can be helpful as tracking the progress can be done more simply with such as "yes or no" type questions, instead of specific data sets that can lead to procrastination or be misleading. The "yes or no" approach makes it easier for the individual and other people in a team setting to see if progress is being made and if steps are being completed.

An example of a PACT goal might be a person's life mission statement and is often strongly influenced by a person's own value systems.

CLEAR (Collaborative Limited Emotional Appreciable Refinable)

CLEAR goals were introduced by Locke and colleagues during the 1980's and were developed for group goals where collaboration is focus and is often used in the workplace or volunteer organisation but can be effective with most group activities.

The C in CLEAR stands for 'Collaborative'. CLEAR goal practitioners believe that goals should involve buy-in from individual members of the group and that all group members should understand the common goal and the process in how to get there.

The L in CLEAR stands for 'Limited'. CLEAR goal practitioners believe that goals should have time and financial boundaries, and that all members should understand what this looks like. Understanding these boundaries is thought to improve the goal being achieved.

The E in CLEAR stands for 'Emotional'. CLEAR goal practitioners believe that goals should have emotional investment from all members. This is thought to assist in providing motivation during the more difficult periods.

The A in CLEAR stands for 'Appreciable', meaning measurable. CLEAR goal practitioners believe that goals should be able to be measured in a way that suits all members of the group, so that progress can be monitored, and so that all members can be held accountable.

The R in CLEAR stands for 'Refinable'. CLEAR goal practitioners believe that goals should allow for adjustments to be made during the process of working towards the goal. This also allows for changes in circumstances, whilst also allowing for continued input from the group members.

A learning example of a CLEAR goal is – Save $5000 by end of April for a family holiday to Western Australia. The family holiday allows for the emotional investment, the money amount is the appreciable/measurable figure, and the location can be refined/changed if need be.

WOOP (Wish Outcome Obstacle Plan)

WOOP goals were first introduced by Oettingen and colleagues as an alternative to the SMART goal framework. It was originally designed for younger people but has been found to be effective for anyone who tends to self-sabotage. This suggests that it may be more helpful than other goal frameworks for people with depression, anxiety, and other mental health difficulties.

The W in WOOP stands for 'Wish' and WOOP goal practitioners believe that goals should allow for challenge and change without whelming oneself. It can be used as a slower, kinder approach.

The O in WOOP stands for 'Outcome'. WOOP goal practitioners believe that goals should assist the person in identifying the best possible outcome, such as a smaller attainable goal or a larger more challenging but still realistic goal.

The second O in WOOP stands for 'Obstacle'. WOOP goal practitioners believe that goals should also allow the person to identify any obstacles that may hinder progress or success, and these can include "real" meaning external obstacles such as other people, finances, or tasks, or can include "imagined" meaning internal barriers such as self-image, confusion, etc.

The P in WOOP stands for 'Plan'. WOOP goal practitioners believe that goals should assist a person in tracking their habits such as a journal, allow for self-care, and allow for smaller goals such as micro-goals to be achieved on a regular basis.

A 'WOOP' goal is designed to help a person manage their inner difficulties to lessen the behaviours associated with their prior self-sabotage.

WISE (Written Integrated Synergistic Expansive)

WISE goals were introduced to assist a person who is setting multiple goals, to more effectively plan their goals to work together or assist each other, instead of the goals hindering each other.

The W in WISE stands for 'Written'. WISE goal practitioners believe that goals should be written down on paper or digitally to allow the person to work towards multiple goals whilst minimising confusion.

The I in WISE stands for 'Integrated'. WISE goal practitioners believe that goals should fit together in some way. This might include time, travel, or any other common element.

The S in WISE stands for 'Synergistic'. WISE goal practitioners believe that goals should be working in the same direction. It is difficult to save money, if a person also has a goal to pay off a debt simultaneously.

The E in WISE stands for 'Expansive'. WISE goal practitioners believe that goals should challenge oneself enough that it motivates the person. The challenge should be a motivator and not lead to whelming oneself. 'Expansive' is a flexible part of the 'WISE' model and should adapt to allow for goals to be met efficiently as possible.

A learning example of a WISE goal is – to pay off all debts including a car and house within 10-15 years, without negatively impacting the family's mental health.

Goal Summary

All goal frameworks have beneficial ideas, and most practitioners of a particular goal framework feel that their choice is the better one for their needs. It is up to the individual to identify if any of the current frameworks are beneficial, or if there are ideas in each of them, they can benefit from. Using any formal goal framework can assist in learning more efficiently and either achieving or understanding a failure more easily. Using a goal framework also assists by giving the relevant person or group responsibility over the outcome as well as clarity and direction.

Key Points & Relevant Personal/Professional Experiences

Types of intelligence IQ/EQ/AQ

The idea of intelligence is controversial and ever changing. I use the idea of different types of intelligence when helping a person identify their areas of strength, especially when their strengths don't meet the traditional academic idea of intelligence.

There are theorised to be at least nine types of IQ (Intelligence Quotient) intelligence which can be an influential factor when people are trying to learn. The nine types are Spatial, Naturalist, Musical, Logic/Mathematical, Existential, Interpersonal, Bodily/Kinaesthetic, Linguistic, and Intrapersonal.

Spatial intelligence often refers to a person's ability to generate, retain, retrieve, and transform well-structured visual images. This can include visualising the outcome such as sculpting or geometry and can also include the ability to understand sizes and spaces without the assistance of measuring devices.

Naturalist intelligence often refers to a person's ability to identify, classify and manipulate elements of the environment, objects, animals, or plants leading to our ability to recognise differences between species and understand how they relate to each other.

Musical intelligence often refers to a person's ability to perceive, distinguish, transform, and express sounds and musical forms. It allows people to create, communicate and understand meaning through sound. This intelligence includes sensitivity to the rhythms, melodies, and tones of a piece of music.

Logic/Mathematical intelligence often refers to a person's ability of scientific reasoning, mathematical calculation, logical thinking, inductive and deductive reasoning, and the sharpness of abstract patterns and relationships. The five traits of mathematical logic are classification, comparing, mathematical operations, inductive and deductive reasoning, and the forming and rechecking of hypotheses. This area of intelligence is often paired with a person's numeracy ability, which refers to the person's ability to use numbers and mathematical concepts in everyday life, such as connections with the mathematical concepts of fractions and addition to a recipe.

Bodily/Kinaesthetic intelligence often refers to a person's ability to manipulate objects and use a variety of physical skills. This intelligence also involves a sense of timing and the perfection of skills through mind–body union. Athletes, dancers, surgeons, and crafts people exhibit well-developed bodily kinaesthetic intelligence. Linguistic intelligence often refers to a person's ability to think in words and to use language to express and appreciate complex meanings.

Linguistic intelligence allows us to understand the order and meaning of words and to apply meta-linguistic skills to reflect on our use of language. Linguistic intelligence is the most widely shared human competence and is evident in poets, novelists, journalists, and effective public speakers.

Existential intelligence often refers to a person's ability to tackle deep questions about human existence, such as the meaning of life, why we die, and how did we get here and often includes spiritual leaders and philosophers.

Interpersonal intelligence often refers to a person's ability to understand and interact effectively with others. It involves effective verbal and nonverbal communication, the ability to note distinctions among others, sensitivity to the moods and temperaments of others, and the ability to entertain multiple perspectives. Teachers, actors, politicians, leaders, and charismatic people often exhibit interpersonal intelligence.

Intrapersonal intelligence often refers to a person's ability to understand oneself and one's thoughts and feelings, and to use such knowledge in planning and directing one's own life. Intra-personal intelligence involves not only an appreciation of the self, but also of the human condition. It is evident in psychologist, spiritual leaders, and philosophers. It is theorised that most people whose strengths include Interpersonal, Intrapersonal and/or Existential intelligence, often have a more developed emotional intelligence.

EQ (Emotional Quotient) also known as emotional intelligence is theorised to be an even stronger predictor or influencer regarding a person achieving the result of their goal. The five types of EQ are Self-Awareness, Self-Management, Motivation, Empathy and Social Skills. Self-Awareness can be briefly explained as a person's ability to understand their own emotions and intentions. Self-Management is the ability to manage one's own efforts and behaviours. Motivation is the ability to find internal and external reasons and use processes to direct oneself towards achieving their goals. Empathy is the ability to tune into and understand others' emotions and situations. Lastly, Social Skills is the ability to interact easily and healthily with other people, often seen as being extroverted and/or charismatic. The five types of EQ are very interactive and are rarely separated as they are in this book, and have strong interactions with the above Interpersonal, Intrapersonal and Existential Intelligence Quotients. Emotional Intelligence and Emotional Quotients are often referred to as 'Social Emotional' skills or learning in the mental health and education sectors. Organisations such as CASEL (Collaborative & Academic Social & Emotional Learning) discuss this further with their framework. Their framework includes five broad, interrelated areas of competence and provide examples for each: Self-Awareness, Self-Management, Social Awareness, Relationship Skills, and Responsible Decision-Making.

Here Self-Awareness refers to the abilities to understand one's own emotions, thoughts, and values and how they influence behaviour across contexts (integrating personal and social identities, identifying one's emotions, etc.). Self-Management refers to the abilities to manage one's emotions, thoughts, and behaviours effectively in different situations and to achieve goals and aspirations (identifying and using stress-management strategies, using planning and organisations skills, etc.). Social Awareness refers to the abilities to understand the perspectives of and empathise with others, including those from diverse backgrounds, cultures, & contexts (taking others' perspectives, showing concern for the feelings of others, understanding the influence of organisations/external systems on behaviours, etc.). Relationship Skills refers to the abilities to establish and maintain healthy and supportive relationships and to effectively navigate settings with diverse individuals and groups (communicating effectively, showing leadership in groups, standing up for the rights of others, etc.). Finally Responsible Decision-Making refers to the abilities to make caring and constructive choices about personal behaviour and social interactions across diverse situations (demonstrating curiosity and open-mindedness, recognising how critical thinking skills are useful both inside and outside of formal learning settings, anticipating and evaluating the consequences of one's actions, etc.).

Finally, more recent research has highlighted AQ (Adaptive Quotient) as the most important indicator of success. This includes our ability to adapt and may also include the speed at which a person, team or organisation can adapt to change.

The benefits of a person having a high adaptability combined with a fast cognitive processing ability and skill can sometimes have a negative effect on a person's memory retention. One tool to manage this possible negative effect is mindful thinking. Mindful thinking involves a person paying attention to one thing, in the present moment and can involve repeating or paraphrasing information, writing information, or reorganising information as the person is learning it.

No type of intelligence is inherently superior, and all people have their own combination of the various interpretations of intelligence. What is more important is how a person is able to utilise their strengths, how the environment supports and allows the person's strengths to be used and the person's goals and values. When a person finds the "right fit" their strengths and values align with the school or organisation they are a part of.

Defining motivation and "the Why"

As mentioned, many of the goal frameworks work on exploring the motivation behind learning at the group level. They discuss briefly how the group narrative influences the individual motivation to achieve an agreed upon goal. Here we will briefly look at the individual aspects of motivation, also known as "the Why". They have been separated here for simplicity and clarity.

Motivation Types

There are three motivation types, Internal, External Positive and External Negative. Internal motivation is also known as inspiration and often leads to a person wanting to learn information or perform a task for their own internal interests or goals. When a person is interested, their internal motivation increases and their want to learn or perform a particular behaviour will increase. This is often a slight increase and can make setting up goals and other motivations easier. The difficulty of relying on internal motivation is that it is often short lived. This can lead to large improvements becoming less likely, because the person might give up, or wait until the next inspiration. Internal motivation is a great time to build structure and begin the goal, and if used correctly, can then be maintained by the other aspects of motivation.

Another type of motivation is known as external motivation. The two types of external motivation I discuss with clients include External Positive and External Negative Motivation. External Positive Motivation is when a person can use or be influenced by positive environmental motivators such as other people (in a team) or an upcoming holiday date. This type of motivation can be helpful in maintaining goals that had been set up during the inspiration stage and can be useful in the continued learning of difficult tasks. The various goal frameworks discussed earlier can be used as external positive motivation tools. External Negative motivation involves the external pressure or threat of an environmental stimulus or person as the motivator. Examples include bills, due dates, work performance indicators, etc. This type of motivator can be used as a beneficial tool, but if relied upon can lead to burnout, disinterest and various other negative emotional and physical responses to the task or information the person is trying to improve or complete.

When a person understands how to utilise the combination of Internal Motivation and External Motivation, it makes it easier for them to achieve their goals. The combination and specific motivators are often contextual and therefore should change or be adapted as such to improve the chances of success.

3 Forgotten Motivation Areas

Three areas often forgotten when discussing motivation and learning are: Value Adding, Routine & Creativity, and Silliness & Fun.

Value Adding

When we value something enough, we often find time for the task or learning. How a person adds value can often be contextual and be strongly influenced by the person's own life experiences. A person's core value such as kindness can be a tool for adding value to a behaviour or learning, as can other examples including – the end goal, interest, pressure, and other powerful emotions such as hope.

Routine

A person's daily, learning and life routines can greatly assist or hinder progress in learning or achieving. A person's sleep and health routines can impact how well they are feeling physically and mentally which will then impact how much energy and motivation they have available for learning or improvement. A person's learning routine can impact how efficient and successful their time spent learning is (as discussed in the 'Illusion of learning' section). And a person's life routine, the behaviour they have maintained over a long period of time can greatly impact their ability to learn new information or tasks or improve on current ones. When a behaviour becomes a habit, the routine of this habit becomes its own motivator.

Creativity, Silliness and Fun

Creativity, silliness, and fun can mean the same thing or have different interpretations, but all can be used to assist in learning. Creativity can include thinking "outside the box" or can mean learning or expressing learnings and behaviours artistically. Adding silliness and fun to a task by reorganising the task can allow a person's brain to lessen the internal obstacles because of the stimulation and endorphins triggered by the silliness or fun aspect. This can include attempting to "moon walk" whilst brushing one's teeth or can be more interactive such as "ice break" activities often used in large team meetings or presentations.

Identifying Obstacles

Part of understanding the motivation is also understanding any barriers, whether internal or external. Some barriers can be both internal and external obstacles such as language, culture, learning differences and age. At first, they seem to be induvial and therefore internal, but the social supports or lack of social supports can strongly influence whether these internal aspects become obstacles or not.

Internal Obstacles can include low self-image, stress, emotional triggers, perception of self, etc. Often our perception including our life history, own emotions and the context of the goal or learning objective influence how the person responds to the idea and the required behaviours. These all can all form part of our internal obstacles and can negatively interact with any external obstacles leading to a person feeling lost, defeated, whelmed, etc., before they even start their learning journey. Once a person understands what their internal obstacles are, they have an opportunity to process or overcome these (often with professional supports) prior to initiating their learning behaviour.

External Obstacles can often lead a person feeling powerless, helpless, and hopeless. Common examples of external obstacles can include institutional discrimination (including racism, gender discrimination and financial discrimination), cost of living, responsibilities such as children or bills, geographic location, language barriers and many others. Whilst identifying external obstacles can seem counter-productive to achieving any learning goals, it can also be helpful if done with the right intent. By identifying any external obstacles, a person is then able to plan ways to overcome these, which might then lead to their learning behaviours being more successful. For example, if a person identifies that a professional institution favours a specific type of professional qualification, they can either choose to study that specific qualification or choose a more supportive institution prior to beginning their learning behaviour.

Once a person has understood and developed processes or skills to overcome any identified obstacles, their learning journey will often be more successful. Suggestions to help with overcoming obstacles include – joining a study or relevant social group, changing institutions, or choosing a more supportive institution, seeking professional assistance such as speaking with a psychologist/careers counsellor/tutor and investing in self-care no matter the learning goal.

Awareness of the Treacherous Trio

There are three common types of emotional filtering that impact a person's ability to learn and interact with other people: Confirmation Bias, Cognitive Dissonance and Motivated Reasoning. These three types of unhelpful thinking can severely impact a person's ability to learn and improve and interact with the world. There is a strong overlap across these three types of thinking, but I have tried to separate these as much as possible to assist a person in understanding them more effectively. Almost everyone has at least one, if not all three of these unhelpful thinking styles depending on the topic. This is because the human brain is developed to look for difference and similarity and is often socially and emotionally driven rather than logically driven. Despite how logical a person is, they will still have some version of social and emotional thinking that colours their opinions and worldview.

Confirmation Bias occurs when a person confirms their own viewpoint as more accurate than information that doesn't fit their viewpoint – "The Earth is flat because the horizon is flat". Cognitive Dissonance is the internal tension that occurs whenever a person holds two cognitions that are psychologically inconsistent – "The Earth is flat, but I accept ALL planets are spherical". Finally, Motivated Reasoning is the tendency to accept what we want to believe with much more ease and much less analysis than what we don't want to believe – "The majority of scientists lie about the earth being rounded, as there was one scientist who said the earth was flat". All three are similar and are used to explain how no-one sees the world how it is, but rather they perceive the world based on their own experiences, expectations, and belief systems.

When a person understands their Confirmation Bias, it can help them to lessen the impact of the bias, which in turn may allow them to improve their ability seek more accurate and relevant assistance in their learning journey. For example, if a person is aware that they have an age bias, they might then be willing to ask older people for assistance, once they have spent time and effort in overcoming this bias. This might also allow for incidental learning to occur as well as improving their social emotional connections and skills.

When a person understands their Cognitive Dissonance, it can help direct their planning phase of their learning to overcoming this internal obstacle. When a person understands why they hold the cognitive dissonance, they can spend energy and time reducing the dissonance and its impact.

Finally, when a person understands what causes their Motivated Reasoning, it allows them to develop more efficient learning plans for themselves or for people they teach or influence. For example, a teacher who uses a meta-analysis on learning in combination with one-on-one conversations with students and their parents, can then use this combination of qualitative and quantitative information to challenge their own beliefs regarding what teaching methods are best for learning difficulties.

We are all human, and we will all continue to have varying degrees of bias, dissonance, and motivated reasoning, however, being aware of our version of these, can lead to better individual outcomes for the individual, and for anyone they influence.

Music, Sound, & learning

Music and sounds have been used for thousands of years to improve a person's health. In approximately the last 100 years many western science studies have examined if music and sounds could be utilised to improve a person's ability to learn. With the understanding of neuroscience and the invention of various brain modelling technologies (such as the fMRI and PET scans) and techniques, scientists have been able to study the impacts of sounds and music more directly.

Playing and Listening to Music

The brain processes language, sound, and the written word, and when done together activates multiple areas across the brain. Recent studies have demonstrated that music activates both the left and right brain hemispheres simultaneously. This can lead to improvements in learning and memory. The sound enters the ears and travels along the auditory pathway that interacts with other areas of the brain that impacts our movement, speech, thinking patterns, speech patterns, knowledge and memory retention and focus. Hearing engages our cognitive, sensory, motor and reward systems in the body, often simultaneously, and more so when the person is playing an instrument.

When a person is learning to play an instrument, their eye sees a symbol, their brain hears the sound and attaches or reinforces a memory to the music and speech sound, the brain instructs the body to make the specific sound, and then the brain listens and attunes to the sound. Some studies suggested that musicians' memory retrieval advantage can be explained by their brain's ability to give each memory multiple "trigger tags", where one memory can be associated with a conceptual tag, an emotional tag, an audio tag as well as a contextual tag. As well as this, some research has found that the brain can become up to 30 percent denser (this is a good thing) in students who learn to play instruments compared to those who don't learn. This greater density also has been found to improve overall brain efficiency, allowing the brain to have greater capacity for daily tasks and learning new information.

The brain's need for efficiency becomes a strength when learning material that has music attached to it, via the brain's pattern recognition ability. The brain looks for pattern in the sound and any information relevant to that pattern is stored more comprehensively, allowing for easier retrieval in the future. The pattern skill of the brain is improved through learning to play a musical instrument – reading sheet music teaches not just musical notation and the connection to the specific sound, but also activates a phonological loop leading to a deepening of sound-word connections. When the brain processes sound, it strengthens the same areas of the brain that are responsible for learning language and learning to read, suggesting that music and reading are complementary. Other ways in which learning a musical instrument can improve a person's language skills include separating speech from noise, improving aural perception, assisting in earlier language acquisition, improving hearing prosody in speech, improving a person's language syntax, learning unique words, improving phonological skills and improving language comprehension.

Learning to play a musical instrument has been found to train the brain in areas beyond learning the specific instrument. Some longitudinal studies have found that when people learnt a musical instrument as a younger child and continued this learning, they were much less likely to develop Alzheimer's or Dementia symptoms in older age. Music researchers such as Anita Collins found – if a person begins learning a musical instrument before the age of seven the minimum amount of time recommended before they can reap the long-term benefits in late adult hood is two years. This minimum becomes three years if the person begins after the age of seven for long term benefits, but the longer a person learns musical instruments, the greater the long-term benefits are regarding learning and music.

Some studies suggested that people who learnt an instrument instead of only listening to music, performed better at sporting and academic tasks than people who listened to music only. Some academic tasks not often linked to music that have improved by the person learning an instrument include – improved mathematical ability, improvement in planning and strategising ability, improved attention to detail and improved simultaneous analysis of both cognitive and emotional aspects of a problem or task. Other executive brain functioning benefits relating to learning a musical instrument include improving the level of attention and focus and assisting with strategy, planning and time management skills. Learning an instrument builds movement maps also known as muscle memory, which has been found to translate to improved body awareness in sports that utilise the same body areas – learning to play a double bass can assist a person in understanding their body, leading to improved muscle control, which can then assist in ball and bat sports due to the brain's mapping of the body. The improved mapping of the body also has been found to improve general fine motor skills required for daily tasks, with people who have played an instrument showing a slowed deterioration of fine motor skills in older age. Sport and music are complimentary to each other. Sport often includes competition which improves a person's ability to focus and shutout irrelevant stimuli, while music allows a person to absorb sensory stimuli in order to understand and differentiate, leading to a greater ability to understand one's internal and external environments. Learning a musical instrument has also been found to improve teamwork and spatial awareness.

There are various benefits of listening to music in learning, and some include emotional processing, focus improvement, destressing, etc. For example, music helps people to process their emotions by consciously choosing their favourite style of music and often subconsciously choosing the required beats per minute. The beats per minute combined with the chosen music style also helps to destress and relax the person. Some studies have found that the impact of listening to music can have similar effects on destressing as remedial massage, at least in the shorter-term. Janata and colleagues used Functional Magnetic Resonance Imaging (fMRI) and found that music assists in memory retrieval by triggering emotions relevant to the historic event, whether formal learning or life event.

The specific type of music does not matter as much as previously thought. Scientists previously thought that classical music was best for calming and high beats per minute music was best for energising. Whilst this is true for some people, there are many people who can have an opposite response to specific music. Rap music and heavy metal music often associated with aggression and energy, can assist some people in calming and focusing. Some studies have found that the style of music might have less impact on short-term focus but can impact how effectively the brain organises the new information.

Regarding formalised learning such as exam preparations, many recent studies have found that music assisted students in learning more material and retaining more information compared to people who did not use music during study preparation. Music has also been found to improve a person's reading ability by assisting with sound recognition which then leads to an improvement of recognising letter and word sounds and sound combinations. Music has had similar effects on sporting related learning such as basketball shooting, where people who listened to music while practicing three-point shooting, were found to have higher percentages compared to people who practiced without music.

Music also strengthens social skills including social connection. There are various examples with the most common examples of how music directly assists with social connection to people known and not known including – sporting anthems, Christmas carols, nursery rhymes and popular music choruses. Music therefore strengthens a person's social emotional learning, and as humans are a social species, this can assist many other areas of human learning. By improving a person's social connection, music can indirectly enhance other socio-emotional skills such as the ability to identify emotions internally and from other people and manage and express emotions constructively. Other social and emotional skill improvements that have been connected with learning a musical instrument include improving a person's overall wellbeing and their insight regarding their wellbeing, increasing positive social behaviours including healthier social engagement, improving non-verbal skills, improving empathy and improving a person's perceived personality (allowing for easier social interaction).

Playing a musical instrument can also increase the volume and activity in the brain's Corpus Callosum. The Corpus Callosum is known as the brain's bridge between the two hemispheres, and improvements in this area lead to better communication between the two brain hemispheres. This strengthening of the Corpus Callosum can then lead to improved emotion regulation, which can then improve a person's ability to calm or focus.

Boys's Music Engagement

This subsection will be drawing heavily from Anita Collins' and colleagues' research as well as various other sources that referenced her research.

Prior to the age of 13, the engagement in music from boys and girls is very similar. However, after the age of 13 (during the ages of 13 to 16 especially), the research demonstrated that in a large majority of schools in Australia and internationally, boys' participation in learning a musical instrument drastically decreased, and if a boy was to continue playing an instrument, it often changed to a gender stereotyped instrument. The research discussed that the primary causational reason for this change is a boy's environment.

There were multiple positive environmental aspects that increased male engagement in playing a musical instrument and these included – success and praise from male role models, regular accomplishment that is noticeable, positive parental support that didn't emphasise perceived gender stereotypes, access to technology and support to create their own music, sense of acceptance from other peers (especially other male peers), school culture regarding how music is discussed and received (and what instruments were taught) and an overall interactive learning environment. Individually the young male had to have an interest and positive attitude towards music, success and acceptance and praise, which could all be generated by the above positive environmental factors.

When the environment was supportive, didn't focus on perceived gender norms, was interactive and small successes were acknowledged or celebrated, the rates of boys' stopping engagement in playing a musical instrument drastically reduced, and in some schools the rates were able to increase.

Sound

New technology utilising sounds such as Audio Bilateral Stimulation (Audio BLS) and Audio Binaural Sounds have also been found to improve the brain's Corpus Callosum. The most basic version of audio BLS involves a basic sound going from one ear to the next. This basic audio BLS example is used in psychology to help a person calm their emotional brain centres and to help them focus, by activating the Corpus Callosum via sound. The Binaural Sound utilises a different approach to activate the Corpus Callosum. The Binaural Sound involves each ear receiving a different sound or sound frequency. The frequency difference between the waves entering the left and right ear that the person may perceive consciously or not helps the brain to calm and to focus. When a person's brain is calmer, the brain has an improved ability to access the frontal regions used in problem solving, learning and movement. These improvements have been measured with the use of electroencephalogram (EEG) in various studies, with similar results across the board.

Summary

As discussed, there are many ways in which music and sound can improve a person's overall health, learning ability and physical ability. There are too many studies to reference, but most have found music is positively correlated with increased performance across most aspects of life. The type of instrument learnt, the choice of listening music type and the beats per minute are all individual, but once the right fit can be found, it can become a long-term positive lift habit. During the ages 13 to 16 the male social brain is very vulnerable to environmental opinions. Knowing what we know about the benefits of playing a musical instrument and what it can offer a person's brain long-term; it is important that boys have the opportunity and encouragement to continue or start learning a musical instrument regardless of the specific instrument.

The more recent formalised types of sounds such as Audio Bilateral Stimulation and Binaural Sounds are yet more examples of how sound can improve a person's overall health and functioning.

Key Points & Relevant Personal/Professional Experiences

Neurodivergence & Learning Introduction

Neurodivergence can simply be explained as 'brain difference'. In more detail, it refers to the neurological differences in the way the brain is formed. It is the belief that neurological differences are not an error but genetic variances in brain development that serves a function in our genetic evolution. One evolutionary theory states that without difference in thinking (neurodivergence) we would not have fire or electricity. This does not ignore the challenges neurodiverse people experience, but it changes the lens in which these differences are viewed. Intelligence is valued in our society so neurodivergent individuals who are gifted in their fields are often celebrated and rarely diagnosed with a disorder. Neurodivergent individuals who are not gifted often require a diagnostic label known as a disorder in order to seek any assistance regarding their difficulties.

In this section I will be focusing more on how the Autistic (Diagnosed label known as Autism Spectrum Disorder/ASD), ADHD (Attention Deficit Hyperactivity Disorder) and Trauma brains may learn differently. There is also a growing body of research discussing the advantages of neurodivergence and how it has theoretically influenced and assisted in our societal and technology advancement.

Autism and ADHD learning brain

Brief Introduction

Everyone knows everyone is different, but there are also some further differences with the Autistic and ADHD brains. For example, neurotypical brains generally use stimulation as a tool to excite the brain. Whereas, for many Autistic and ADHD brains, stimulation can be a helpful tool for calming and focus, if the correct stimulation is used.

Research has found that thirty-eighty percent of people who have been diagnosed ADHD would also meet the diagnostic threshold for ASD, and twenty to fifty percent of people who were diagnosed ASD would also meet the diagnostic threshold for ADHD. For simplicity most of this chapter will combine the ASD and ADHD learning differences, however, this section could be its own book with the amount of information now available.

Autism as a diagnosis, is a complex, neurological disorder characterised by deficits in communication and behaviour often seen as deficits in social-emotional skills. Some studies utilised an EEG (electroencephalogram) and their results suggested that autistic children have deficits in the number of mirror neurons which might explain some of the development delays and some of the brain differences. Other common differences and difficulties Autistic people may experience include poorer Interoception, Proprioception and Exteroception, greater need for Stimming, Relationship and Communication differences and a greater Emotional Intensity when triggered. Many people with diagnosed ASD are often encouraged to seek professional mental health assistance and can occasionally be prescribed mood stabilisers with mixed results. The most common difficulty faced by people who have been diagnosed ASD regarding seeking mental health assistance is not feeling heard or understood by neurotypical approaches and professionals.

ADHD as a diagnosis is another common complex neurological disorder that is characterised by difficulties regarding regulating attention, sense of time (also known as time blindness), planning and prioritising, working memory, meta-cognition depth and amount (too much of both), starting and shifting tasks, self-regulation and adapting to changes. Many ADHD adults are also encouraged to seek mental health assistance, alongside a prescribed medication. However, ADHD people also report that the most common difficulty regarding seeking mental health assistance is not feeling heard or understood by neurotypical approaches and professionals.

Another common difficulty for neurodivergent people is masking. Masking in this context is when the person's brain hides part of their real self, often without their own knowledge. It serves as a survival response to help the person feel they fit in. However, it can often lead to difficulties with anxiety and other mental health related difficulties, as well as impact their ability to learn. Once the person becomes comfortable in themselves, it becomes easier to remove the masking need and behaviours.

However, for many Autistic and ADHD people, the brain difference can become a strength once the individual and their support people understand how to use the brain difference as a strength. This approach doesn't undo any difficulties the person might have, rather helps the person to achieve their goals and live a better quality of life.

Differences and Strengths

When a person is interested in a topic, the brain often allows for more resources to be used, thereby making attempting, or completing the task easier. The same is true for the Autistic and ADHD brains, however, this is heightened and known as fixated thinking or hyperfocus.

The difference between fixated thinking, hyperfocus and being interested, is the intensity at which the person experiences that interest. When a person is interested, their internal motivation increases and their want to learn or perform a particular behaviour also increases. This is often a slight increase and can make setting up goals and other motivations easier. Fixated thinking is more common with the neurodivergent brain and is when a person experiences a more intense interest about a behaviour, topic, or theme. This can be helpful as it allows for an even greater amount of internal motivation but can come at the cost of other areas of functioning, including daily functioning or social functioning. Fixated thinking often lasts many years, sometimes a lifetime and a person can experience fixated thinking in combination with hyperfocus. Both Fixated thinking and Hyperfocus can be known as being passionate about a topic or outcome.

Hyperfocus is the greatest of the three intensities and allows the person's ability, quality and/or quantity to be greater than their normal functioning. This is a strength, often called a superpower, as during hyperfocus the person can initiate tasks, set up structure for goals and start multiple tasks or learn the basics for multiple topics at once. The weakness of hyperfocus is it is often short lived, often up to six months. This then leaves a person with multiple tasks started but not finished, with the person struggling to use any form of motivation or goal framework without external assistance, leading to feeling whelmed or burnout.

There is growing research around working memory challenges and challenges feeling connected with others, especially in group contexts, and the ability to perspective take, which often is more impactful in the female presentation of ADHD and ASD. This is often seen once the young person reaches middle school. However, this can often be improved by the young person spending time with one-on-one conversations with supportive peers and adults, which improves their ability later in life when working in small to medium sized groups. This can be important to address as working memory difficulties can negatively impact the young person's identity development and social connectedness.

The Autistic and ADHD memory can also be different. Firstly, the discussed fixated thinking and hyperfocus, can assist in memory of information and of ability for the specific interest topics, during the interest period. However, daily memory functioning can be impacted negatively as well. The busy brain pays less attention to one task at a time, and this leads to the information or behaviour not being retained in memory.

There are many ideas that neurodivergent people can use to improve their memory retention and some include– choosing to focus for five to ten seconds on the task, speaking the task or information out loud, adding association and value (such as movement, interest and motivations), writing the task, using adapted versions of power cards (often utilising a person's interest topic or character), slowing a task down to allow for more conscious attention on the task and the use of the 'Eisenhower Box'. The Eisenhower Box can be explained as a simple decision matrix that is used to help a person prioritise a task or list of tasks based on their urgency and importance. Another idea often practiced by neurodivergent people involves movement. Many neurodivergent people have reported that by combining movement when they learn, their ability to focus and remain calm, increases. The research supports this idea further, by discussing that the use of the Proprioceptive and Vestibular systems in movement can promote focus in some people.

Recent neurodivergence related nutrition research has also found that nutrition and exercise play an important role in the regulation of endorphins and focus. The research has suggested that neurodivergent people benefit more than their neurotypical peers with higher levels of Proteins and Omegas and benefit more from exercise.

Trauma brain learning differences

Trauma can be defined as "any event where a person feels helpless, hopeless and/or powerless", which can include direct abuse, vicarious trauma, neglect, or other forms. Trauma impacts a person's brain and body at multiple levels. Trauma effects the entire body leading to multiple physical and psychological difficulties and disorders.

When a person experiences trauma it can rewire their brain. When a person experiences trauma at a young age (pre-12 years of age) it can rewire their brain impacting not only focus, but also impacting – how and when endorphins are released, memory, emotional regulation, learning ability, the levels of cortisol and dopamine in the body that are available, and impact a person's motivation and ability to trust other people including teachers, coaches and instructors. Simply put, this rewiring of the brain leads to a the "fight and flight" state (sympathetic nervous system being in control) becoming the baseline (or normal) instead of a response to contextual stressors (in "healthy" brains the parasympathetic nervous system also known as the "rest and digest state" is in control and is baseline).

The abnormal amount of cortisol released in a traumatised person effects various brain areas needed for learning, memory and emotional regulation including the hippocampus (involved in learning and memory and converting short-term memories to permanent memories), and frontal cortex region. This abnormal cortisol response also over activates the Amygdala (involved in fear, emotion, and memory), increases anxiety, triggers aphantasia (lack of cognitive visual ability which impacts memory storage and retrieval), triggers various emotional regulation difficulties, triggers Alexithymia (poor Interoception leading to poor understanding of one's own emotional experience), triggers insomnia and other sleep disturbances, worsens memory, overstimulates epinephrine and norepinephrine (leading to poorer motivation regulation), leads to poorer behaviours (such as "class clown" or aggressive behaviours) in classroom and other social settings and worsens learning capability overall.

There are many ideas that people in positions of teaching can implement to support the traumatised brain to learn effectively. Some of these include – group and individual learning programs, emotion regulation psychoeducation for teacher and students, journaling ideas and emotions, drawing ideas and emotions, channelling negative emotions into constructive goals, having an emotionally safe person and environment such as a teacher or mentor, and having other supports in place or at least ideas in how to engage in those supports. Other supports include regular psychological assistance, social clubs such as sports, music, or tabletop gaming as well as regular sleep and eating habits.

Learning Disorders

Learning disorders are a group of neurodevelopmental disorders that manifest during formal schooling, characterised by persistent and impairing difficulties in learning foundational academic skills for reading, writing, and/or mathematics. These are diagnosed when there are specific deficits in an individual's ability to perceive or process information efficiently and accurately. The official definition states that there must be significant impairment in the specified scholastic skill, and this impairment should not be due to sensory/motor deficits, poor teaching, lack of adequate stimulation, or any such external causes. This is a good definition, however, many external causes such as trauma can lead to a learning disorder developing as a trauma response. Learning disabilities can range in severity and may affect only one specific skill or a combination of skills. They are usually present from birth or early childhood and can persist throughout a person's life. Some people with learning disabilities may need accommodations to succeed academically and professionally, while others may be able to overcome their challenges with extra support and effort.

Research has suggested that approximately 10 percent of school aged children experience some form of learning difficulty, although this is often thought to be an under representation when compared to what teachers and instructors observe. The most common learning disorders diagnosed and observed in the western schooling system include – Intellectual Developmental Disorder (where a person experiences deficits in general mental abilities and impairment in everyday adaptive functioning compared to other people their own age), Language Disorder (difficulties in acquiring, using, comprehending and producing language compared to other people their own age), Speech Sound Disorder (difficulties in production of correct sounds), Auditory Processing Disorder (difficulties in understanding information provided verbally or through sounds), Stuttering difficulties, Social Communication Disorder (greater difficulties with the – social use of language, understanding and following social rules and adapting to social rule and language changes), Autism Spectrum Disorder, Attention Deficit Hyperactivity Disorder, Dyslexia (difficulties in reading, writing, and spelling), Dyscalculia (difficulties understanding number-based information and math) and Dysgraphia (difficulties with writing ability, including problems with letter formation/legibility, letter spacing, spelling, fine motor coordination, rate of writing, grammar, and composition).

As with most difficulties, if a person receives the right support, they can overcome and/or manage their difficulties and still achieve their goals. Many people considered successful in our western media (such as Albert Einstein, Alexxis Wineman, Bill Gates, Breanna Clark Charles Darwin, Elon Musk, Eminem, Emma Watson, Greta Gerwig, Howie Mandel, James Carville, Johnny Depp, Justin Timberlake, Satoshi Tajiri and Simone Biles) have various learning difficulties and disorders but have still been able to achieve their goals. As well as the various supports available for children, there are also many supports for adults with learning difficulties available such as the 'Reading and Writing Hotline' in Australia. Personally, I have been able to use my differences in learning as a strength but have also had to create extra processes that other people often don't have to in order to be effective in my professional and personal tasks.

Irlen Syndrome

Irlen Syndrome, also referred to as Meares-Irlen Syndrome, Scotopic Sensitivity Syndrome and Visual Stress, is a visual perception processing disorder, and is not an optical problem. It is a problem with the brain's ability to process visual information, often affecting specific colour wave lengths. This problem has a strong genetic component and is not able to be identified with optical assessments, standardised educational assessments or medical tests. In Australia a diagnosis of Irlen Syndrome can be suggested by professionals that have previous training in education, psychology, Occupational Therapy, speech therapy or other education or medical related fields and have registered with the AAIC (Australasian Association of Irlen Consultants).

Irlen Syndrome is considered controversial despite first being described in the early 1980s. This is because there is still not enough data and evidence to conclusively demonstrate the symptoms are separate to other mental and physical health conditions. Despite this, many people have benefited from seeking assistance. Symptoms of Irlen Syndrome include – sensitivity to light, reading difficulties, distortions to specific coloured print, spelling problems, delayed learning, concentration difficulties, behavioural problems, handwriting problems, depth perception difficulties, eye strain, headaches and migraines and greater levels of fatigue after schooling or academic work.

Irlen syndrome can be treated using tinted glasses or contact lenses, and coloured overlaps for books and screens for technology. This method works by filtering out specific light wavelengths to correct the defect in visual pathways. Individuals with Irlen syndrome will need to attend testing to determine the severity of the syndrome and if colour technology can eliminate the difficulty. The correct colour overlay for the individual will then be decided. Once the prescribed tinted glasses or contact lenses have arrived, individuals with Irlen syndrome often see a reduction in light sensitivity, headaches and fatigue and often report improvements in reading, depth perception, concentration, driving, and computer use ability.

Key Points & Relevant Personal/Professional Experiences

Human Body Basic-Complex from a Eastern Centric

Eastern approaches emphasise balance, energy flow, prevention and holistic health. Many ideas in Eastern Centric models fall under the heading of Traditional Chinese Medicine, however, it is much more difficult to separate the different frameworks and practices due to the overlaps, intertwined histories and because of the nature of the Eastern Centric approach. Many ideas discussed in the previous psychology sections have origins in the Eastern Centric health practices. The origins of Eastern science, particularly in China, India and Japan used holistic approaches stemming from spiritual based philosophies like Taoism, Bushido, Confucianism, and Ayurveda. Eastern approaches integrate this connection by emphasising the role of energy flow and energy balance in maintaining overall health.

Traditional Medicine

It is thought that traditional Chinese Medicine began between the 1940's and 1950's from physicians who attempted to bring together the many streams of Ancient Chinese Medicine and apply them in the modern academic world. This unfortunately led to a loss of the foundations of Ancient Chinese Medicine despite the best efforts, as eventually it was realised that the models were not able to be used under the more westernised medical and academic model. As a side effect of Traditional Chinese Medicine's attempt, it ignored the non-material elements and underpinnings of Ancient Chinese Medicine. Traditional medicine utilises holistic practices that integrate various disciplines like medicine, philosophy, and spirituality. Qi gong, spiritual practices and movement practices such as Tai Chi are still utilised in some "traditional medicine" approaches.

Limitations

The Eastern medicine's focus on prevention, balance, and treating the root cause rather than just symptoms is much better for a person's health longer term. However, when a person has not been practicing the required behaviours and ideas to achieve balance, or if they are born with genetic diseases such as cancer, ignoring the Western Medical model can lead to a higher mortality rate when the difficulties are severe such as 'Stage 4 Cancer' (Metastatic Cancer).

The core limitations include – Acute Care solutions are lacking, poorer understanding of the mechanisms behind how treatments work and subsequent lack of empirical evidence, time intensive treatments are often required (lifestyle vs quick fix), diagnostic precision is reduced as it often examines the body as a whole which can lead to misdiagnoses, limited understanding of genetic influences over the efficacy of treatments, cultural and spiritual clashes with modern living, lack of specificity regarding terms and ideas such as "finding balance", and the improvement of the whole body might mask an underlying cause of a severe disease such as genetic based cancer (inherited risk).

Tai Chi Practice for Health

What is Tai Chi

Tai Chi is considered an Internal art and has key principles including Outward Movement, Body Structure and Internal and key concepts including Jing, Song, Chen and Huo. Outward Movement refers to the improvement of balance and coordination and internal strength through controlled movements. This controlled movement appears from the outside to have a slow, smooth and continuous flow like water flowing in a river against a gentle resistance.

Body Structure refers to maintaining a supple, upright body that is well aligned and in as straight a vertical line as possible. Various injuries or weaknesses may make this more difficult. One example of this would be when a person bends their knees, their body wants to change from vertical to lessen the pressure on the leg muscles. With practice, a participant can become vertical or close to vertical as their body adjusts to the Tai Chi movement patterns. The second part of Body Structure involves being aware of each step as you transfer weight. The transference of weight consciously from one leg to the other allows for more smooth movements whilst maintaining a vertical posture.

The term 'Internal' in Tai Chi refers to the internal components of the human body, with the mind being a large focus. By integrating the mind into Tai Chi practice, the participant can improve their balance and brain body awareness. This internal awareness also involves controlling the muscle tension to allow for gentle, somewhat relaxed movements and joints, and allows the mind to be focused on the movements being practiced instead of the many distractions modern life has.

Jing can be roughly translated as mental quietness or serenity. When a participant focuses their mind on posture, body awareness, breathing, loosening of joints, and relaxing their mind has less ability to focus on the modern life distractions. For some this can be the hardest part of practicing Tai Chi after the basic movements are learnt, as the participant may then find themselves focusing on other life tasks such as cooking dinner. By practicing internal arts such as Tai Chi, a person can learn to have some control over their stress mind, to help induce the 'Jing State'.

Song can be roughly translated as relaxation and a sense of loosening and stretching out. For people who can visualise, this can be a useful tool as the participant can mindfully focus on loosening their joints by gently expanding them from within the body. This can then lead to a more relaxed state as the body's tension is released.

Chen roughly translates as sinking. This is used when referring to sinking your Qi to the 'Dan Tian'. The Dan Tian in Tai Chi practice is the central point of everything and is an area that is three finger widths below the belly button. Exhaling can facilitate the sinking of Qi to the Dan Tian which helps the body and mind relax and achieve Jing and Song states. In Tai Chi practice, it is believed that Chen enhances stability, Song and Qi cultivation.

Huo refers to agility or the ability to move nimbly. Agility is developed through regular practice with proper body posture, weight transference, control of movements, loosened joints and strong internal strength. In Tai Chi practice, it is believed that Huo aids in Qi cultivation and improves flexibility.

Tai Chi has many health benefits and is often discussed with a practice known as Qi Gong.

Common Types of Tai Chi

There are many types of Tai Chi practice including specific types for health, as well as types with a martial focus. The five most common types practiced today include Yang style, Chen style, Wu style, Sun style and Wu Hao style.

Yang style was founded by Yang Luchan in the 19th century. It features slow, flowing and large movements with an emphasis on grace, balance and relaxation. It has a strong focus on health improvement and meditation, and less martial focus.

The Chen style is known as the oldest Tai Chi style and was created by the Chen family in Chenjiagou village. It alternates between slow, flowing and fast movements with explosive actions, emphasises spiralling energy and coiling movements and includes jumps, stomps, and intricate footwork due to its greater focus on martial, strength and agility applications.

The Wu style was created in the 19th century by Wu Quanyou and his son Wu Jianquan. It features smaller, more compact movements, subtle postural adjustments with relaxation over strength and focuses on soft, fluid transitions and a higher stance. Its primary focus is internal energy cultivation and balance.

The Sun style was created by Sun Lutang in the early 20th century and features elements of Tai Chi, Xingyiquan and Baguazhang. It features agile, light footwork and smooth transitions, and movements that flow forward in a continuous graceful manner. Its primary focus is longevity, health and energy (Qi) flow.

The combined Wu Hao style was originally developed by Wu Yuxiang and later refined by Hao Weizhen. It features small, precise and controlled movements and emphasises mental concentration and posture alignment. Its primary focus is internal energy refinement and mindfulness.

Dr. Paul Lam's Tai Chi for Health

When working in my first psychology job, I was fortunate enough to have the opportunity to complete Teacher training in Dr. Paul Lam's Tai Chi for Health program. The program discussed the benefits of Tai Chi, how to be an Effective Teacher, Safety and Risk assessment, their Stepwise Progressive Teaching Method, Tai Chi Principles and many other tools regarding teaching the Tai Chi program. The lessons learnt in the course can be applied in most areas of professional practicing from helping a client one on one, to facilitating effective workshops. This section will be drawing heavily from the course, as well as other Tai Chi resources.

The most common benefits of using Tai Chi, experienced by practitioners and teachers include – improving health, more effectively managing arthritis, diabetes and other chronic conditions, developing patience, tranquillity and inner balance, being part of something greater than oneself.

Many studies have found, and recent studies are finding that Tai Chi has many physical benefits. One of the focuses during the 'Tai Chi for Arthritis' training was 'fall prevention'. When teaching or practicing the sequence of moves, a person may gain improvement in their self-confidence, awareness of their body and joint and muscular health the person decreases their risk of falling and improves their chances of recovery if they do fall. Increasing awareness of fall prevention not only benefits the individual, but also positively benefits the families of people with arthritis as well as lessening the burden on the public health system.

To get the most out of Tai Chi practice, it is important to have an effective teacher. The first aspect of an effective is Attitude and this includes – The teacher's passion for Tai Chi as a healing art, The teacher's relationship with the participants, being positive in your own expectations, how you speak and, in the feedback, you give the participants, constructively correcting mistakes, expecting positive outcomes for the participants and using positive energy such as having a genuine smile while teaching.

The second aspect is the skill level of the teacher specifically regarding Tai Chi. Having the ability and knowledge to increase or decrease the difficulty level of what is being taught can drastically influence how participants learn. This can also influence their own level of passion for Tai Chi and may influence them to want to teach Tai Chi themselves. This leads to the Teaching skills of the teacher. This is just as important as the ability to do the moves, and some have argued more important. Teaching the way, the participants best learn is a skill in its own right, and when a teacher can combine visual instruction, with clear verbal instruction and with clearly defined movements to practice, people have the flexibility to learn how they learn – visually, auditorily or kinaesthetically.

Communicating effectively is the next aspect and involves Listening, Speaking Clearly, Recognising Feelings and Applying Tai Chi Principles. Being an effective listener involves being able to understand what the participants are saying before responding, and ensuring you wait for the participant to finish speaking before finishing their sentences or answering their questions. Speaking Clearly involves communicating with our body, feelings and with clear instructions, and being able to adjust how you speak to suit the learner's language and Tai Chi ability. Recognising feelings involves recognising the participants feelings based on their language and body language, but also being aware of your own feelings and how they may influence how you see the situation.

Applying Tai Chi principles involves understanding the foundational principle of Tai Chi namely, Harmony/Balance or better known as Yin and Yang. Once this is understood, then applying the principles of control, smooth and continuous movements, and allow for Tai Chi to have a rhythm. Risk assessment by the teacher is ongoing, as any injury can be a setback for the participants. Risk assessment involves communicating with the participants to assess their ability levels, and being able to adjust exercises to fit the participants' needs. When you find out a participant does have an injury, be careful not to overstep by giving medical advice, ensure any advice suggested is relevant specifically to the Tai Chi practice and within the teacher's own abilities and professional training. This will decrease risk of injury and increase the participants' ability to continue their Tai Chi development and practice.

Lastly Facilitating enjoyment is very important in the role of a teacher. This is best achieved through helping the participants find the intrinsic enjoyment of Tai Chi, guiding them through the initial awkward phases, plateau phases and rough patches and using methods such as the 'Stepwise Progressive Teaching Method'.

Qi Gong Understanding

The biggest difference between Qi Gong and Tai Chi is the focus. They both focus on the human body physically and can have spiritual aspects, however, Qi Gong normally focuses on the internal body systems more specifically and can be explained as a form of movement and mind using intention and mindfulness to guide the body's Qi. Qi Gong is often used to assist in a particular area such as the mind, body or spirit. To confuse it further, Tai Chi practitioners often use Qi Gong in their practice, and rarely are the two separated as they are in this book.

In this section I will be drawing heavily from the 'White Tiger Qi Gong' courses I have studied (see appendix), as well as several other Qi Gong resources referenced in the Appendix. It is noted however, that despite there being a strong focus on internal spirituality in Qi Gong, my interpretation of the spiritual aspect of Qi Gong will have a strong physical and mental health focus. It is also noted that Qi Gong is often referenced as a healing art but has been used in martial arts for thousands of years for both healing and destructive purposes and intent. However, as stated this section will be focusing more on the physical and mental healing aspect of Qi Gong. Studies have found at least thirteen physical and mental health benefits of Qi Gong including improving – blood pressure, balance, mild anxiety and depression, quality of sleep, muscle strength, bone density, quality of life, immune system, inflammation, cognitive performance (focus), arthritis and cardio fitness.

Fascia lines correlate strongly with the majority of the Meridian lines practiced in Chinese medicine. It is believed that each organ has a fascia layer covering it and that they act as energising chambers for the organs. Some qi gong practitioners and traditional kung fu practitioners believe that the body's qi is stored in the fascia layers where it works like a cushion to protect the organs.

There are various areas within Chinese Medical Theory, but it can be summarised through the Yin and Yang Principles, the five-element approach, the three Treasures, and Meridian lines.

The idea of Yin and Yang comes from the Chinese version of creation, namely 'The Dao', loosely meaning 'Created Duality'. It was first written in about the sixth century BCE by Lao Tzu (who was a Daoist philosopher) in his book 'I-Ching'. The main aspects of Yin and Yang include – the idea of opposites always being relative to each other, they consume each other to maintain and create balance, and they inter-transform into each other (once one reaches its peak it slowly begins to turn into the other). Yin energy comes up from the earth and Yang energy comes down from the sun and sky. Nature Yin is material – produces form, grows, is matter, contracts, descending and below; where nature Yang is – immaterial, produces energy, generates, is energy, and expansion. Body Yin is – inferior (below), anterior-medial, front, structure, body and organs, front side that we need to protect; where body Yang is – superior (above), posterior-lateral, back, function, head, skin muscles, back side that has protection and is strong.

Activity Yin is – cold, quiet, wet, soft, inhibitions, slowness, substantial, conversion, storage and preserves; where activity Yang is – heat, restless, dry, hard, excitement, rapidity, non-substantial, transformational and change. Disease Yin is – chronic disease, gradual onset, lingering pathological, cold, sleepiness, pale face, likes hot drinks, likes to curl up; where disease Yang is – acute disease, rapid onset, rapid pathological, heat, restlessness, red face, likes cold drinks, lots of bed covers. The Yin organs include Heart, Lung, Liver, Spleen, Kidneys, Pericardium, Conception (Ren). The function of the Yin organs is to store vital substances such as Qi, Blood, Essence, Body Fluids, and to store only pure refined substances it receives from the Yang organs after transformation of food and air. The Yang organs include Small Intestine, Large Intestine, Gall Bladder, Stomach, Urinary Bladder, San Jiao/Triple warmer, Governing (Du). The function of the Yang organs is to empty and refill, they receive, move transform, digest and excrete. Too much or too little of one, will impact all five elements.

Qi Gong discusses a concept known as the 'Dantian'. This can be defined as the body's energy centres, and there are three Dantians in the human body (Upper, Middle, Lower). The Upper Dantian is associated with the Pineal Gland, is the forehead between the eyebrows (sometimes referred to as the 'Third Eye'), and this is where the body's spirit/Shen is refined and converted into 'Wu Wei' (emptiness). The Middle Dantian is associated with respiration, and the health of the internal organs and the Thymus Gland, is level with the heart and this is where the Qi (vitality) is refined and turned into the Shen. The Lower Dantian is associated with the 'Golden Stove Storage' area of the life force, is located 3 finger widths below the navel and processes the body's Elixir into Jing and is where Vitality begins in the body. These three are also known as the body's 'Three Treasures'.

From the Daoist perspective, the first of the 'Three Treasures' is known as Qi. According to Daoist practice, Qi is the shared matter with the universe that – gives use life and vitality, is our breath, immaterial and material (constantly changing form), nutrient substance that nurtures the body and activates life activity. The Qi Essence is the basic constitution strength, that allows for growth, reproduction and development and is the basis of kidney Qi and is the basis of marrow.

The next Qi is known as Pre-Heaven Qi and comes from the parents, promotes growth and the development of the human body. Post-Heaven Qi is known as the nutrient Qi and is inhaled from air through lungs and dispersed through lungs. Yuan Qi is strongly related to Essence Qi, is dynamic, is the basis of kidney Qi and facilitates the transforming of Qi and blood. Gu Qi is the Qi of food and is produced by the spleen. Zong Qi derives from the food Qi with the air and is transformed into Gathering Qi, which then nourishes the heart and lungs and enhances and promotes lung function. Zen Qi is the last stage of transformation of Qi and is transformed using Yuan Qi and circulates the channels and nourishes the organs and originates in the lungs. Ying Qi nourishes the internal organs, and closely relates to blood and flows with the blood in the blood vessels and channels. Wei Qi is a coarser form of Qi and flows in the outer layers of the body. It adjusts the opening and closing of the pores, has its root in the lower burner with the kidney, is nourished by the middle burner in the stomach and spleen and is dispersed by the upper burner in the lungs. Central Qi connects to the Yuan Qi in the spleen and stomach and connects to the post-Heaven Qi derived from food. The many functions of Qi can be summarised as – Transforming, Transporting, Holding, Raising, Protecting and Warming.

From the Daoist perspective, the second of the 'Three Treasures' is known as Shen. Shen is the appearance of thinking and consciousness as well as the internal Zang Fu essence. It is the heart and mind combined.

Finally, the third of the 'Three Treasures' is known as Jing. Jing is – the constitution and physical energy and is inherited from our parents. It is the material basis for the physical body/infrastructure, nourishes, moistens, and fuels the body, is related to reproduction, is the basal root of the body's energy and is stored in the kidneys and the Dantian.

There is thought to be three main causes of disease – internal, external, and other. Internal causes are related to the emotions when they are prolonged or intense that the imbalance occurs such as anger, sadness, excitement, grief, fear, shock, etc. External causes include wind, cold, damp, dryness, summer heat and fire. Other causes of disease include exercise, diet, constitution, over working, fatigue, sex, trauma, parasites, poisons, and incorrect treatment.

The five elements are another cornerstone of Qi Gong practice. The five elements are Fire, Earth, Metal, Water and Wood. The Fire element is thought to create earth and control metal. In the human body it is the heart and small intestine and generates the spleen and stomach and moves in an upward direction. It is also relevant to our tongue sense, bitter taste, colour red, laughter, joy and love, summer, and the hot environment.

The Earth element – is thought to create metal and control water. In the human body it is the spleen and stomach and nourishes the lung and large intestine, house the Yi and is the centre point of reference for the five elements. It is also referred to as the "provider of all" as it is responsible for creation, transforms food into Qi and balances Yin and Yang. It is also relevant to our Lips and mouth sense, muscle tissue, sweet taste, colour yellow, singing, worry and pensiveness, late summer (harvest) and the humid and damp environment.

The Metal element – is thought to create water and control wood. In the human body is the lungs and large intestine and nourishes kidney and bladder and is contraction. It is referred to as the defensive system, turns Yang Qi into Yin Qi, and is also relevant to our nose sense, skin tissue, pungent taste, colour white, crying, grief, autumn and dry environments.

The Water element – is thought to create wood and control fire. In the human body is the kidney and bladder and nourishes the liver and gallbladder and has downward energy. It is referred to as the development and growth element, moving with fluidity. It is also relevant to our ear sense, bones, salty taste, colours blue and black, groaning, fear, winter, and cold environments.

The Wood element – is thought to create fire, and control earth. In the human body it is the liver and gallbladder and nourishes the heart and small intestine and has expansion energy. It is referred to as the planning and vision element and is also relevant to our eye sense, tendons, sour taste, colour green, shouting, anger, spring, and wind environments.

The five elements and Meridians are intertwined throughout the human body according to ancient Chinese Medicine and according to some Traditional Chinese Medicine. I will quickly discuss the difference between Traditional Chinese Medicine and Ancient Chinese Medicine, before returning to the five elements and meridians. It is thought that traditional Chinese Medicine began between the 1940's and 1950's from physicians who attempted to bring together the many streams of Ancient Chinese Medicine and apply them in the modern academic world. This unfortunately led to a loss of the foundations of Ancient Chinese Medicine despite the best efforts, as eventually it was realised that the models were not able to be used under the more westernised medical and academic model. As a side effect of Traditional Chinese Medicine's attempt, it ignored the non-material elements and underpinnings of Ancient Chinese Medicine. What is now considered Ancient Chinese Medicine began between approximately 200BCE-200CE and was the first systematic approach to healing after shamanic healing and moved closer to nature in its approach. It included connecting with resonance from the natural source energy and aimed at helping the student in developing a deeper understanding of energies and self-healing.

Meridians are the pathways in the body (sometimes referred to as channels) that form the anatomy of Chinese Medicine. Qi and blood circulate to the organs internally and externally via these pathways. Nutrient Qi flows inside the meridians and Defensive Qi runs outside the meridians. Diseases of internal organs will find their way into the corresponding meridians, which then can have a more global negative impact. Blockages to the meridians occur if the network of channels is disrupted, this can affect the local area as well as affecting – the organ relating to the meridian, and the Qi, Jing and Shen flow. A person needs to open and clear meridians, to allow for the energy to flow freely. There are Fourteen important meridians – each of the ten major organs have their own associated meridian, the Pericardium and the San Jiao have their own meridians and the Ren and Du have their own meridians. The meridians penetrate to the Yin and Yang organs and there are three Yin and Yang meridians on the upper extremities and three on the lower extremities. The meridians run approximately symmetrically and run vertically and bilaterally.

There are four fire meridians in total. The Heart fire meridian connects with the small intestine and lungs and is responsible for – clearing heat, unbinding chest, benefiting voice, relaxing muscles, regulating blood flow, and improving heart rhythm. The Small Intestine fire meridian connects with the gallbladder, bladder, ren, heart and stomach and is responsible for – clearing heat, reducing swelling, benefiting shoulder, arms and neck and lessening pain. The Pericardium fire meridian connects with the Sanjiao and is responsible for – soothing Shen, aiding sleep, and dreams, clearing heat from Qi, improving nutritive and blood levels, harmonising stomach and intestines, unbinding chest, regulating Qi. The Sanjiao/Triple Heater fire meridian connects with all burners and pericardium and is responsible for – clearing heat, improving constipation and ear issues, activating meridian channels and lessening pain.

There are two earth meridians in total. The Spleen earth meridian connects with the oesophagus and spreads across the tongue and is responsible for – regulating the spleen, lessening bleeding, restoring consciousness, harmonising middle Jiao, harmonising the spleen and stomach, resolving dampness, harmonising liver, and kidneys, regulating menstruation, regulating intestines and promoting digestion. The Stomach earth meridian enters the stomach and spleen and is responsible for – lessening pain, harmonising stomach, and spleen, nourishing blood, clearing fire, and reviving Yang.

There are two metal meridians in total. The Lung metal meridian connects with the middle Jiao, diaphragm, lungs, and throat and is responsible for – lessening coughing, wheezing, and transforming phlegm, regulating water passage, benefits throat, clears heat from lungs and moistens lungs. The Large Intestine metal meridian connects with the lung and large intestine and is responsible for – helping to improve constipation and tooth aches, inducing childbirth, expelling wind, clearing heat, reduce swelling, regulating ears, nose and throat, adjusting sweating and plays an eliminating role.

There are two water meridians in total. The Kidney water meridian connects with the kidney, bladder and Ren channel and is responsible for – tonifying the kidney as a base of Yin, Yang and Essence, activating Qi, benefiting lungs, strengthening lumber spine and throat, regulating lower Jiao, warming intestines and harmonising stomach Qi. The Urinary Bladder water meridian connects with the spine and lumber region and is responsible for – working with the Vagus nerve, clearing heat from eyes and warming uterus.

There are two wood meridians in total. The Liver wood meridian curves around the stomach and intersects the Du Channel and is responsible for – moving liver Qi, nourishing liver blood and Yin, regulating menstruation and lessening stiffness in the body. The Gallbladder wood meridian connects with the liver and gallbladder and is responsible for – detoxifying, benefitting the head, improving headaches, shaking and tumour growth, spreading liver Qi and helping sinew and joints.

The Ren (conception), Du (governing) and Dai (girdling) meridians are pathways that do not have acupuncture points. The Ren meridian is part of the primary and extraordinary meridians, runs through the central line of the body, has its own channel and is also part of the primary channels. It is responsible for – tonifying Essence, assisting in conception, warming the spleen, nourishing original Qi, calming spirit and grounding. The Du meridian is part of the primary and extraordinary meridians, runs through the posterior central line of the body and is responsible for – calming the spirit, nourishing the brin, tonifying kidneys and Essence, reducing anxiety and promoting sleep. The Dai meridian connects the upper and lower body, runs along the 'Belt Line' of the body and is responsible for assisting with – issues in the middle aspects of the body including lumbar weakness and muscular weakness and issues in the lower extremities.

As well as helping people improve their overall health, in more recent times, Qi Gong has been used to help people recover from some mental health related difficulties. What we consider mental health is still physical as I will discuss in a later section, but we call it mental health as the brain is very complex, and our understanding of the brain still has a lot of room for improvement. According to Chinese Medicine, what we call high levels of anxiety corresponds with the spleen system and is connected to the element of earth. An imbalanced spleen system leads to various digestive issues and impacts our thoughts such as overthinking. The previously discussed fascia information is also relevant when discussing Qi Gong and mental health, as it has been suggested that poor mental health can be found as tension in the fascia. Qi Gong discusses using grounding movements along with the other principles discussed to help a person connect with the earth element directly. These movements focus on twisting and dynamic movements to soften the fascia by removing the emotional tension in the fascia, and the twists can be classified as "Co-activation of functional opposites that create spirals in the fascia compartments".

Qi Gong discussed that being stressed or staying in the Sympathetic Nervous System for too long can impact our body in various ways including – changing skin colour (pale), changing fluids such as urine, increasing our brain waves to the Beta 14-30hz more frequently, emitting Wei Qi and burning up the Yang Qi supply, weaking the immune system, depleting Jing, shortening life span, decreasing libido, increasing the risk of high blood sugar levels and type 2 diabetes and leading to an addiction of the negative emotional state.

It is believed that our emotions are chemical consequences that form feedback of our past experiences, that can impact the now and increase our risk of future stress. This can be known as an 'Emotion Loop' and involves – our thoughts driving our feelings, our feelings then driving our thoughts, then the loop hardwires our brain into the same patterns which conditions our body to the past. Then those thoughts cause a biochemical reaction in the brain that release chemical signals, the signals can then make the body feels exactly the way the person was just thinking. This then causes you to generate more thoughts that make you feel the same way you were just thinking. The simplest way to stop the loop is through – focused intention with an elevated emotion we want to replace the previous emotion with, which can then lead to transformation.

The last area of Qi Gong explored here is the idea of healing sounds. The idea was formally created in 420-589CE by Tao Hongjing, following this, in 1386-1644 various body movements were formally introduced by Hu Wenhuan and Gao Lian. The exact pronunciation of the healing sounds is less important and can vary depending on dialect origins, but it was reported that the common thread of the healing sounds based on the five elements of Chinese Medicine and associated body organs. The healing sound for the heart was suggested to be 'Haa', the lung healing sound was 'Ssss', liver healing sound was 'Shoo', spleen healing sound was 'Whoo', Kidneys healing sound was

'Chway' and the tiple warmer healing sound was 'Shee'. The idea of healing sounds is also explored in yogic practice.

One area that is not specifically associated or taught in Qi Gong practice is known as the Kuji-Kiri or nine syllables/seals. I have included it in this section as it involves Qi cultivation and Chakra awareness and activation. It traces its historic origins to Japanese ninja and samurai practice and each of the nine seals have their own mantras the practitioner would use to focus or channel their mind/spirit/energy. These nine seals include Rin, Pyo, Toh, Sha, Kai, Jin, Restu, Zai and Zen seals. These seals were often used to assist in personal cultivation of Qi as well as the activation of personal chakras. However, there was still a lot of mythology and mystery regarding their use, and many thought they were used as magic spells and as a form of weaponry.

The Rin Kuji is thought to channel power throughout the individual's body to help create focus and generate energy. It is thought to be connected to the fire element in Qi practice and the Root Chakra. The Pyo Kuji is thought to be the energy direction Kuji and is associated with the Sacral Chakra. The Toh Kuji is known as the Harmony Kuji where the person is in harmony with themselves and their environment and is associated with the Solar Plexus Chakra. The Sha Kuji is thought to be the healing Kuji through increasing the individual's own vibration and is associated with the Heart Chakra. The Kai Kuji is thought to be the Premonition of danger or the Intuition Kuji. The Jin Kuji is thought to be Awareness Kuji. The focus of this Kuji is not on the potential for danger like the Kai Kuji, but instead is the awareness of other people's thoughts and possibly emotions. The Jin Kuji is associated with the Third Eye Chakra. The Restu Kuji is thought to be about the perceived control of time and space and is also associated with the Third Eye Chakra. The Zai Kuji is thought to be concerned with Elemental Control. Finally, the Zen Kuji is thought to be Absolute Enlightenment whereby the individual has overcome each of the internal challenges of the other eight, has no hand signals and must be uncovered individually. One possible healing art that utilises Kuji practices is known as Reiki, although this has not been included in this book.

This overlap of Qi and Chakras is interesting as is the history. The Kuji-Kiri's history can be found through the Hindu and later Buddhist spiritual practices, which was later adopted and adapted further for use in the Japanese military and martial practices of the Samurai and Ninjutsu. The Qi element of the practice finds its origins in the Buddhist spiritual practices and the Chakra focuses originate in the Hindu spiritual practices. This overlap is very useful as it demonstrates the overlap of ideologies and health practices across time and cultures and highlights how interconnected or eclectic our human body should be for overall health.

Key Points & Relevant Personal/Professional Experiences

Yoga Understanding

Yoga originates from traditional Indian medicine practices and can be defined as a system of practices that are used to balance the mind and body through exercise, meditation, breath work and developing insight into the person's own emotions and health. Many people also practice yoga as a form of individual spiritual practice. There are many different types of Yoga, with the most common ones including Hatha Yoga (Sun and Moon or Will or Force), Yin Yoga (Restorative), Vinyasa Yoga (Sequence Yoga), Power Yoga (Muscular Endurance), Bikram Yoga (Hot), Ashtanga Yoga (Energetic/Physical), Kundalini Yoga (Spiritual, Sound Healing) and Yoga Nidra (Sleep). As yoga has a long history of practice there are variations in the understanding of what yoga means and how to distil the practice of yoga. Like most traditional practices, the separation of yoga into types came much later and is often used for people who are new to yoga to assist them in choosing what fits their goals the most. Traditionally yoga was not just a practice a person completed once a week, but a lifestyle. Separating yoga into types runs the risk of undermining this philosophy, and as a yoga student, I felt it best to leave this separating to the yoga instructors and yogi's.

Some yoga practitioners discuss the idea of the 'Eight Limbs' of yoga. The eight limbs include Pranayamas, Pratyahara, Asanas, Dharana, Niyamas, Dhyana, Yamas and Samadhi. Pranayamas discuss the mindful and controlled breathwork that allows the person to clear the mind and calm the body. Pratyahara is the conscious withdrawal from the outside world by tuning out external stimuli and directing all attention inwards. Asanas are the physical yoga postures that help a person connect their body, mind and spirit through strength, balance and focus. Dharana refers to focused concentration that occurs by disciplining the mind to observe our thoughts objectively and slowing down the thinking process. Niyamas are the personal duties and spiritual observances to maintain a "pure soul". Dhyana is meditative absorption, the uninterrupted flow of continuous concentration. Yamas are the ethical principles that guide the person's behaviour towards the world around them. Finally, Samadhi is also known as enlightenment and is achievement of a state of bliss and peace by seeing life and reality for what it is, the union of the mind and body.

My focus as a yoga student and fitness trainer has always been relating to the physical exercise component, as such I will be focusing on the physical and mental benefits of yoga, with minimal focus on the formal spiritual practice, although many people report spiritual benefits of yoga without formally practicing the chakras, etc. The easiest way I have found to explain yoga's physical benefits when compared to other exercises and sports is – "improving one's strength through body control and stretch". This definition exemplifies the physical benefits of yoga but fails to encapsulate the two other main reasons why some people are drawn towards yoga, these being breath and spiritual healing/insight development.

Yoga and Body Systems

Yoga improves our physical health by improving many our body systems directly including the – Skeletal System, Muscular system, Nervous System, Cardiovascular, Respiratory, Digestive System and brain health. It has also been demonstrated to reduce stress and improve epigenetic health (gene expression).

Yoga improves the Skeletal system by stimulating the release of synovial fluid and improving bone density. Yoga improves the Muscular system by improving the strength and endurance of our supporting/smaller muscles around our joints, as well as placing our larger muscles under healthy levels of strain. Many yoga related poses also improve the core strength which reduces pressure in the spine. This can lead to muscular-skeletal health improvements, especially for people who work desk jobs and sit hunched during most of their workday.

Yoga improves the Nervous system by helping to teach a person about their parasympathetic state and providing the practitioner tools they can use when in a sympathetic state. It has also been found to increase the endorphin related hormones, decrease cortisol and stimulate the Vagus nerve. Yoga improves the Cardiovascular system by assisting in lowering blood pressure and better utilise oxygen through breath training.

Yoga improves the Respiratory system by assisting in increasing lung capacity and reducing breaths per minute which can strengthen the respiratory muscles, improving the flow of the lymphatic system which assists in removing toxins and reducing stress.

Yoga improves the Digestive system by decreasing cortisol, decreasing unhealthy cholesterol, boosting healthy cholesterol and lessening the severity of IBS and constipation. Yogic breathing practice has also been demonstrated to assist the brain directly through increasing levels of Gamma-Aminobutyric Acid (GABA) in the brain, developing and strengthening the Interoception regarding emotions and allowing a person to slow down which may positively influence mental health. As a result of all these benefits, it makes sense that our immune system also benefits, and some studies have suggested that the combination of exercise, breath work and development of Interoception, all contribute to this improvement. Recent research has also shown promising results in reducing the speed of glaucoma deterioration.

Yoga Breath Work, Chakras, and more

As mentioned, an important part of yoga practice is the breath work. The two most common breath practices in yoga are Kapalbhati and Ujjayi Pranayama. Kapalabhati can be translated as 'Shining Skull' and is a method used to warm up via breath. It involves controlling the breath by sharply exhaling while pumping you stomach in and out. The inhalation is passive, while the exhalation is forceful and sharp. This is theorised help the lungs clear any waste from the air passageways.

Ujjayi Pranayama is often referred to as an 'Ocean Breath' and is used to calm the brain and create internal heat. As well as learning various ways of breathing, the person often learns various positions or sequences to help them reach their emotional, spiritual or physical goals. There are many examples of yogic breath work, and some of the other examples will be discussed in the 'Psychology of Body Brain Connections' section.

Another important part of most yoga practice involves a basic understanding of what is known as Chakras. Chakras can be defined as wheels or disks that allow the main energetic channels of the body to flow through and from. There are more than 100 Chakras, and with the seven main Chakras/Energy Centres located at approximately the Root, Sacral, Solar Plexus, Heart, Throat, Brow and Crown. Some yoga instructors believe that the seven chakras allow for the 72000 energetic channels called Nadis to carry vital life force energy, often referred to as Prana throughout the body. There are three major Nadis – Ida, Pingala and Sushumna, and they run up and down the spine in a DNA-like helix, and it is theorised that the Chakras form where the three Nadis interact. The biggest different between the Nadis and the Meridian lines, and the Nadis and our nerve systems is that the Nadis are not physical, but more energetic or spiritual channels. This makes it easier to understand spiritually, but harder for it to be understood from the western scientific method.

Another concept of yoga that is useful to understand for physical and mental health reasons is known as the four Bandhas. According to yogic teachings, the four Bandhas can be used to engage, employ and control the body's energy system and to direct this energy to the parts of the body the person wants to and assist the brain centres, Nadis and Chakras. The four main Bandhas include the Root Lock/Mula-bandha, Throat Lock/Jalandhara-bandha, Lifting of the Diaphragm Lock/Uddiyana-bandha and accessing all three locks simultaneously/Maha-bandha, and the two minor Bandhas include the Hand Lock/Hasta-bandha and Foot Lock/Pada-bandha.

The Mula-bandha is activated by exhaling while engaging the pelvic floor and drawing it upwards towards the navel. It is used to activate deep core strength and strengthen the entire pelvic floor area including the muscles that support the pelvic organs. The Jalandhara-bandha is activated by extending the neck while lifting the heart, then dropping the chin to the chest, while the tongue presses into the roof of the mouth. It is used to tone the muscles of the neck and assist in controlling the stream of energy through the nerves and energy channels of the neck. The Uddiyana-bandha is activated while in seated the position. The person will have their feet straight in front of them at hips width. From there, the person will slowly angle the body forward from the waist while keeping a soft joint (small bend) in the knees. The palm of the hands will be placed on to the knees. Next the person takes a deep inhale while pushing the stomach forward, and then use a forceful exhale to empty the lungs. The abdominal muscles are tightened (drawn in towards spine). The position or pose is held for until the next inhalation and process is repeated. This bandha is used to strengthen and tone the abdominal muscles, while practicing meditative, controlled breathing to assist in energizing the body.

The Maha-bandha is achieved through the use of the three major bandhas together (in succession). The Jalandhara-bandha is completed, followed by the Uddiyana-bandha and finally the Mula-bandha. The person releases this series of locks in reverse when they are ready to allow for controlled flow of the body's energy. It is believed that this practice assists in strengthening the autonomic nervous system and pelvic region, assists in anxiety and purging related difficulties, supports the intestinal functioning, assists the body's immune system, assists in thyroid regulation, strengthens internal organs, promotes core strength and energises the body.

Some schools of yoga also discuss the idea of healing sounds in relation to the body's own energy fields (also known as resonance) and chakras. Yogic practitioners who use healing sounds believe that it can directly influence the body's own energy fields and assist in realigning the body's chakras.

Herbalist Understanding

There are a lot of different herbs that can be used to help a person recover from an injury or illness or maintain better overall health. Herbs can have multiple effects and can be used as the primary or as support ingredients, depending on the goal or problem. Some types of effects herbs can have include Adaptogen, Adjuvant, Alterative, Amphoteric, Anaesthetic, Analgesic, Anti-Allergy, Anticatarrhal, Anti-Emetic, Anti-Inflammatory, Antimicrobial, Anti-Rheumatic, Antispasmodic, Antitussive, Astringent, Bitter, Calming/Relaxing, Cardioactive, Cardioprotector, Cardiotonic, Cholagogue, Decongestant, Demulcent, Diaphoretic, Diuretic, Emmenagogue, Expectorant, Gut Healing, Hepatic, Hypnotic, Hypotensive, Immunomodulator, Immunostimulant, Lymphatic, Nervine, Synergistic (pairing), Warming, and others. Some herbs can only be used short term, some are safe to use long term, some herbs are known as restricted herbs due to either their potency or possible side effects and herbs differ in how quickly they assist the body.

As herbs have so many possible healing abilities, it is no surprise that there are many physical and mental health ailments and difficulties that can be supported by or treated with herbal remedies. I have focused primarily on the herbal effects as there is too much information regarding herbal use to fit in this type of book. Herbs have been used for thousands of years, and research from at least the last fifty years has found that they may be useful for various mental health presentations such as PTSD, Anxiety, Depression, Sleep, Cognitive Health, Physical Recovery. It is also important to remember that some herbs may be contraindicated with prescribed medication, or may other side effects, so check with a trained herbalist/dietician (who has extra training in herbs) prior to consuming medication and herbs simultaneously. Some herbs are best used when fresh and many are useful when dried. There are many ways in which to use herbs including sprays, tinctures, lozenges, syrups, creams, teas, infusions, capsules, baths, salves, suppositories, recipes and more.

Separating Herbs into Basic Function

Traditionally, herbs are used synergistically and rarely separated. Often herbs are chosen for how they assist a person, with most herbs serving multiple purposes. Here the herbs are separated for easy understanding.

Adaptogen herbs

Adaptogen herbs can be used to help the body manage or adapt to a chronic condition, are known as metabolic regulators and are often used as a secondary effect with many other herbal remedies. Other roles Adaptogen herbs can assist with include – helping to address debility and potential true exhaustion (adrenal burnout), supporting the body to manage prolonged pain, assisting with managing severe stress, assisting in the treatment of Fibromyalgia, supporting the immune system and helping to guard against allergic reactions, assisting the digestive system, assisting in management of gastrointestinal pain, assisting in management of insomnia and anxiety, assisting the anti-inflammatory, antioxidant, antiviral, expectorant and demulcent properties of other herbs and foods, reducing the allergic response to stress, assisting with liver health, assisting energy levels, supporting thyroid recovery and used as a primary or secondary herb in general and adrenal tonics. There are many examples of adaptogen herbs including Ashwagandha, Astragalus, Brahmi (Bacopa Monnieri), Codonopsis (Dang Shen), Damiana, Ginseng, Gotu Kola, Guduchi, Hawthorn Blossom, Holy Basil, Hops, Korean (Panax) Ginseng, Liquorice, Passionflower, Nettle Seed, Rehmiana, Reishi, Rhodiola, Saw Palmetto, Schisandra, Shatavari, Shiitake, Siberian Ginseng, Tulsi, and Valerian.

Adjuvant herbs

Adjuvant herbs are used to enhance the production of antibodies to enhance the immune response, are used to increase the efficacy of the blends they are in (acting like an accelerator), promoting movements of the constituents from the digestive tract into the bloodstream (to enhance absorption), and some act via the stimulation of the nervous system and circulation. The many examples of Adjuvant herbs include – Andrographis, Angelica, Ashwagandha, Astragalus, Bayberry, Cayenne, Cinnamon, Damiana, Echinacea, Ginger, Panax Ginseng, Picrorrhiza, Poke Root, Prickly Ash, Rosemary, Shatavari, Wood Betony and Yarrow.

Alterative herbs

Alterative herbs are used – to enhance the metabolic and eliminatory processes, when a person's body is out of balance (often due to chronic disease, stress, inflammation or autoimmune diseases), for skin conditions, to help address toxicity, to slow the degeneration of joints, to help cleanse the body of toxins and to support the eliminatory organs. Alterative herb examples include – Birch, Black Cohosh, Bogbean, Burdock, Celery Seed, Cleavers, Dandelion Leaf and Root, Echinacea, Figwort, Fringetree, Fumitory, Garlic, Golden Seal, Mahonia (Oregon Grape), Nettle, Poke Root, Red Clover, Sarsaparilla, Uva-Ursi and Yellow Dock.

Anaesthetic herbs

Anaesthetic herbs are often used to help numb the throat. They can be used in various forms including a spray, syrup, gargle and lozenge form. Example herbs include Clove, Peppermint, Propolis and Myrrh.

Analgesic herbs

Analgesic herbs are mostly used to manage pain, and this includes – General pain relief, easing of diarrhoea related pain, headaches and aching muscles, lessening of muscular tension around the joints, managing stress and as external warm compresses around the ear and jaw. Examples of Analgesic herbs include Belladonna, Californian Poppy, Cramp Bark, Datura, German Chamomile, Henbane, Hops, Jamaican Dogwood, Lavender, Meadowsweet, Passionflower, Peppermint, Valerian, Wild Lettuce and Yellow Jasmine.

Anti-Allergy herbs

Anti-Allergy herbs are used to support the immune system's response to allergens either as primary or secondary herbs and can be used internally or externally. They are used as they help to dampen the immune response and it is theorised, their action on the Mast Cells supports the immune system. They are also useful when vulnerable populations such as young children or elderly adults have a respiratory tract infection or digestive infection. Example herbs with this action include – Albizzia, Baikal Skullcap, Feverfew, German Chamomile, Lemon Balm, Nettle, Plantain, Wild Yam and Yarrow.

Anticatarrhal herbs

Anticatarrhal herbs are often used when there is an excess of mucous, associated with the inflammation of the surround mucous membranes. The mucous is often located in the back of the nose, throat or sinuses and occasionally can be found to impact bowel movements. These herbs often are used as they either help to dry the mucous or make the mucous watery (through a warming process) to allow for it to be expelled more easily. Examples of these herbs include Cayenne, Cranesbill, Echinacea, Elderflower, Elecampane, Eyebright, Garlic, Golden Rod, Goldenseal, Ground Ivy, Herb Robert, Hyssop, Irish Moss, Marshmallow (Flowers, Leaves and Root), Mullein, Peppermint, Plantain Ribwort, Sage, Thyme, Uva-Ursi, Volatile Oils and Yarrow.

Anti-Emetic herbs

Anti-Emetic herbs are helpful to manage nausea and when the digestive system is infected by mucous dripping into the system. Example of helpful herbs include – Aniseed, Black Horehound, Fennel, Ginger, Henbane, Lobelia, Meadowsweet, Peppermint and Spearmint.

Anti-Inflammatory herbs

Anti-Inflammatory herbs have three main classes – Volatile Oils, Salicylates and Steroid Precursors. Herbs that contain volatile oils often help to regulate inflammation via inhibition of the formation of certain Leukotrienes and via the inhibition of the peroxidation of Arachidonic Acid. These are often better suited for managing inflammation in the respiratory system and digestive tract and occasionally are used for external inflammation.

Salicylate herbs are best used for inflammation in the joints and for inflammation across the musculoskeletal system when injuries or infections occur. Inflammation can also occur follow long periods of physical tension in the body or long periods of spasmodic actions that may lead to injuries. Steroid Precursor herbs often are used to help the body to make steroidal compounds to manage inflammation such as in autoimmune disease inflammation. Some herbs can have multiple anti-inflammatory pathways they assist with.

Some examples of Anti-Inflammatory herbs include – Angelica, Burch, Black Cohosh, Black Haw, Blue Cohosh, Bogbean, Celery Seed, Chickweed, Cleavers, Cornsilk, Couch Grass, Cramp Bark, Cranesbill, Devil's Claw, Dill, Elderflower, Fenugreek, German Chamomile, Golden Rod, Goldenseal, Hawthorn, Herb Robert, Horse Chestnut, Irish Moss, Lady's Mantle, Lavender, Lemon Balm, Lime Blossom, Liquorice, Marigold, Marshmallow (root, leaves and flowers), Meadowsweet, Mullein, Nettles, Peppermint, Plantain (Ribwort), Sage, Shepperd's Purse, Slippery Elm, Spearmint, Wild Yam and Yarrow.

Antimicrobial herbs

Antimicrobial herbs are often used as secondary herbs depending on the type of infection and if they are being used internally or externally, and they can be used in most if not all body systems. Example of when they are used as primary herbs include damage in the digestive mucosa that leads to infection and to support specific types of infection. Often, they are used as secondary herbs to assist with other herbal actions including – Anti-inflammation, Anti-septic, Antispasmodic, Astringent, Bitter, Carminative and Immune related actions. Examples of these herbs include Aniseed, Bearberry, Caraway, Cayenne, Cinnamon, Clove, Cranberry, Echinacea, Elecampane, Elderberry, Garlic, Gentian, German Chamomile, Ginger, Goldenseal, Hops, Juniper, Lemon Balm, Liquorice, Mahonia (Oregon Grape), Marigold, Marjoram, Myrrh, Pau d'arco, Peppermint, Pine, Plantain (Ribwort and Greater), Rosemary, Sage, St John's Wort, Thyme, Usnea, Uva-Ursi, Wild Indigo, Wormwood and Yarrow.

Anti-Rheumatic herbs

Anti-Rheumatic herbs are used to help treat the conditions of heat, pain and swelling in the joints. These herbs have various effects including Anti-inflammatory, Promoting blood flow, Diuretic, Antispasmodic, Alterative and other effects. Useful herbs from this section include Angelica, Bayberry, Bearberry, Birch, Black Cohosh, Bladderwrack, Blue Cohosh, Bogbean, Burdock, Cayenne, Celery Seed, Cleavers, Cramp Bark, Dandelion (Leaf and Root), Devil's Claw, Feverfew, Ginger, Horseradish, Juniper, Mahonia (Oregon Grape), Meadowsweet, Mugwort, Mustard, Nettle, Parsley, Poke Root, Prickly Ash, Rosemary, Wild Yam, Willow, Yarrow, and Yellow Dock.

Antispasmodic herbs

Antispasmodic herbs are often used to relax the musculature by lessening the spasms in muscle fibres via the autonomic nervous system. This doesn't affect the Central Nervous System but does help to ease pain. Examples of herbs with this effect include Angelica, Aniseed, Belladonna, Black Cohosh, Black Haw, California Poppy, Caraway, Catnip, Celery Seed, Chery Bark, Cramp Bark, Damiana, Datura, Dill, Elderflowers and berries, Fennel, Fenugreek, Feverfew, German Chamomile, Greater Celandine, Ginger, Henbane, Hops, Hyssop, Lavender, Lemon Balm, Lime Balm, Liquorice, Lobelia, Marjoram, Motherwort, Mugwort, Passionflower, Red Clover, Rosemary, Sage, Skullcap, St John's Wort, Thyme, Wild Carrot, Wild Lettuce, Wild Yam, Valerian and Vervain.

Antitussive herbs

Antitussive herbs help to reduce coughing which can lead to improvements in sleep and lessening of pain with Wild Cherry Bark being the most recommended herb.

Astringent herbs

Astringent herbs are used for a lot of different reasons. They are used externally to help stem bleeding, to help recovery of broken and weeping skin, to reduce inflammation, to help tone veins and to make the skin more receptive to other herbs (most useful when there are open scars and spots that have been recently squeezed). When Astringent herbs are used internally, they can assist by reducing secretions from mucous membranes, heal the bladder wall, act as an anti-diarrhoeal, bind tissue to improve tissue integrity and reduce inflammation. Astringent herbs are recommended for shorter term use only. Examples of Astringent herbs include Agrimony, Bayberry, Cranesbill, Elderflower, Eyebright, Hazel, herb Bennett, Herb Robert, Lady's Mantle, Meadowsweet, Nettle, Oak, Plantain, Shepperd's Purse, Tormentil, Witch Hazel and Yarrow

Bitter herbs

Bitter herbs have an active ingredient that stimulates our taste buds leading to reactions in our digestive system, preparing the body to digest food. Bitter herbs also have various other uses in the body including increasing appetite in people who don't have one, supporting the liver, maintaining body sugar levels, helping to manage Leaky Gut Syndrome, assisting to fight inflammation in the body, helping the body to fight infections in the digestive system, assisting the body's skin health, helping the body during convalescing stages of colds and flu, strengthening the person's digestion to ensure the body gets the best nutrition and supporting the liver during hormonal fluctuations. Herb examples include Agrimony, Angelica, Bearberry, Bogbean, Catnip, Centaury, Dandelion Root, Gentian, German Chamomile, Ginger, Golden Seal, Lemon Balm, Mugwort, Purslane, Sage, Spearmint, Thyme, White Horehound, Wormwood and Yarrow.

Cardioactive herbs

Cardioactive herbs are often for short term use only as they contain Cardiac Glycosides which can have a negative impact on mental and physical health if used for too long. Cardioactive herbs have many uses including promoting the urine to assist with Oedema, inhibiting the reabsorption of water in the kidney and promoting blood flow to the kidney. Herb examples include Broom, Bilberry, Cayenne, Figwort, Garlic, Ginger, Ginkgo, Hawthorn Berries and Flowering Tops, Horse Chestnut, Lemon Balm, Lily of the Valley, Lime Blossom, Motherwort, Prickly Ash, Rosemary and Yarrow.

Cardioprotector herbs

Cardioprotector herbs can be used longer term, although short term use is still recommended. These herbs are used to assist in the management of hypertension, to promote the production of urine to assist with Oedema, inhibit the reabsorption of water in the kidney and to promote blood flow to the kidney. Herb examples include Broom, Bilberry, Cayenne, Figwort, Forskohlii, Garlic, Ginger, Ginkgo, Hawthorn Berries and Flowering Tops, Horse Chestnut, Lemon Balm, Lily of the Valley, Lime Blossom, Motherwort, Prickly Ash, Rosemary and Yarrow.

Cardiotonic herbs

Cardiotonic herbs can be used longer term, although short term use is still recommended. These herbs are used to strengthen the cardiovascular system, promote healthy elasticity of the system, promote the production of urine to assist with Oedema, inhibit the reabsorption of water in the kidney and to promote blood flow to the kidney. Herb examples include Broom, Bilberry, Cat's Claw, Cayenne, Figwort, Forskohlii, Garlic, Ginger, Ginkgo, Guggul, Hawthorn Berries and Flowering Tops, Horse Chestnut, Lemon Balm, Lily of the Valley, Lime Blossom, Motherwort, Prickly Ash, Rosemary and Yarrow.

Cholagogue herbs

Cholagogue herbs are used to promote the flow of bile from the liver and to assist the digestive system. Cholagogue herb examples include Artichoke, Barberry, Dandelion Root, Fringe Tree, Fumitory, Gentian, Goldenseal, Greater Celandine, Lemon Balm, Mahonia (Oregon Grape), Rosemary, Sage, Wild Yam and Yellow Dock.

Decongestant herbs

Decongestant herbs are often paired with Anticatarrhal herbs due to their overlapping effects. Decongestant herbs are used to – assist the respiratory system, relieve excessive mucous and catarrh in the upper respiratory tract, manage sinusitis, manage blocked ears and hay fever, assist the body in the loosening of the mucous through liquefying the mucous, reduce the secretions from the mucous membranes and to maintain healthy skin. Herb examples include Aniseed, Elderflower, Garlic, Ground Ivy, Eyebright, Plantain, Golden Rod, Goldenseal and Mullein.

Diaphoretic herbs

Diaphoretic herbs are used to assist the immune system and help to manage fever. Herb examples include Catnip, Cinnamon, Elderflower, Ginger, Horseradish, Lime Blossom, Peppermint and Yarrow.

Diuretic herbs

Diuretic herbs have a side effect of removing electrolytes from the body which needs to be observed due to possible impacts on muscles including the heart. Diuretic herbs assist the body in various ways including – promoting the production of urine to assist with Oedema, inhibiting the reabsorption of water in the kidney, promoting blood flow to the kidney, flushing the urinary system to remove infections, encourage other herbs to make contact with the mucous membranes, remove excess fluid from the body (helping the cardiovascular system, menstrual cycle and lessening congestion with the reproductive organs) and removing waste products to lessen the chance of waste excreting through the skin. Herb examples include Agrimony, Bearberry, Birch, Burdock, Broom, Buchu, Celery Seed, Cleavers, Cornsilk, Couch Grass, Dandelion Leaves, Elderflowers and Berries, Hawthorn, Horsetail, Juniper, Lily of the Valley, Lime Blossom, Parsley, Pellitory of the Wall, Saw Palmetto, Uva-Ursi, Wild Carrot and Yarrow.

Emmenagogue herbs

Emmenagogue herbs have been found to be very dangerous for pregnancy, so as always, medical advice is recommended. Emmenagogue herbs assist with stimulating menstruation, reducing excessive bleeding during menstruation, assist in regulating hormones and can be used to strengthen the uterus in preparation for trying to conceive and prepare for labour. Herb examples include Agnus Castus, Black Cohosh, Black Haw, Blue Cohosh, Condurango, Cramp Bark, Fenugreek, Feverfew, Gentian, German Chamomile, Ginger, Goldenseal, Hyssop, Lavender, Lime Blossom, Marigold, Motherwort, Mugwort, Nasturtium, Parsley, Partridge Berry, Pasque Flower, Pennyroyal, Peppermint, Poke Root, Raspberry Leaf, Rosemary, Rue, Sage, Southernwood, Tansy, Thyme, Valerian, Vervain, White Horehound, Wormwood and Yarrow.

Expectorant herbs

Expectorant herbs have several types of effects including Relaxing, Stimulating and Amphoteric, with secondary types of Expectorant herbs including soothing Demulcent and Aromatic Expectorant herbs. Relaxing Expectorant Herbs can include Demulcent, Antispasmodic and Anti-inflammatory herbs that – are high in volatile oils, high in mucilage that can exert a demulcent action on the gut (and respiratory system), help reduce spasm in the bronchial tubes and make mucous watery (so it's easier to expel) to help a dry congested cough. Examples of Relaxing Expectorant herbs include – Aniseed, Cherry Bark, Goldenseal, Grindelia, Hyssop, Irish Moss, Lobelia, Liquorice, Lungwort, Marshmallow (Flowers, Leaves and Root), Thyme and Vervain.

Stimulating Expectorant herbs – helps to thin mucous and irritate bronchioles to encourage coughing, are used to clear lungs of large amounts of mucous and congestion (such as bronchitis and chest coughs) and are high in saponins, alkaloids and volatile oils. Examples of herbs include Anise, Caraway, Cowslip, Daisy, Elecampane, Fenugreek, Ipecac, Primrose Root, Sweet Violet and White Horehound.

Amphoteric Expectorant herbs can be stimulating and relaxing and are often used in addition to other treatments. Examples include Mullein, Elderflower, Elder Berries and Garlic.

Other ailments that the various types of Expectorant herbs can assist with include – lingering colds, immune support and in various paediatric conditions. Other Expectorant herbs include – Fennel, Lobelia and Sundew.

Gut Healing herbs

Gut Healing herbs are used to – assist the body in managing inflamed bowel conditions, helping the digestive system's interaction with the immune response, assist in managing leaky gut issues and autoimmune issues, assisting in combating malnutrition and dysbiosis, address intestinal damage and assisting the body in managing allergies that may stem from the gut. Herb examples include Aloe Vera, Agrimony, Bayberry, D'Arco, German Chamomile, Liquorice, Marigold, Marshmallow Root, Meadowsweet, Plantain, Slippery Elm, Wild Yam and Yarrow

Hepatic herbs

Hepatic herbs have many uses including promoting healing and regeneration in the liver, supporting the liver in its detoxification and eliminatory processes by stimulating bile production and bile flow, managing long term constipation, assisting the digestive system's interaction with the body's immune response, supporting the liver during hormonal fluctuations, supporting the liver in the breakdown of hormones and supporting the liver during the menstrual cycle. Herb examples include Agrimony, Artichoke, Barberry, Burdock Root, Celery Seed, Centaury, Cleavers, Dandelion Root, Elecampane, Fennel, Fringetree, Fumitory, Gentian, German Chamomile, Goldenseal, Lemon Balm, Mahonia (Oregon Grape), Milk Thistle, Motherwort, Prickly Ash, Schizandra, St John's Wort, Turmeric, Wild Yam, Yarrow and Yellow Dock.

Hypnotic herbs

Hypnotic herbs contain alkaloids and are normally used to promote sleep. Other reasons they may be used include managing stress, anxiety, panic or over-stimulation by encouraging the parasympathetic system, encouraging deep sleep, assisting in the management of insomnia and supporting the nervous system by assisting the person to manage the side effects of autoimmune related diseases such as Rheumatoid Arthritis. Herb examples include California Poppy, German Chamomile, Hops, Lime Blossom, Motherwort, Mugwort, Oats, Passionflower, Skullcap, St John's Wort, Valerian, Vervain, Wild Lettuce and Wood Betony.

Hypotensive herbs

Hypotensive herbs are used to help manage high blood pressure by relaxing the muscles that circle the blood vessel, calcium channel blocker activity and via the ACE inhibitor activity of certain procyanidins and flavonoids. Herb examples include Black Cohosh, Black Haw, Blue Cohosh, Cramp Bark, Fenugreek, Forskohlii, Garlic, Hawthorn, Lime Blossom, Mistletoe, Motherwort, Nettle, Passionflower, Siberian Ginseng, Skull Cap, Valerian, Vervain, Yarrow and Yellow Jasmine.

Immunomodulator herbs

Immunomodulator herbs assist the immune system by – stimulating and addressing imbalances in the immune system, modulating the immune system's response, normalising the immune system response longer term, stimulating and suppressing aspects of the immune, enhancing the activity of T-suppressor cells (which may assist in combating tumours) and possibly stimulating the body's killer cells and macrophages. Herb examples include Aloe Vera, Andrographis, Ashwagandha, Astragalus, Baikal Skullcap, Brahmi, Cinnamon, Codonopsis, Dong Quai (Chinese Angelica), Echinacea, Garlic, Gotu Kola, Holy Basil, Marshmallow, Pau d'arco, Plantain, Poke Root, Rehmannia, Reishi, Rhodiola, Shiitake and Thyme.

Immunostimulant herbs

Immunostimulant herbs help to stimulate the immune system if a person is debilitated due to chronic health issues or other severe mental or physical issues such as exhaustion. These herbs also help the body to fight infection (especially in the upper respiratory tract), assist the body in non-specific stimulation of the immune system, assist in combating flus, and help people break the cycle of poor recovery. Herb examples include Aloe Vera, Andrographis, Astragalus, Brahmi, Cinnamon, Codonopsis, Dong Quai (Chinese Angelica), Echinacea, Garlic, Gotu Kola, Holy Basil, Marshmallow, Pau d'arco, Plantain, Poke Root, Rehmannia, Reishi, Rhodiola, Shiitake, Thyme and Wild Indigo.

Lymphatic herbs

Lymphatic herbs main role is to assist the body in draining/channelling away fluid and preventing too much storage of flood. Lymphatic herbs are also used to – clean the fluid and interact with the immune system by neutralising potentially harmful particles and microbes, helping the immune system through assisting the lymph nodes when they are swollen and tender, helping the tonsils when they are inflamed, red, swollen or congested, helping to clear congestion around the mucous membranes and supporting the lymphatic system in managing inflammation. Helpful herbs include Bladderwrack, Astragalus, Cleavers, Burdock, Echinacea, Figwort, Liquorice, Panax Ginseng, Poke Root, Marigold and Wild Indigo.

Nervine herbs

Nervine herbs are used to manage physical illnesses caused by high levels of stress, tension and other mental health difficulties such as anxiety. Some Nervine herbs also come under their own section known as Anxiolytic (used to treat anxiety). They are used to relax the nervous system, strengthen the nervous system and address the stress causes of illnesses such as IBS. Other uses include improving sleep, lessening panic attacks, assisting in wound healing, assisting the immune system, managing restlessness, assisting in management of convulsions in epilepsy, lessening tension headaches, lessening stress related hiccups and assisting in management of depressive symptoms. Research so far, has found that they don't suppress the REM phase of sleep (whereas many pharmaceutical sleep aids do), are rarely addictive and rarely interrupt natural body brain communication. Herb examples include Brahmi (Bacopa Monnieri), Black Cohosh, Blue Cohosh, Black Haw, Black Horehound, California Puppy, Catnip, Cramp Bark, Damiana, German Chamomile, Ginkgo Biloba, Gota Kola, Holy Basil, Hops, Kava, Lavender, Lemon Balm, Lemon Grass, Lime Blossom, Lobelia, Meadowsweet, Motherwort, Mugwort, Oats, Passionflower, Pennywort, Red Clover, Rose, Rosemary, Siberian Ginseng, Skull Cap, St John's Wort, Valerian, Wild Lettuce, Wild Oats and Wood Betony.

Synergistic herbs

Synergistic (pairing) of herbs refers to herb pairing that enhance each other's effects, and this is referred to as working synergistically. Synergistic pairs include – Cleavers and the Viola Species, Agrimony and most other herbs that act to assist the digestive system, Angelica and White Horehound & Elecampane in the respiratory system, Black Pepper & Turmeric, by significantly Enhancing its Absorption in the gut, Marshmallow and Solomon's Seal & Slippery Elm for activity on the Joints, Prickly Ash and Yarrow by Enhancing Yarrow's effects on the Capillaries and Peripheral Circulation, and Skullcap and Passionflower by enhancing each other's Anxiolytic and Nervine Effects.

Everyone including professionals have their favourite herbs for various presentations. However, some research suggests there are herbs that have high accessibility, multi-use and have the most research regarding effectiveness and safety. According to some research the top five herbs for Mental health are Bacopa, Rhodiola, Kava, Liquorice and St. John's Wort; and the top five herbs for overall physical health are Turmeric, Chamomile (preferably German Chamomile), Milk Thistle, Basil and Cinnamon. Alongside all the above herbalist uses and options there is a supplementary practice known as Aromatherapy.

Aromatherapy is often used alongside herbalist practices and often involves using essential oils (volatile oils) to engage aroma (smell) to help alter consciousness to alter mental and physical health. One theory on how aromatherapy may work suggests that the binding of the chemical compounds in the essential oils may bind or interact with the olfactory bulb, which then in turn, triggers the brain's limbic system. As a result, there are many benefits, however, there may be a mental health related risk if the person has previous traumas associated with smell, the aromatherapy may accidently trigger this, even if the person is unaware. Some benefits of using aroma therapy either as its own practice or alongside other approaches include – bringing pleasure or influencing mood, reducing pain, assisting sleep and relaxation, assisting focus and learning, influencing perception of self and of own health, it may assist as an antibacterial (through cleaning) and as an anti-inflammatory. Aromatherapy can be mixed with other liquids such as carrier oils (coconut or almond oil), diffused into a mist, made into a plaster on the skin or directly inhaled when mixed with heated water.

Key Points & Relevant Personal/Professional Experiences

The Mind in Eastern Thought

The idea of the human mind being studied scientifically rarely occurred in most Eastern health practices. Instead, the mind, body and spirit were often merged and fluid. The majority of Eastern practices viewed the mind through a spiritual lens with the understanding changing based on the type of spiritual lens chosen.

It is always difficult to summarise spiritual practices as each reader has their own emotional interpretation of a belief system, especially if it a system the reader practices in their life. Here we are focusing specifically on interpreting what is meant by 'The Mind'. The major Eastern Cultural interpretations of the mind included Taoism, Buddhism (mind is impermanent and subject to the three poisons), Tai Chi and Ayurveda and cultivating Qi, Yoga and Chakras, Hinduism and seeing the mind as Manas (the subtle body), Confucianism (emphasising the mind's role in cultivating virtue and fulfilling social responsibilities) and finally mindfulness. Meditation and mindfulness form major parts of the majority of Eastern practice with each practice interpreting its role slightly differently. However, the differences regarding specifically the mind, have been found to be minimal with the similarities often being far greater, with meditation and mindfulness thought to be useful for the cultivation of inner peace, discipline and clarity.

Human Body Basic-Complex Integration of Western Centric and Eastern Centric

Recap

Thus far we have discussed that Western Centric ideas often focus on specialisation which gives us a brilliant depth of understanding about that specific area or function of the body. While Eastern Centric ideas tend to be much more holistic, providing less depth of the specific area, but greater understanding of the connectedness between areas in the human body. As you will see in the final case studies the integration of both Western and Eastern practices almost always shows the best outcomes. Even Western Surgery practices have connections to Eastern Medical practices from the year 108 CE when the Chinese surgical pioneer Hua Tuo practiced organ transplants and surgeries.

Again, the separation of Western and Eastern centric ideas were often caused by culture, political and spiritual differences and not because of efficacy of difference. This is easily evidenced by the use of psychology in the current Western medical model. General practitioners and many other medical specialists now understand the importance of an eclectic approach. A large portion of current psychology has been based upon many Eastern practices, although credit has rarely been given in that direction.

Holistic Health

Sleep, Thought and Our Brain

Our brain operates with at least five different frequencies, all of which have their own associated states. Each frequency is bidirectionally connected to impacts in functioning when they are too high or too low.

The Delta frequency is from 0.5-4 hertz and is associated with deep dreamless sleep, automatic self-healing, immune system function and collective consciousness. When the Delta waves are too high the person might experience learning problems, and inability to think and severe ADHD-like symptoms. When the Delta waves are too low the person might experience poorer sleep and feel the inability to revitalise the brain and rejuvenate the body.

Theta frequency is from 4-6.5 hertz and is associated with deep mediation, light sleep, REM sleep, the dream-like state between sleep and awake, intuition, memory and vivid visual imagery. When the Theta waves are too high a person might experience ADHD and depression symptoms. When the Theta waves are too low the person might experience increased in stress and anxiety, and poorer emotional awareness.

Alpha frequency is from 7-12.5 hertz and is associated with calmness, open focus, relaxed thinking, reflective thinking, creative thinking, visualization and effortless learning. When the Alpha waves are too high the person might experience daydreaming, an inability to focus and might feel they are too relaxed. When the Alpha waves are too low the person might experience anxiety, higher stress, insomnia and OCD related difficulties.

Beta frequency is from 13-38 hertz and is associated with normal waking states, daily activities, close focus, alert/working state, five physical senses awareness. When the Beta waves are too high the person might feel too much adrenaline or anxiety, have a higher-than-normal arousal level, higher stress and an inability to relax. If the Beta waves are too low the person might have ADHD-like symptoms, daydreaming, depression and poor cognitive ability.

Lastly, the Gamma frequency is 35-40 hertz or greater and is associated with peak focus and concentration and problem solving. When the Gamma waves are too high the person might experience anxiety, stress and higher arousal levels. When the Gamma waves are too low the person might experience learning difficulties, and ADHD and depression symptoms.

It has been suggested that there are ages when the brain frequencies develop. Delta frequency is developed from 0-2 years of age, Theta from 2-6 years of age, Alpha from 6-12 years of age and Beta from 12 years of age and older.

As humans, we often forget that we are still animals and that we are just as affected by the sun and planet as any other species of animal on earth. Natural light stimulates the serotonin in our body which, in turn assists with positive/happy moods. Artificial light is rarely full spectrum and light, and even when it is, it can impact our circadian rhythm which in turn can be a risk factor for cancer, depression, earlier death, PMS, PMDD, menopause, andropause, dementia, insomnia, mood disorders type 2 diabetes, and other. Recent western scientific research provides the knowledge to explain how the sun and earth interact with our bodies. The sun has an eleven-year cycle which impacts the level of UV light we receive, and the cycles are correlated with various physical and mental health difficulties.

UV light is a type of electromagnetic radiation, and we normally receive this from the sun. UV light is filtered out from the earth by the ionosphere, and stratosphere. The three types of UV light are UVC, UVB and UVA. UVC light doesn't reach earth and approximately half of the UVB light from the sun reaches earth. All the UVA light reaches the earth. Visible (VIS) light represents forty-two percent of the total sunlight reaching the earth's surface, Infrared (IR) light represents forty-eight percent of the total light from the sun reaching the earth's surface, Microwaves can either be absorbed or reflected out into space by the Ionosphere and Radio frequencies reach earth's surface and enable earth-to-space communication.

UV, VIS and IR frequencies are thought to be key components in human evolution and have had substantial impact on human physiology, as they impact our circadian rhythm, and overall wellness. The amount of UV, VIS and IR light we experience depends on the time of date, our latitude, altitude and time of year. The light frequencies change throughout the day within a particular latitude, altitude and time of year, and the main reason for this is the sun's elevation. At sunrise, the VIS and IR light are present while UV is not and stay present until sunset. When the sun elevation is greater than or equal to twenty degrees UVA light appears, when the elevation is greater than or equal to thirty degrees all light frequencies are present, when sun elevation drops below thirty degrees UVB light disappears and when sun elevation drops below twenty degrees UBA light disappears. All of these different light frequencies interact with our eyes and body.

Circadian rhythm is one of the body changes that is greatly influenced by the available light frequencies. Our natural Circadian rhythm dictates that our light and dark cycles are synchronised with the sun and the earth, and health issues may arise when this doesn't happen. Circadian rhythm is the organisation of our molecular and quantum processes in the human body in response to the environment including the natural world. This also includes the control of our gene expression, biochemical reactions such as hormonal changes, tissue and organ growth and repair, Hypothalamus, the Suprachiasmatic nucleus and the eye.

One of the main hormones that is greatly influenced by light is Melatonin. Melatonin is very important and is used for more than just sleeping. Melatonin beings with the interaction of UV light and the amino acid Tryptophan in the eye, which then catalyses the conversion of Tryptophan into Serotonin. Serotonin is then stored in the gut and is released at night from the gut and made available to the Pineal Gland. From there it is converted to Melatonin in the Pineal Gland. For this natural process to happen the Melanopsin and Neuropsin receptors in the eye and the Retinal Pigment Epithelium must not detect blue light after sunset, and digestion should be absent in the gut at night. Apart from sleep, Melatonin also reduces body temperature and reverses the DC electric current in the brain.

Different light frequencies eventually cause the release of Growth Hormone, Thyroid Stimulating Hormone, Adrenocorticotropic Hormone, Follicle Stimulating Hormone, Melanocyte Stimulating Hormone, Luteinizing Hormone and Prolactin. Light also impacts the Pituitary Gland which functions as a bridge that also includes the Hypothalamus and works to connect the Autonomic Nervous System to the Endocrine and the Immune systems. To help wake us up and counter Melatonin, Cortisol is naturally triggered as a healthy response. However, the function of Cortisol can change when in stressful situations. Natural morning sunlight, assists the body in creating Vitamin D. For this to happen we need approximately forty-five percent skin exposure when the sun is at approximately forty-five degrees. If this is done successfully, the body will produce Vitamin D which serves many functions including – helping the kidneys to hold onto as much of the Melatonin Sulphate as possible, promoting a health gut and helping the body to improve and maintain healthy Bones, Intestines, Immune system, Cardiovascular system, Pancreas, Muscles, Crain and control of Cell Cycles. A lack of sunlight may also cause a phenomenon known as Sundowning which has several negative impacts on the body including decreases in melatonin in the body, increases in agitation, confusion and anxiety in the late afternoon and evening, deterioration of the Suprachiasmatic Nucleus (SCN) and may worsen symptoms of or increase risk of dementia.

Due to many causes and scenarios in the modern human world, artificial light is often used and overused. Whilst this serves many positive functions, it can have a negative influence on the human body including – altering electron and proton flows to the Mitochondria, negatively impacting gene expression, leading to Leptin or Insulin resistance, lowering Oxytocin resistance, increase the cravings for carbohydrates, increase dehydration, and increasing the risk of Cataracts, Diabetes, Anxiety, Depression and Multiple Sclerosis. Cortisol is also often impacted by the modern world but also plays a secondary role in assisting the circadian rhythm in waking us up.

Sleep performs an important role in our brain health where it serves as a natural detoxification process. During quality sleep many changes happen that include – our brain's cells shrinking, allowing the cell space to expand by more than 60%, flushing waste into the bloodstream via the glymphatic system into the liver to detoxify, washing out Beta-amyloid plaque twice as fast compared to sleep state and increasing flow of the cerebrospinal fluid. Most people follow a monophasic sleep pattern where they sleep for one period and wake for one period. This is useful for most people, however, there is a small percentage of people that find monophasic sleep, less helpful. For this small percentage of people, polyphasic sleep may be helpful. There are variations, however, if the person has multiple periods of sleep and wake in a 24-hour cycle, it can be classified as polyphasic sleep.

It is believed that 'Thought' is formless energy until attention is added. This means that our emotions are the sensations we experience from subtle physiological responses which occur subconsciously before we then consciously have the experience. Whilst we can't control this, we can influence this process through various types of body training that involving developing our internal body awareness through various practices such as mindfulness, meditation, yoga, etc. The idea that emotions and thoughts are energy can be discussed using the yogic framework including the seven yogic Chakras.

Chakras and Neurology

Using a neurophysiological lens, the seven yogic Chakras have been found to have strong anatomical correlations with the 'Western' medical understanding of the human body, with the Chakras being situated over the locations autonomic Ganglia (clusters of nerve cell bodies projecting from the spinal cord to other nerve cells, which in turn project to their target organs) of the Spinal Cord. The seven Chakras/Energy Centres are Root, Sacral, Solar Plexus, Heart, Throat, Brow and Crown.

The Root Chakra is associated with the colour red and is associated with various physiology including – Large Intestine, Rectum and Adrenals. The Sacral Chakra is associated with the colour Orange and is associated with various physiology including – Prostate, Uterus, Testes and Ovaries. The Solar Plexus Chakra is associated with the colour Yellow and is associated with various physiology including – Stomach, Spleen, Pancreas, Liver, Gallbladder and Small Intestine. The Heart Chakra is associated with the colour Green and is associated with various physiology including – Heart, Lung, Thymus and Immunity. The Throat Chakra is associated with the colour Blue and is associated with various physiology including – Lungs (volume of the voice), Speech Organs and Thyroid. The Brow Chakra is associated with the colour Purple and is associated with various physiology including – Hindbrain, Midbrain, Eyes, Pituitary and Pineal Glands. The Crown Chakra is associated with the colour White/Purplish White and is associated with various physiology including – Neocortex and Pineal Gland. Chakras have also been found to correlate with the static electric fields along the spine, which may have a correlation to the spinal autonomic ganglia. It is believed that if a particular Chakra or static electric field is out of resonance with the others, it can be considered "out of phase".

Human Health and Earth

Regarding the earth's impact on our individual health, there is a phenomenon known as the 'Schumann Resonance'. The Schumann Resonance is the negative electrical charge of the earth, with a frequency of 7.83. The surface of the earth is electrically conductive, possessing a continuously renewed and limitless supply of free electrons. The earth's surface and the ionosphere form a resonating cavity charged by broadband electromagnetic impulses such as lightning strikes. This results in a negatively charged surface of the earth known as the Schumann Resonance. The easiest way to access this helpful charge is to make physical contact with the earth directly for at least fifteen minutes. This may lead to several benefits including – the reduction of electric fields induced on the body, reduction of overall stress levels and tension, improvement in the Autonomic Nervous System, and may be anti-inflammatory. In the modern world however, there are many Non-Native Electromagnetic Fields (EMF) which may impact our health negatively such as increasing our risk of disease. The low frequency examples include – house wiring, lighting and microwaves; and the radio frequencies include cordless phones, mobile phones, Wi-Fi, etc.

Resonance is also discussed by professionals who identify themselves as holistic healers when discussing healing through sound. Healing Sounds have been used by many cultures for thousands of years, from Ancient Egyptians, Native American tribes, Indian cultures, Ancient Greek cultures, and more. The "western" scientific approach started investigating healing sounds in the early to mid-1800's. It is thought that humans have a natural resonance (of 9-16 Hz), and that our emotions also influence this natural resonance. Sound healing is theorised to work by influencing these resonances to help a person relax, focus, develop insight, improve sleep, lessen pain and for other. There are different types of sound healing including Sound Baths, Guided Sound Meditations, Chanting, Vibroacoustic, Acutonics and Binaural Beats. As a result, there are many different tools that people and sound healing practitioners use including Tibetan Singing Bowls, Crystal Singing Bowls, Tamburra, Bamboo and Native American Flutes, Bells, Steel-Tongue Drums, Gongs, Rattles, Shakers, Frame Drums, Chimes, Tuning Forks and Rainsticks.

Immune and Allergies

An allergy is an over-response of the body's immune system, in its effort to protect the body against what it perceives to be a threat. When the immune system's resistance is down, sensitivities are increased, and allergies develop. There is a chemical in the body known as Histamine. Histamine is stored in cytoplasmic granules along with other amines (i.e. serotonin), proteases, proteoglycans, cytokines/ chemokines, and angiogenic factors and rapidly released upon triggering with a variety of stimuli. Mast cell and basophil histamine release is regulated by several activating and inhibitory receptors. Histamine released from mast cells and basophils exerts its biological activities by activating four G protein-coupled receptors, namely H1R, H2R, H3R (expressed mainly in the brain), and the recently identified H4R.

The Histamine's jobs include dilating the blood vessels so that extra lymphocytes can arrive quickly, and speeding up the metabolic rate of all the cells in the area so they can have the energy to protect themselves from foreign bodies and defeat the foreign bodies. Most of the time this is helpful, and causes only minor inflammation, however when there is an allergic reaction too much histamine is released and the body over-responds to certain antigens causing an allergen (and as a result an allergic reaction). Causes can include food, poor mental health (prolonged stress etc. can cause an autoimmune response), stings, environment (dust, grass, etc.), overexposure at young age, genetic expression, migration of allergies to different body locations and body systems, medical conditions, addictions (to substances, pain, foods, allergen producing substances), and an overdosing of vitamins and medication and other causes.

Lifestyle choices such as food and exercise can often assist with minor allergies, however, doctors, dieticians, psychologists, naturopaths, and other trained professionals can all be helpful. Whilst medical approaches should normally be step one of the person's journey, other approaches such as finding and treating the cause of the allergy should also be attempted with a trained professional.

Psychoneuroimmunology Understanding

Psychoneuroimmunology (PNI) can be defined as the relationship between the brain, our thoughts and emotions and our immune system. It primarily focuses on the interaction of our conscious thoughts and emotions and how they can directly influence our neurology and immune system. The mind-body is not mystical or magical as it is measurable in terms of a chemical response that is self-activated. This idea was first investigated in the 1950s by various doctors trying to understand the mind's manifestation from the western scientific cell-based approach. An emotionally induced illness is not imaginary due to the mind-body connection. The PNI research was demonstrated in 1975 and has been studying the discussed interconnections ever since. It is noted that the predominate theory behind the PNI area of study is no longer accepted by modern day immunologists, however, a lot of the PNI research is still useful regarding self-improvement and self-healing.

The 'PNI Global Awareness' training information defines spirituality as the personal development that can be defined as a person who uses all of their internal resources effectively. I like this definition as it can apply to everyone regardless of any formal spiritual or religious backgrounds and can encourage self-responsibility of one's health.

Whilst PNI research has a strong focus on internal healing, it does not dismiss the organic nature of illnesses. Some organic causes for illness include bacteria and germs, genetics, and accidental injury.

PNI research acknowledges that traditional practices, alternative medical practices and holistic practices are effective at alleviating the symptoms of many illnesses. However, PNI research suggests that these approaches may be missing important information and approaches. PNI research discusses that the releasing of emotional suppression is required to ensure that the associated physical counterpart of the emotional pain is also released, often through physical intervention such as massage, acupuncture and other approaches. It also notes that helping professionals should be aware that they may accidentally compromise a person's level of overall wellness if they work with the mind and body as separate. This is because it is the direct relationship between how and where emotions are physically manifesting in the body that can determine the likelihood of change success. This success is therefore dependent on individual improvement, external support regarding emotions and thoughts (friends and or professional) and physical manipulation of the body's negative emotional manifestation.

A strong focus in PNI research is known as Biochemical Perception. Biochemical perception highlights what a person can do to change the negative biochemical responses to stress. How a person perceives an event, directly impacts our immune system, thereby affecting our emotional and physical health. This provides an understanding of the importance of managing internal and external emotional conflict. The biochemical perception is also about how our internal environment is affected by stress, and that our perception of this can influence whether the stress increases or decreases. Emotions have a direct impact on our immune system as the body communicates with the brain via bidirectional communication. Francisco Varela has previously defined the immune system as the body's brain, as the immune cells travel in the bloodstream throughout the body, they contact almost every other bodily cell. Every cell within the body responds to the way we think. The emotional aspects of a person influence their physical manifestation as evidenced by how stress modulates the activities of the nervous, endocrine, and immune systems.

The physiology of hopefulness can help the body to fight disease, whereas longer term emotional stress quietly harms the immune system and other system in the body. Nerve proteins known as neuropeptides affect our emotions as well as our physiology. A feeling in the mind will translate as a peptide being released somewhere in the body, as peptides regulate every aspect of the body including digestion and immune system responses. Neuropeptides' neuronal signalling of molecules influence the activity of the brain in specific ways.

Different neuropeptides are involved in a wide range of brain functions, including analgesia, reward, food intake, metabolism, reproduction, social behaviours, learning and memory. When we change the way we think, we can change the way we feel and this creates a perceptual change, which in turn allows for a deeper level of self-governance around our thinking. Every emotion has connection with a physical counterpart, and every ailment has an emotional attachment.

A researcher and author Candance Pert discussed that the body and mind are one and that what a person thinks and how they speak, directly impacts the state of the body's cells. The spleen, every lymph node, and all floating immune cells are in close communication with the brain. Emotions live and run every system of the body, and are in bidirectional communication with the nervous, endocrine and immune systems. Our emotional state is directly affected by perception, suggesting that negative mind will lead to an unhealthier body.

Our perception changes, life changes, etc. trigger an epigenetic response, meaning they change our genetic memory and gene expression. Genetic memory can be altered through the process of positive thinking and visualization (for those without Aphantasia), which stimulates a positive emotional state and adjusts to a negative one. Generating pleasant feelings helps a person to gain a sense of control, build hope, and increase the ability to generate and experience love, laughter, empathy, joy, confidence etc. The body's goal is homeostasis; however, the responses are not always accurate, and a stress response may be activated when there is nothing to fear, dependent on the emotions and thoughts a person is experiencing in the moments prior, during and following. Whilst the goal is to generate positive emotions and thoughts, to assist the body's health and recovery, we also don't want to suppress the negative emotions and emotional awareness. If we ignore our needs and suppress our emotions, our subconscious mind will alert us to the fact that something is wrong, which may result in a physical manifestation of emotional strain and medical illnesses. This highlights the ever-increasing importance of self-interventions.

Self-care is an umbrella term in this section will be focusing on what the individual can do to improve or maintain their health. However, it is important to remember that most of us don't live in silos and that the environment and people around us may either contribute to unhealthy levels of stress or be of assistance in managing unhealthy levels of stress. Self-care and self-efficacy can include choosing to be supported while remaining independent, managing our own perception of life, building emotional resilience, learning stress management techniques, learning relaxation, meditation and mindfulness techniques, promoting hope and happiness, proactively managing our internal emotional environment, understanding the power of our consciousness and taking appropriate levels of responsibility for the influence we have had and continue having on our health.

These ideas are useful to generate longer term health that in turn promotes natural chemicals in the body to assist in stress management. To further assist with self-efficacy, affirmations have been found to be a powerful wellness tool. Their aim is not to override the mind-body connections, but to relax, visualise (if possible), and generate within oneself an environment that is conducive to wellness. If the belief is health, safe and doesn't impact the person financially, the placebo effect can be of great benefit regarding some of these ideas, as for some people, the placebo effect allows them to build internal awareness of their needs. As stated throughout the book, poor or inadequate nutrition, a lack of emotional support, financial challenges and a lack of hope or purpose in life are all risk factors and, in some cases, causes for illness. Self-care and self-responsibility are important aspects of illness recovery. Self-care can be smaller things such as a longer shower, large things such as a holiday, and everything in between that assists a person to gain some mental and physical health benefit. Self-responsibility is taking an appropriate level of responsibility for any negative and positive outcomes that the person had control over. Assertive communication is another overlooked part of self-care. It allows a person to feel heard, connected and valued and therefore can lessen the number of negative thoughts and emotions a person holds. It also allows for the person to set healthier interpersonal boundaries and say no to taking on too many tasks. Assertive communication also lessens the need for aggression as the assertive communicator will often have less feelings of powerlessness or whelm, and less need to use aggression to process their negative experiences. Self-care and self-responsibility don't have to mean doing more, it can include finding time for oneself to relax.

The psychoneuroimmunology information has a strong overlap with various sections of this book including the holistic areas of health, as well as a strong overlap with psychology and the tools that will be discussed in the psychology sections.

Key Points & Relevant Personal/Professional Experiences

Psychology Tools as examples of the Integration between Western and Eastern Centric

There are many skills and tools a person can learn to assist in the management of the impacts of stress, trauma, AOD (Alcohol and Other Drugs) misuse and poor nutrition. Earlier I noted that most of the tools discussed can be traced back to various practices including yoga, tai chi, Qi gong and martial arts. This section will discuss different tools and skills including tools that are considered cognitive tools, breathing related tools, somatic and movement related and various other types of tools.

Mindfulness and meditation are the most well-known tools associated with psychology today. Mindfulness has its origins in meditation but there are some differences. Meditation and mindfulness are tools that can assist with accumulating positive emotions and processing away negative emotions; however, they don't just happen. Mindfulness and meditation are used to help calm the body, letting thoughts pass without judgement. This can be done as self-practice or practiced initially, with a professional. We don't want to ignore the negative or disturbing, rather find ways and learn tools to process, often with the assistance of a trained professional. Moving from a negative projection of self to a more positive projection is of benefit and can be achieved by a range of mind interventions that respect the need for interlinking the body with emotional wellness. Emotions generate like emotions (fear generates fear, hope generates hope, etc.), so acknowledging the negative emotions and working towards generating the positive emotions is the goal. The mindfulness definition I teach clients is "paying attention, to one thing, in the present moment, without judgement". This simple but slightly vague definition allows it to be used in various contexts with various tools such as eating, showering, lying down, muscle contractions, etc. It can be used in formal settings or added on to something the person is already doing such as showering.

Mindful eating involves a person holding food such as a biscuit or raisin in their mouth. The idea of the exercise is to develop insight and improve the person's Interoception as well as having the shorter-term benefit of grounding the person. It can evoke various emotions and when done in a professional setting can be useful in exploring thoughts such as control, patience, and emotions such as frustration or relaxation.

One example of emotional mindfulness is known as RAINe (Recognise, Accept, Investigate, Non-identify and evaluate). The person takes a moment to identify an emotion they are experiencing, then goes through the other stages with the end goal often being a calmer state and improved insight. Another tool similar to this is known as the visual shape and colour activity. If it is established that the person doesn't have aphantasia or alexithymia, then the professional and person proceeds to the first step. The person identifies an emotion they are experiencing, then they find where it is in their body, they attach a shape and/or colour to that emotion location, then move the shape and/or colour to one of their feet, next they notice how the start and finish locations feel, notice if the shape and/or colour has changed and finally they notice if the emotion has changed. This is often abstract for many people initially; however, many people have reported positive outcomes.

There are many other types of visual mindfulness, and these can include building a vision of success using the brain's principle that if imagination can be real, visualising a mind palace, visualising the negative thing drifting away such as on a boat or in clouds, visually adding a comedy element to a negative trigger, or visualising a target either physical or metaphorical. Some of the visual mindfulness tools can overlap with meditation, which is often thought to be a deeper mindfulness tool. Research has suggested that meditation may assist by boosting the immune system, reducing stress, dealing with negative emotions, lowering blood pressure, reversing heart disease risk, lessening substance use, managing weight, managing eating disorders, and improving sports related performance. Mantras are another tool that can be used in meditation and as daily mindfulness practice. Mantras can be simple such as personal mantras (I am kind), professional mantras such as (being assertive and kind helps meet the targets) and many others.

Other cognitive tools that may assist a person in managing stress including learning new things (brain training), doing old things a new way (brain training), reframing and the locus of control. Learning new things can be exciting and rewarding. If the person can focus on the direction of the new change instead of focusing solely on the achievement at the end, the journey becomes part of the excitement. Doing boring tasks in a different way can also help people to calm, refocus, and have more energy such as brushing your teeth with the opposite hand while moon walking. The locus of control and reframing often work well together. Reframing is changing the words we use with self-talk, talking about tasks and between people. Reframing changes our perception of the event, feeling or goal, which increases the chance of success. The locus of control is focusing on the aspects we have control over, such as when we shower, what food we choose to buy, etc. Sometimes there are negative events or memories where a person feels they are stuck and can't change anything, and this is when the reframing becomes important. Instead of "I am stuck in a job I hate" it might be "while I'm looking for work elsewhere, I will spend my time practicing healthy boundaries". Cognitive-based mindfulness such as gratitude journals or mindful reframing, improves front brain activation used in reasoning and problem solving, and is often the most beneficial when practiced regularly in low to medium stress states.

There are many forms of breathing practice that can be used to help a person slow down, calm, relax and focus, or even just build body awareness. Diaphragm breathing (also known as belly breathing) is a type of breathing that doesn't just use the diaphragm but also uses the vagal nerve to lessen the physiological response to stress and can be practice by almost anyone. The three types of breathing I like to use for myself and for people I help include ultradian breathing, humming breath and straw breathing, as all three have a lot of scientific research to support the positive effects and have been practiced in various forms for thousands of years. Ultradian breathing makes use of the brain's natural ultradian rhythm (brain hemisphere dominance changing in 90–120-minute cycles, by shifting contralateral nostril dominance). This communication is bi-directional and can be manipulated by choice. By closing the left nostril, we can increase left hemisphere activation and vice versa. Humming breath is very easy to learn. Recent studies have found a strong correlation between humming and decreased anxiety as the humming reportedly does several things – Increases Nitric Oxide which is helpful for blood health, the Rhythm activates the Vagus Nerve and calms the brain, it slows the speed of our breathing which calms the physiological responses and as a result calms the Central Nervous System. Various yoga practices have utilised the humming breath among other sound-based practices as a mindfulness and medication tool. The recent research now supports the humming breath, and the majority of the research suggests variations of the 'Mmmmm' sound to be the most effective at stimulating the Vagus Nerve. The straw breathing is also very easy to learn and can involve an actual straw or pursed lips. Breath research found that the average person will have 8-20 breaths per minute, a stressed person will often have more than 20 per minute, and research suggests the healthiest range is 8-12 breaths per minute. By pursing the lips or exhaling through straw after inhaling through the nose, the breaths per minute may decrease allowing for slower more full breaths.

The final type of breathing I practice comes from Pilates. It involves slow inhales and exhales whilst activating the transverse abdominus (TA). This is helpful as it strengthens some of the core muscles, slows breathing and helps build awareness. It is also helpful in martial arts regarding lower core muscle strength. One weakness of the Pilates' breath is that does not relax the body as much as other breathing practices.

One area of psychology that has seen a recent resurgence is the area of somatic and movement related psychology. This often involves movement or touching along with other forms of mindfulness. Common examples of movement that can be used for mental and physical health include Tai Chi, Qi Gong, Pilates, Yoga, Walking and any exercise that is safe and the person enjoys. Some research has found that when a person is physically moving forwards, it can stimulate the dopamine response and has a larger release when the person is focused on a goal.

People store stress, distress, trauma, and other negative experiences in their body – this may be improved through 'Body Orientated Psychotherapy' (Light touch massage, deep touch massage, movement related exercises without touch, energetic massage, joint manipulation, fascial massage and manipulation, lymph and nervous system massage, acupuncture, etc.). The Language of the body is touch and movement (body narrative), language of mind is words. Other body work such as progressive muscle relaxation, proprioception related exercises, acupuncture and sensory grounding can all assist with calming the body, and lessening stress held in the body.

Basic examples of proprioception include using a stress ball, having your feet on a balance board while seated and walking. The use of a balance under the feet while seated, in a therapy of medical appointment can assist in calming the person and improving focus. The body may find it difficult to maintain higher levels of stress with slow and flowing movements, so the balance board can be effective. A stress ball under a heel while seated can allow a person's natural fidgeting behaviour of the leg shake to become more beneficial longer term. Often people will leg shake to get rid of energy (often from nervousness, or adrenaline). Whilst this is useful short term, the leg shake often increases in speed and can lead to an increase in stress. The stress ball allows the leg to shake and absorbs some of the energy being generated thereby lessening the loop of stress created by a speedy leg shake.

Body-based Mindfulness such as PMR or sensory grounding, improves regulation (less reactivity) of reptile and mammal brains (bottom-up). Progressive Muscle Relaxation (PMR) can be done in full (often called a body scan) and is a very effective tools to relax the body before sleep, or it can be taught and practiced with one body part (often the forearm or quad controlled flex), and this can be used for in the moment tension reduction and stress reduction. This is a very useful tool for people who find the more traditional types of mindfulness related practices too abstract, as it provides almost instant physical feedback, and is practical or 'hands-on' type activity. Whilst often used by children, rocking can be beneficial with high stress difficulties for adults as well. Rocking may increase sleep spindles which are associated with improvements in sleep and can generate touch and feelings of being cared for which is a basic evolutionary need. Self-massage such as massing the ears (Auricular Contact) may assist in in activating the Vagal nerve as assist in calming to the surface and known as a Vitality Point in some health paradigms. Deep Massage and gently pulling the ear lobes and outer ear may also assist in relaxing and energising and may release tension in the TMJ.

There is a movement type of practice known as Tension and Trauma Release Exercises (TRE). The TRE are a series of exercises designed to mildly stretch and stress the leg and psoas muscles (attaches – femur, pelvis, lumbar spine). Tightness in psoas leads to increased pain in neck, shoulders and lower back. Chronic contraction of the psoas increases the body's arousal or fight and flight state, leading to an increase in stress. The TRE activate the Central Pattern Generators up the spine leading to the tremoring response. This response is used by the body to lessen the arousal levels at all three levels (reptile, mammal and front brain). One side effect of the TRE practice is neurological exhaustion. When a person practices this for the first time, or after a long time between practice, they may experience physical and mental exhaustion, due to the body's arousal state and release of tension. As a result, many people who self-practice TRE often do so before bed.

Sensory grounding is often taught as an observational tool, where the person identifies five things they see, four then can hear, etc. However, I use principles taught in the fitness world as well as the sensory and OT related workshops attended, to teach a more practical and somatic sensory grounding practice. We have anywhere from 8-50 senses depending on how they are defined. However, in psychology we initially discuss our five basic senses with people, and these can be used to help us relax/distract/ground and are also how our memories (good and bad) can be stored. The person identifies what their favourite taste, touch, sight, sound and smell are, and then they try and work on having a practical tool for at least two of these answers that they can carry on their person. Examples include a trail mix for taste, soft scrunchie or wrist band for touch, favourite photo or video saved on their phone for sight, music playlist or podcast saved on their phone for sound and favourite cologne or essential oil for smell. This version of sensory grounding practice enables a person to have a tool that they can use in the moment without having to try and use their frontal brain regions when they are struggling.

One practice that some people find helpful is known as Skin Brushing. According to research skin brushing can assist a person's lymphatic health, skin health, immune system, lessen congestion from allergies, lessen dissociation, may assist in managing mild to moderate depression, anxiety and stress, can be a self-care activity and can be used as a mindfulness activity. There are various versions however, the research suggests that there are specific pathways that should be followed for maximum benefit, so check with a trained professional first.

The final somatic related tool is known as either Saccadic Eye Movements or Saccade Stacks. Saccadic Eye Movements have been practicing in various forms in several spiritual practices such as in Buddhist meditations. However, it was officially introduced in a type of psychological therapy in 1989, and the thumb variation that I use and teach, I learn from the AMN academy holistic health course. Saccade Stacks are a variation of bilateral stimulation and can be done using pens (which is what most of the videos on the internet will use in their demonstrations), but this can also be done using your own thumbs. The Saccade Stacks help our 2 brain hemispheres communicate via the corpus Callosum. Short term this can be used to improve a person's ability to access their emotional experiences, and long term can strengthen a person's Corpus Callosum. Originally this used to be done by the professional tapping on a person's head, or having a person follow the professional's pen, but limitations such as the client not liking their head touched, were found. Saccade Stacks also has the positive side effect of improving physical performance in fitness related tasks via neurological firing prior to performing the exercise.

There are many other tools that people can self-practice or practice with a professional that don't fit neatly into one type. The first one discussed is known as Animal Assisted Therapy (AAT). AAT often involves a trained mental health professional and their trained animal companion interacting with a person or group to discuss and improve mental health. A lot of research has found that the presence of a trained animal in the room assists in rapport building and calming for many people. However, it is noted that it is the professional's responsibility to ensure any protentional people seeing them are aware of the animal's presence as some people have phobias and allergies towards specific people. The most common animals used in AAT include dogs, cats and horses (equine therapy).

Rapport is a tool of its own, that may be forgotten about in many medical settings. Rapport is simply described as people feeling emotionally safe. There are various psychological studies, biochemistry studies and even magnetic resonance studies that have examined rapport either directly or indirectly. Most studies found that when a person feels emotionally safe, they are more likely to be honest, have better cognitive functioning and retain more information. They are also more likely to have better healing or recovery outcomes.

I will only briefly list some of the more technological advanced tools that can assist a person's mental and physical health, which should be discussed with a trained professional before using to applying to use. These include Cranial Electrical Stimulation (CES) (using a microcurrent to stimulate specific brain areas and releasing neurotransmitters), Photobiomodulation (PBM) (using red or near-infrared (NIR) LED light directly to the brain trans-cranially and intranasally) to stimulate, heal, regenerate or protect tissues), Hyperbaric Oxygen Therapy (HBOT) (inhaling 100% oxygen in a hyperbaric chamber that is pressured) and Heart Rate Variability Training (training or encourage a higher variability in the heart rate, although this area is still being studied).

Bilateral Stimulation is a practice of helping our two brain hemispheres communicate via the corpus collosum and research has suggested by this doing this a person can have better insight into their own emotional experiences longer term as well as help them calm in the short term. This can be done with walking, through with the previously mentioned saccade stacks and with audio sounds known as audio Bilateral Stimulation (BLS). BLS is a very easy to use practice that can assist in insight development longer-term but also assist shorter-term in lowering the level of arousal a person is experiencing. By wearing headphones and listening to a program or app that has a simple tone going from ear to ear, the person can lower their arousal level. BLS is also an area that moves nicely into the area of sound therapies.

Sound therapies are used to assist in activating or reactivating the parasympathetic nervous system. As well as BLS, other examples include vibrating music tables, binaural music/beats, tuning forks, humming, vowel sounds, singing, etc. Very similar in theory but different in practice to BLS is Binaural Auditory Beats, where each ear is presented with a different tone entering the ear simultaneously, the brain then combines/reorganises the two different sounds and reconciles the difference into one coherent sound which helps to relax the body, lowering state of arousal. Sounds are used to restore patterns of vibration in the body through the conscious lengthening of a sound by using breath and voice, often a vowel sound, and often used alongside other tools such as yoga or movement. Often sound related therapies are used for pain management, and managing insomnia, PTSD, stress, pre- and post-surgery and pain addiction. The use of music and formal music-based programs such as the 'Safe and Sound Protocol' can be used to assist the Vagal system and assist in longer-term improvement in arousal management.

We often use sound therapy incidentally when we speak to other people. Many languages including English are dependent on hearing the harmonics of the word which can be adversely impacted by middle ear difficulties and by background sound. Emotions are expressed with different harmonics. Practicing overt communication of positive emotions utilises the harmonic element of language to further enhance positive emotion and thereby can improve mental health. This understanding of sound, emotion and tone also helps us to understand the importance of interacting with other people. This interaction is known as social health and not only assists in lessening avoidance, processing emotions, building connections, etc., but can also directly assist people in managing urge related behaviours and disorders by allowing a person to "ride the urge" until the urge lessens or dissipates.

Another tool that many people use as part of their daily routine is formally known as hydrotherapy. Formal hydrotherapy often involves specially designed baths where the water temperature can be controlled, along with sounds and smells, to assist in relaxing a person. This can be somewhat emulated with relaxing showers at home. The use of water and temperature can assist in managing pain, improving illness recovery, boosting mood and assisting various body systems such as the digestive and immune systems. When water is heated, it can help drive blood to the surface, when cooled it can help stimulate and drive the blood deeper into the body, and the alternating temperature can assist in stimulating blood flow and help move oxygen around the body. This can also be used with hot and cold packs when hydro-related practice is not viable. People such as Wim Hoff and practice such as Tumu breathing have used the idea of temperature to assist in illness recovery and even emotional insight development. For people who have access to baths and enjoy a bath instead of showers, adding Magnesium Sulphate, or Apple cider vinegar in water can assist in illness or tension improvement.

Nutrition has already been discussed in some detail but is again relevant to mention. Ensuring healthy levels of nutrients, fatty acids and minerals assists the whole body in manage stress and trauma related arousal. A lot of research has continued to highlight the benefits of omega 3's. Along with nutrition healthy exposure to natural light, especially early natural light has been suggested to improve overall health and assist in the management of brain injuries such as TBIs.

As discussed, the circadian rhythm is a very important aspect of our health and an area known as sleep hygiene discussed several of the elements that can be used to improve quality and quantity of sleep. When a person is in bed for more than 30 minutes and are still unable to sleep, some people find benefit from journaling their thoughts, this can be a list, story, or verbatim what they are thinking and can help to tell the brain to stress less as it is recorded and may assist the person in accidently processing some of the emotional cause of the thoughts. Sometimes when a person is in bed for more than 30 minutes and can't sleep, it can because they have too much physical energy, from either stress or adrenaline, or from not doing enough movement during the day for their body. In these cases, getting up and walking around or performing other non-stimulating activities can help a person feel tired. The 30 minutes is only an average, and some studies suggest 20 minutes, either way, the short period of time awake if left unchanged, can quickly change into a person still being awake four hours later.

Other sleep hygiene tips can include ensuring the room is dark enough, the bed comfortable enough, the room temperature being cool or warm enough, eating enough, (for some people, if they don't eat enough, their body will wake during the night, impacting the sleep rhythm), limiting stimulants (sugars, caffeine, energy drinks, trans-fatty foods, etc.) before bed, practicing a regular routine helps the brain understand when to increase or decrease melatonin production (can be as simple what time a person goes to bed and wakes, or it can be detailed i.e., teeth, shower, toilet, read for 'X' minutes), managing screen use (using night time or orange light filters to lessen the blue and white artificial light), limit any mentally stimulating tasks such as stimulating games, articles, videos, etc., and the use of showering to assist in routine and melatonin management (relaxing shower at night and refreshing or colder shower in morning).

Finally seeking professional assistance for mental health is of great benefit, as even psychologists see psychologists. Research has supported the idea that when a person looks into the eyes of another person and discuss difficult topics, over a short period of time, both people's brain wave become very similar, activated by mirror neurons which, in this context can impact a person's emotions and empathy. It has also been suggested that the emotion mirror neurons are stronger than motor mirror neurons. When a person's motor mirror neurons are activated our skin cells and pathways help us understand it is not happening to us. Emotion mirror neurons don't have a skin barrier or defence, meaning greater emotional brain-brain influence, often called empathy. This is often a positive except for when it leads to manipulation/vicarious trauma, etc. There are many, many other tools used by professionals in therapy that I have not included here on purpose. The majority of the information in this book can be used by a person to assist themselves, whereas many of the tools I have left out the book often can be done incorrectly leading to a worsening of the difficulties.

There are many other therapies and practices that a person may gain benefit from that are not discussed in this book. Some examples include Acupressure or acupuncture, Alexander technique, Art therapy, Chiropractic medicine, Dance therapy, Energy Medicine, Environmental medicine, Feldenkrais method, Massage therapy, Reflexology, Reiki and Tibetan medicine. If a practice is safe, healthy and helpful, often it is okay to practice. If a person is unsure, they should seek the opinion of a qualified professional in the area they are wanting to explore.

Ethical Considerations

We have established that the eclectic approach is best, utilising the strengths of the Eastern Centric practice combined with the specialisation strengths of the Western Centric practice.

However, there are several considerations that must be considered. Firstly, culturally sensitive practice is a must. For example, when using mindfulness and discussing humming breath in psychology I specify my own qualifications and cultural biases, so the client has the option to explore this further. A GP can't teach yoga if they are not qualified but can recommend basic mindfulness breathwork that they have learnt through continuing professional development skills or similar. The GP can also refer a client to local yoga instructors that the GP feels would benefit the person.

When working within the medical model it is also important to continue using evidence-based practice. Although there are many great ideas that come from the Eastern Centric field, there are some that still lack the approval of various governing bodies such as AHPRA. As such a professional must be aware of this and not recommend anything that does not have clear evidence under their field's model whilst keeping within their scope of practice.

Finally, it is still important that the individual has the right to agree or disagree with professional opinions and treatment options. The professional and their field will dictate in writing what these options, boundaries and communication pathways are. However, generally, the professional suggests a treatment idea or intervention and the individual then chooses to accept, challenge or ignore the professional.

Key Points & Relevant Personal/Professional Experiences

Brief Dip into Health and Martial Arts

Brief Introduction

There are many books about the benefits of martial arts, so I will only provide a summary in the following subsections.

Some of the first records of martial arts being formalised, dates to approximately the 20th century BCE, where murals have been found in ancient Egypt depicting wrestling techniques. Many cultures across recorded human history have had the need to defend themselves as well as the need to move at a group level. The changing needs, belief systems and cultural practices influenced what was taught and what was considered effective. In more recent times, many researchers and martial arts enthusiasts have attempted to list the known martial arts from around the world, and along with online training options, the world of martial arts have become more global and accessible than ever before. Some people include distance weapons training as a type of martial art, however, due to my own personal background, I will be focusing on systems of cultural and self-defence practice that either originated or have a strong focus on self-defence and close quarters weapons. As such guns, bows and other such longer distance weapons focused martial arts will not be included.

I am passionate about martial arts because of the physical, mental and social health benefits I have directly gained, as well as those I have seen my clients gain.

Physical Health benefits of Martial Arts

Martial arts offer people physical and mental health benefits and some martial art practices also include spiritual health benefits. Since martial arts involve moving the body, most if not all the benefits listed here can also be true regarding exercise in general. As such some of the following points will be revisited again in the fitness section of this book.

The key physical health benefits of martial arts include improved cardiovascular health, enhanced strength and muscle tone, increased flexibility and mobility, improved coordination and balance, assistance with weight management, improved bone and joint health, improved reflexes, boosted immune system, enhanced posture and postural awareness, mind-body awareness and injury prevention.

Improved cardiovascular health occurs from the often higher-intensity movements that most martial arts include, that lead to enhanced heart health and endurance. Enhanced strength and muscle tone stems from the warm-ups and the practicing of techniques such as upper body strikes, lower body strikes, and grappling that all work to improve muscular strength and improve overall muscular definition. Increased flexibility and mobility arise from warm-up stretching as well as general movement of the body. Better coordination and balance occurs from repeated practicing of sequences such through katas/patterns, sparring and other technique based movements. The pathways in the brain continue to develop and metaphorical blueprints form, leading to improved body awareness and improved motor skills. Weight management or weight change occurs from moving the body, people can lose fat, gain muscle changing the distribution of the body's overall weight. Bone and joint health can improve from the weight-bearing exercises like stances and movements that can strengthen the bones and joint cartilage through something known as Wolfe's law.

Improved reflexes can occur because of the better body awareness and is most evident in situations that involve sparring or reactive drills. The immune system can improve because of the regular exercise supports. Enhanced posture and postural awareness occurs from the improved mind-body awareness as well as the improvements in physical strength. Finally, if done correctly, martial arts can serve as injury prevention as a side-effect of all the above. However, many people can receive injuries through accidents or improper techniques or training so it is often best to have a skilled instructor.

Mental Benefits of Martial Arts

The benefits of martial arts go well beyond the physical. Unfortunately, in the world of mixed martial arts such as UFC (Ultimate Fighting Championship), the many mental benefits can be forgotten about, as it is often the physical that is sold to the people.

Discipline, focus, reliance, humility, self-confidence, mindfulness, self-discovery, person growth, and connection are all mental health related benefits of martial arts. With the right guidance a person can learn through exercise about themselves. The most common way of testing this is through katas/patterns and sparring. These are not just used for physical fitness but are used to help a person understand their limitations, and understand which of these limitations are actual (injury, medical disease, etc.) and which are perceived (not strong enough, not capable). Visualisation is also a tool that can develop as the person practices a sequence of moves or as the person shadow spars (sparring an imaginary opponent).

Many older martial arts such as the various school of kung fu and karate as well as martial arts such as Kalarippayattu help a person focus inwardly through visualisation and mindfulness techniques. The simplest mindfulness techniques arise from breath work. Gaining an understanding of how-to breath to relax, to improve fitness and to reduce the mental aspect of pain can help a person grow an understanding of their internal self. Visualisation can also be used when practicing breath work, and is helpful in relaxing the body, recovering and changing the relationship with the mental aspect of pain. An example of this in martial arts and in psychology for emotional and physical pain involves the following – identify the emotion and emotion location or pain location, then attach a colour or shape, next slowly move this colour or shape towards a foot of healthy lower body part, finally notice the changes in the body. Even when a person notices minimal changes, they are often calmer because of the activity and breath work attached to it. The idea of flow is also relevant in martial arts in breath work, movement and in life. Understanding that we can't control everything, but we can control some of ourselves is an important lesson learnt in many martial arts that is useful for life.

The concept of an "inner warrior" often taught to kids with anxiety, is very relevant in the practice of martial arts. All people are capable of going further, achieving more, or being happier, but they first need to understand themselves better. This involves using all of the above martial arts points and then focusing it on a goal such as recovery, or activity achievement.

Movement in general, but especially martial arts, have been used to assist in the recovery or management of various mental health related difficulties such as anxiety, depression, PTSD, ADHD, and ASD. For anxiety, depression and PTSD, the movement and breathwork gained from martial arts practices can be used to reduce physical tension in the body, improve the natural release of endorphins, improve blood flow and lead to improvements in sleep and nutrition. For ADHD and ASD, martial arts have been used to improve body awareness leading to improvements in proprioception and interoception, develop social skills, and improve focus and the natural release of endorphins.

Community, Belonging, and Social Support

Since most martial arts involve training with people other than the instructor, it can often lead to improvement in psychosocial health and social skills. People are involved in a similar interest area, with different goals and different life experiences. They then learn how to defend themselves, develop internal awareness and as a secondary effect, they learn how to interact with others in a healthier way. The level of social health gained depends on the individual who is training, the other people there, and the guidance of the instructor.

Like any group activity, this can often lead to development of friendships which is important for humans as a social species. And a person doesn't have to be an extrovert to benefit from this social interaction. The differences in the people training can also further improve the mental health benefits of going with the flow, building resilience, and positively challenging oneself. In good martial arts schools, the culture and social environment also involves unofficial mentorship and an exchange of differences further strengthening the cycle and social health benefits.

Examples of Martial Arts

This subsection focuses on only the martial arts I have trained in face-to-face. I have dabbled in, and self-studied various other styles, but decided to remove them for this version of the book, based on feedback. I will be focusing more on the idea and/or philosophies of the martial arts regarding distance, attack, and defence, etc., from my understanding and experience.

People often ask what the best martial art is and some trained martial artists debate about what the best style is. Instead of focusing on what the best style or best martial art is, it is often better to identify what the purpose of training is. Is the training for fitness, self-defence, sports & competing, for personal growth, for internal healing or purely as a social activity. One of my instructors once told me that there are only so many ways the body can move. We are all limited to this notion and to the body's kinetic chains. It is often the practitioner of a martial art, not the martial art itself, and the purpose they train for, that determines if the martial art or style is "good".

Specific blocks, attacks, and other moves have not been discussed in this section for various reasons including not wanting to weaken the complexities of the martial arts, and not wanting to give information that may be unsafe (out of context). Almost all martial arts have their own idea regarding breathing techniques and the use of breath in attack, defence and healing purposes. They will often also have their own ideas about the best warm up routine specific to the focus of the martial art. The breathing techniques and the specific warmups will again not be included, but it is important to highlight this.

Itosu Shito Ryu Karate

Itosu Shito Ryu Karate – My first exposure to martial arts was Itosu Shito Ryu Karate at the age of twelve. When I learnt this style of karate, there were three main parts – Kata, Bunkai, and Kumite. It is reported that this style of Karate may have the most kata among the many Karate styles, because the founder of Shito Ryu Karate (Kenwa Mabuni) was greatly influenced by two legendary karate masters – Ankō Itosu and Kanryō Higaonna.

Itosu kata employ more powerful, explosive and linear techniques with long stances, whilst Higaonna kata involve shorter fighting methods with more emphasis on circular movements and the use of both hard and soft techniques. Following Kenwa Mabuni's death in 1958, the style of karate fragmented with many schools having their own variations of the katas and Bunkai.

The majority of the katas could also be taught using a partner activity known as Bunkai. Bunkai symbolises the process of breaking down the movements of a kata to understand its self-defence application and is often referred to as the essence of kata. The Itosu Shito Ryu Karate Kumite had aspects of self-defence with a strong sporting influence. The sporting influence can be seen by the larger stances, the almost gliding movement of the competitors and the importance of controlling your strikes. The most common strikes in this style of Karate include, various punches and kicks, and can include leg sweeps. An extra training drill that was added to the training was known as Tan Gan Ho. Tan Gan Ho was the innovation of Sensei Fujimoto Sadaharu, which was taught to Shihan Kelleher and then my Karate instructor. Its purpose was to teach eye training, foot work development and arm Kumite development. Some of my most treasured sporting and martial arts memories came from my time training in this style of Karate. The main philosophies I took from this style were control of self through breath, muscle control, and control of self even when using aggression.

Rhee Tae Kwon Do

Rhee Tae Kwon Do – my exposure to Rhee Tae Kwon Do came in my mid-teens. Rhee Tae Kwon Do came to Australia during the 1960's and was founded by Chong Chul Rhee. It is still seen as one of the traditional styles of Tae Kwon Do, and currently has no affiliation with the ITF (International Taekwondo Federation) or the WTF (World Taekwondo Federation). Rhee Tae Kwon Do gently highlighted to me the importance of fitness in martial arts. The philosophies I was exposed to during my training had a stronger focus on the fun aspects of kicking and the different distances involved with the different kicks learnt. There was some focus on hand strikes, but I felt kicking was still the primary focus. Their self-defence revolved a lot around striking and the kicking distance both in attack and defence. There were also various forms/patterns that helped a person practice the strikes into sequences often associated with your grading rank. The main skill I learnt from this martial art was the useful application of various kicking attacks and defences using the legs and the relevant distances required.

Wing Chun Kung Fu

My exposure to Wing Chun began in my late-teens into early adult hood. The instructor ensured a strong focus on self-defence whilst keeping the principles of Wing Chun in the foreground. Wing Chun originated during the Qing Dynasty in Southern China and was introduced to Australia during the 1880's but became more well-known during the 1960's and 1970's.

During my training, I found that there was a strong focus on the importance of fitness and how our physical fitness can influence our ability to defend ourselves and others. I found the primary focus of Wing Chun was Directness and Efficiency practiced through linear and simultaneous attack and defence principles. One noticeable difference regarding strikes, is that modern Wing Chun does not include kicks above the waist, as these are understood to putting the practitioner into unnecessary risk. The Wing Chun punch is often referred to as chain or roll punching, is very quick and linear, which allows the practitioner to maintain control over their centre and influence their opponent's centre of attack and defence. Various individual activities were used to teach the basic striking principles, and partner and group activities were used to teach and then test the striking and distance principles whilst under physical pressure. Weapon defence was also regularly taught, where the person could refine the Wing Chun techniques under pressure against various blade, blunt and other weapons. Forms were also used to ensure the person understood the structures of attacks and defences and were often associated with your grading rank. The biggest difference I noticed between the Wing Chun forms and other styles, was Wing Chun form was practiced with minimal floor movement required. My favourite aspect of Wing Chun was the effectiveness of attack, whilst minimising damage to self as the defender. The use of simultaneous attack and defence and the use of subtle angles allowed for this.

Muay Thai (Bob Jones – BJC)

My exposure to Muay Thai also began in my late-teens into early adult hood. The instructor ensured a strong focus on self-defence whilst keeping the principles of Muay Thai in the foreground and exploring some of the sporting elements of Muay Thai. Muay Thai has its origins in a traditional martial art known as Muay Boran. During the 1930's some of the variations of Muay Boran began to become regulated into a sport now known as Muay Thai. Muay Thai is known as the "art of eight limbs" as it uses both hands, both legs, both knees and both elbows. Despite Muay Thai now being used primarily as a sporting martial art, it can still make for a very effective self-defence martial art, as I was fortunate enough to experience. Muay Thai primarily relies on strikes from three ranges – kicking, punching and the knee range, but does make use of several sweeps and occasionally throws. Fitness and body conditioning are very strong focuses in Muay Thai, with Muay Thai practitioners being renowned for their high levels of cardio, toughness and "pound for pound" fitness and ability. My favourite aspect of Muay Thai was the simplicity of the martial art, and how quickly a person could learn the basics, and still be considered effective in its use.

Zen Do Kai Karate

Zen Do Kai Karate – my exposure to Zen Do Kai began in mid-adult hood. The instructor again ensured a strong focus on self-defence whilst keeping the principles of Zen Do Kai in the foreground. Zen Do Kai Karate was invented by Bob Jones, with the first school opening in 1970, with a strong focus on assisting people working in the security industry. This is evident when the various attacking and defending principles are discussed and can be seen in the various kata that form part of the Zen Do Kai Curriculum. Various strikes, throws and basic grappling techniques and principles are taught, and training includes individual techniques as well as partnered and group activities where the techniques can be practiced and refined. Weapon defence was also regularly taught, where the person could refine the Zen Do Kai techniques under pressure against various blade, blunt and other weapons. My favourite aspect of Zen Do Kai was how well rounded the martial art was in both practicality and skills learnt.

Pressure Point Knowledge

The term Pressure Point means the application of pressure to the surface of the body that is sensitive, which can increase or decrease pain. When used to heal, pressure points are used to slowly relax or release tension from a given area. When used in self-defence, the use of the sensitive or Pressure Points cause pain in the specific and sometimes referred area of the body, which may cause a person to stop the attack or be physically manipulated. Pressure Point use in martial arts has a long and varied history.

The majority of self-defence martial arts such as Wing Chun and Zen Do Kai Karate, make use of the vulnerable parts of the human body to gain advantage in attack and defence. Some of the most well-known schools of Pressure Point use in martial arts are Aikido, Hapkido, Ninjutsu, Kyusho Jutsu, Dim Mak, Ju Jutsu and many others. Many security and military systems also make use of this knowledge.

The main barrier to Pressure Point use as self-defence is that it often requires pain tolerance to be low enough for the opposing person to respond. However, this can be overridden if a person has had training, is in a heightened state of aggression or under the influence of substances. Also, individual body difference can make the use of Pressure Points as a primary form of self-defence dangerous as some people have cartilage, fat and muscle differences that can further impede the effectiveness of its use.

Pressure points can also be used in healing practices with some styles of martial arts such as Kyusho, Dim Mak, Kalaripayattu, Tai Chi and many others, using Pressure Points as a way of healing the self or another person.

Key Points & Relevant Personal/Professional Experiences

Importance of Exercise and Physical Fitness

Defining Exercise and Fitness

Throughout this book, the benefits of exercise have been explored.

Exercise is a structured, planned, and repetitive physical activity designed to improve or maintain physical health and fitness. It involves deliberate movements targeting specific muscles or body systems, with the chosen type changing based on the individual's starting health, goals, and genetics. Examples of exercise include running, weightlifting, martial arts, yoga, and swimming. Fitness is a side effect of exercise and can be defined as the ability to perform daily (or goal) activities efficiently and effectively, with enough energy and physical capability to handle unexpected challenges. There are various types of fitness including Cardiovascular Endurance (The capacity and efficiency of the heart and lungs' to supply oxygen during sustained physical activity), Muscular Strength (The muscles' ability to exert force), Muscular Endurance (The muscles' ability to sustain repeated contractions over time), Flexibility and Mobility (The range of motion in joints and muscles during static holds and movement), and Body Composition (The proportion of fat, muscle, and other tissues in the body). At the cellular level, exercise also assists the body's power cells through a process known as mitochondrial biogenesis (the process of creating new mitochondria), which enhances the muscle's capacity to generate energy and sustain prolonged activity.

There can be multiple reasons why a person has difficulty participating in formal exercise including time, energy, stress, etc. When this occurs, changing the person's mindset can be helpful. One such example is focusing on movement and moving more throughout the day instead of pressuring oneself to complete formal exercise. A research group developed an acronym known as NEAT standing for Non-Exercise Activity Thermogenesis, meaning to move more. For people who are unable to do formal exercise, increasing your NEAT may be beneficial and easier to achieve. Examples on how to increase your NEAT include parking further away from a shopping entrance, taking stairs, if possible, instead of escalators and elevators, mindful fidgeting, throwing a ball to your pet, etc.

Pilates Understanding

Pilates was Invented by Joseph Pilates after he overcame his own health and medical difficulties by self-study including learning from 'Eastern' and 'Western' anatomy and fitness theories and paradigms both ancient and modern. During World War one he refined his skill and understanding of the human body and after various jobs in fitness, martial arts and other areas, he moved to the United States of America. In 1925 he met his partner Clara and together they created 'Contrology' and following his death in 1967, Joseph and Clara's teaching method became known as 'Pilates'. Clara's work with the human body and fitness following Joseph's death, allowed for non-athletes to benefit from the 'Pilates Method' due to her own nursing experience and her different teaching ability and method. It is often suggested that Clara's ability to teach the complex movements and theory to untrained athletes, is what allowed for the popularity of the Pilates Method to spread.

Today's Pilates Method continues the previous work, and focuses on 'Intersegmental Stabilisation', otherwise known as 'Core Stability'. The simplest way to explain Pilates to non-practitioners is through the term "Strength through Core". The three fundamental principles of the original Pilates philosophy are 'Whole Body Health', 'Whole Body Commitment' and 'Breath'. The principles of Modern Pilates are Relaxation, Concentration, Alignment, Centring, Breathing, Coordination, Flowing Movements and Stamina, with the terms "muscle control" and "body awareness" encompassing many of these elements. In Pilates, Core Stability, is more than just a six pack, it includes the joint and muscle health along the spine, otherwise known as spinal stability and can include retraining movement patterns.

Relaxing helps the person begin their body-mind condition journey which then leads to a better awareness of the body. This helps a person alleviate some of their physical expression of stress whilst lengthening and strengthening their body. Concentration follows on from the concepts of Relaxation and furthers this through use of visualising which helps the build the neural networks in the brain-body connection journey.

Alignment is the concept of the whole body being involved with every movement, where one movement or alteration will affect the whole body. This also assists with Postural Balance and enhance the overall sense of wellbeing. Centring refers to the "Powerhouse" meaning core stability, and this is achieved through holding the pelvis in neutral position whilst activating the Transverse Abdominals. Pilates Breathing emphasises the use of breathing to help keep the bloodstream "pure" during exercise, which oxygenates the blood and eliminates noxious gases. It is believed that breathing in the Pilates way, helps to expand the thoracic muscles and the ribs to enable the lungs to help the person reach their full potential.

Pilates has the aim to improve a person's Coordination through guided experimentation of exercises. Flowing Movements in Pilates refers to the "flowing motion outwards from a strong centre". In Pilates it is believed that movement is a sign of life, and that flowing movement gives the sensation of harmony and balance. The final principle in Pilates is Stamina. Stamina in Pilates refers to the gradual refining of the core muscles, through increasing the number of repetitions and/or building on reducing the resistance of the exercises, dependent on the person's goal.

Pilates also looks at Motor Control and the relevant Local Stabilisers and Global Mobilisers. Motor Control is now used when speaking of spinal stability as well as other areas of musculoskeletal stability.

Motor Control is the balance between movement and stability and includes our Central Nervous System (CNS creates a stable foundation for movement of the extremities through co-contraction of targeted muscles). Pilates focuses on understanding and improving the Local Stabilisers and the Global Mobilisers in most areas of the body, especially when discussing Motor Control. Local Stabilisers in Pilates refers to the muscles close to the joint, are often postural, are predominantly slow twitch and are type two muscles; whereas Global Mobilisers in Pilates refers to the muscles that are superficial, phasic, are fast twitch and type one muscles.

Contemporary fitness and exercise programs often include Pilates or Pilates inspired exercises as part of their programming due to the overall body benefits. The many progressions and regression in most of the Pilate's exercises make it an accessible form of fitness for most of the population. This combined with the idea that it can be taught very differently also allows for different types of fitness goals from cardiovascular fitness to rehabilitation to strength related goals, to be achieved. There will many Pilates and Pilates inspired exercises in the final chapter of this book.

Resurgence of Calisthenics and its Advantages

Brief History of Modern Calisthenics

Modern calisthenics is also known as "street workout," in today's culture. It is a form of bodyweight training that combines traditional calisthenics with dynamic movements, freestyle elements, body weight muscular control and body weight strength exercises.

The word itself originates from the Greek words kallos (beauty) and sthenos (strength), where ancient Greek warriors and athletes practiced bodyweight exercises to prepare for battle and competitions. During the 19th and 20th century calisthenics began to see resurgence. Friedrich Ludwig Jahn, was a German gymnastics pioneer who developed and organised calisthenics as part of physical education. During the early 20th century calisthenics became a staple in military training programs worldwide due to its simplicity and effectiveness in building functional strength. During the 1930's to 1960's, gymnastics-inspired calisthenics gained popularity in schools and fitness programs, further emphasising basic movements to improve health and flexibility. During the 1970's and 1990's environments in lower income communities around the world, but especially in the United States of America were drawn to calisthenics as it offered the many benefits exercise brings, without the financial outlay that had become accepted by many, associated with gyms. As a result an street workout community began to spread around the world, fuelling its popularity.

Today there are national and international competitions where calisthenics athletes compete in various competitions either focusing on tricks such as the three-sixty muscle-up or body control exercises such as the human flag.

The foundational exercises of Calisthenics can be separated into push, pull, core, leg, isometric and dynamic movements. Push-ups and Dips are the foundational push exercises, Pull-ups and Rows are the foundational pull exercises, Plank and Leg Raises are the foundational core movements, Squats and Lunges are the foundational leg movements, Wall Sit and L-Sit are the foundational Isometric (body control) exercises, and Burpees and Mountain Climbers are the foundational Dynamic full-body movements.

Review of the Basic Science of Calisthenics

Joint health had previously been taught as keeping a slight bend in the joints ('Soft Joints') when performing exercise. However, recent research and understanding suggests that during most calisthenic type movements, it is detrimental to have a Soft Joints as it impacts the tendon and muscle health at the end ranges and insertion points. So, keeping locked joints during calisthenic holds actually strengthens the arm and tendons, although the person has to be careful of hyperextension.

A tight muscle is a muscle that is over facilitated, and a weak muscle is one that is inhibited in its facilitation. By looking at muscles in this way, we can change how we see muscle tightness and change the treatment accordingly, to include mobility, various forms of stretching and strengthening of the weaker muscles. Our Skeletal Muscles contain Muscle Spindles which provides moment to moment information on length and change of length in muscle tissues and play a key role in proprioceptive flexibility. This information is then sent to interneurons in the spinal cord and then the brain stem and cerebellum and basal ganglia which in turn form part of the unconscious proprioception. Another important proprioceptor that influences this proprioceptive flexibility is the Golgi Tendon Organ (GTO). The GTO live at the Muscle Tendonous Junction which is responsive to tension in the muscle which can then reduce type 1a muscle and turn down the volume on the Muscle Spindle to increase flexibility. The term flexibility can be defined at strength at end ranges. Injury can have a negative impact on flexibility, and it is often the pain that has the largest negative impact. The pain we are experiencing can be discussed as part of the Nociception response.

Nociception refers to the Central Nervous System and the Peripheral Nervous System's processing of noxious stimuli, such as tissue injury and temperature extremes, which both activate the Nociceptors and their pathways. Often this is the body's responses to keep us safe from further damage, however, the Nociceptors can be triggered by nerve misfiring and other unhelpful reasons. This leads to a subjective experience of pain a person feels. Improving our Proprioception can assist the body in overriding some of the unhelpful effects of the Nociceptors, as can improving our overall brain body connection.

One simple exercise that can improve muscle control and strength output, that was adapted by the AMN academy is known as Saccade Stacks. Originally researched and used in psychology to help people manage and unlock mental health difficulties, the fitness version is known as Saccadic Eye Movements. AMN academy's research has found the Saccade Stacks can be used to train the person's brain, can increase the motor output of the body, and can be completed without a second person being needed (by using the person's own thumbs).

As mentioned in the 'Muscular System' section, core strength is very important to overall health and is a strong focus in Calisthenics and body weight training. Most exercises require a strong core physically and the ability to activate it mentally. Once a person can activate their core and safely warm up the body prior to formal training to increase mobility, they are often ready to begin Calisthenics.

Suggestions to Improve Skills – Scaling

Progressive Overload, Leverage and Angles, Isometric Training and Plyometrics are all examples of scaling. Scaling is used to help people achieve various calisthenics goals safely.

Progressive Overload occurs when a person increases the number of repetitions they perform a particular exercise or when they are able to add weight to the exercise. A common example of progressive overload in calisthenics involves increasing the number of pull-ups or adding a to your ankles when performing pull-ups. The progressive overload develops strength and muscular endurance leading to a greater ability to perform more difficult exercises such as clap pull-ups.

Leverage and Angles can be used to increase the difficulty of exercises. A common example of this includes adding declines and inclines. When a normal push-up becomes too easy for a person, they can raise their feet, resting it on a bench. This can causes the exercise to become more difficult as the upper body has to lift more of the body's weight, and is called an incline push-up.

Isometric Training put simply, means holding an exercise for longer. Common examples include the plank, and the dead hang. By increasing the amount of time the exercise is held, it improves muscular endurance and can be used to improve strength at end range such as in the dead hang.

Finally, plyometric exercises such as Burpees can be scaled by changing the type of burpee such as adding a push-up, increasing the height of the jump into a tuck jump, increasing the speed of the transition movement and adding repetitions. Plyometrics such as box jumps are often used to improve a person's explosive strength, which is required for performing tricking calisthenic exercises such as the clap pull-up or three-sixty muscle-up.

Strengths and Weaknesses of Modern Gyms

Modern gyms have become a cornerstone of fitness culture, offering a wide range of facilities, equipment, and programs designed to help individuals achieve their health and wellness goals. With state-of-the-art machines, diverse classes, and professional guidance, these gyms cater to a variety of fitness levels and preferences. However, despite their many advantages, modern gyms also face certain challenges, including issues related to cost, overcrowding, and an overemphasis on aesthetics over function.

Strengths of Modern Gyms

The modern gym offers many benefits for people of various levels of fitness and experiences. The improvements in technology have also allowed for the social environment and all-day access to become a realistic option, allowing for people with busy schedules to meet their fitness goals.

Access to Advanced Equipment

The modern gym offers equipment that provides support to people recovering from injuries, people wanting to target specific muscle groups, and people wanting to improve general fitness. The modern gym is equipped with pin-machines, cable machines, free weights including Dumbbells, Barbells and Kettlebells, as well as a variety of cardio-machines such as the treadmill or rowing machine. As well as the equipment, the modern gym offers a social space as well as offering temperature control, which is often important in geographic locations that have extreme heat or cold. There is also high-tech equipment such as heart rate monitors and scales that measure and estimation of body fat percentage and bone density.

Variety of Classes and Programs

Most gyms offer special classes where an instructor either in person or via video, guides a class through a series of exercises. This can be range from yoga and Pilates to high-intensity interval training (HIIT) and spin classes, catering to different fitness levels and interests.

Professional Guidance

Most gyms also offer personal training as either one-on-one or as small group options. This allows people who are new and require extra guidance, or people who train better with a professional there, to reach their fitness goals. These professionals can include gym instructors (often holding a minimum certificate three in fitness), personal trainers (often holding a minimum certificate four in fitness and personal training), physiotherapists and sports exercise physiologists. These professionals can often offer various tailored fitness plans and dietary advice depending on their qualifications.

Weaknesses of Modern Gyms

Like all things, there are weaknesses to the modern gym with the three most common including cost and accessibility, wait times and emphasis on aesthetics over function.

Cost and Accessibility

Gyms can be expensive, ranging from casual to annual contracts, that range from five dollars a day into the thousands a year. This can become a barrier for many people who have no fitness background but want to improve their physical health.

Overcrowding and Wait Times

Many gym owners and managers have advised that gym business models often run with an expected fifty percent attendance rate. However, during peak times which vary depending on the gym, there can often be overcrowding. This overcrowding occurs because of the business model, meaning there is not enough space of equipment during peak times. During these peak times the machines or equipment a person requires can often be unavailable, negatively impacting the person's ability to train, and in some cases have led to injury and physical altercations.

Overemphasis on Aesthetics over Function

With the rise of gym equipment that support muscular isolation training, aesthetic goals became easier to achieve. Now people could train their biceps and ignore their lower body if they wanted to. This led to an increased aesthetic obsession both in the gyms and in society as a whole. This is societal aesthetic obsession is highlighted when watching movies that include heroes, where instead of a larger frame, the male hero now requires a visible six-pack and vein popping muscles. This also led to less focus on function, with some larger muscular athletes being unable to perform basic tasks such as toileting, without struggling.

Fitness Across the Lifespan

The Importance of Fitness Across All Ages

Being healthy is important and being fit can be seen as a type of health. Being fit means something different to everyone and also is different for people across their life. Fitness habits formed in childhood and adolescence assist in laying the foundations for a healthy and active life, including the development of strength, flexibility, and cardiovascular health.

The fitness goals and strategies also change depending on a person's age. When the person is a child, being active and having fun are the primary goals; during the teenage to middle age years, goals become more specific such as running further or maximising strength and muscular growth; and in older adults maintaining mobility and physical independence becomes the primary goal.

Fitness in Childhood and Adolescence

Most of the time, children learn best through play, and exercise is no different. Promoting exercise that involves play can variations of team sports and games involving movement or mixed reality technology. Keeping a child active helps their brain health, and contributes to the development of motor skills, strength, and social interaction. As a child moves into the adolescence age bracket, more structured play is often encouraged or required.

Team sports, martial arts, or structured fitness programs (including gyms, gymnastics, calisthenics, swimming, etc.) all contribute to a healthier young person. The young person has to feel they are gaining some form of benefit for them to want to continue. For most adolescents, social connection is the main driver behind engagement, but of others it is finding the exercise they enjoy. Despite all of the health benefits, if the adolescent doesn't gain something of value (from their perspective) they will often disengage.

Fitness in Young Adulthood

Young adulthood is often the optimal time for peak physical performance, and this can vary from ages sixteen through twenty-five for most people. During this time performance related goals become more common, although the social aspect is still important for many. Fitness routines become important as the person begins to balance adult responsibilities with fitness and health related goals. The use of professionals such as personal trainers or coaches can become more important to help with the development of routine.

Fitness in Middle Adulthood

As a person progresses towards middle adulthood, their number of responsibilities can often increase. Often the person has extra career or family responsibilities to manage and social roles pressuring them resulting in their own health and fitness goals becoming negatively impacted. For some, the routine established during their younger adulthood becomes helpful and they are able to adjust this to fit their new life responsibilities, however, for others, they are unable to maintain their previous health and fitness goals.

As well as the increasing responsibilities, the loss of physical ability can begin to negatively affect the person. The slowing of the metabolism, the reduction in strength and cardio gains, and the reduction in flexibility can all negatively impact a person's ability to begin or maintain a health and fitness routine.

Again, speaking with a fitness, nutrition and even mental health professional can be valuable and sometimes required here, to help develop life routines and life balance, to enable the development of realistic health and fitness goals and routines.

Fitness in Older Adulthood

As we age the reduction in our physical health increases. For most people in older adulthood, their fitness and health goals change from competition and gaining, to maintaining. The importance shifts to the preservation of mobility, balance and strength to help the older adult maintain independence. The type of exercise also shifts towards lower-impact functional exercises and can include more water related exercises.

Maintenance is difficult during this age as the medical difficulties have often increased, sometimes dramatically, and injury and illness occur more frequently. The change in ability and identity also negatively impact the person's motivation. Social can become almost as important as it was during the teenage and young adult years, to help to reduce the impacts of these physical health changes.

Often older adults benefit most from a support team including family and friends, but also physiotherapists, nutritionists and mental health professionals.

Integrating Technology, Data and Virtual Coaching into Health and Fitness

Modern technology was previously used to enhance elite athletes understanding and performance. Today people can purchase technology that provides a lot of information.

Wearable technology is one such example. Smart watches (such as the Omniwatch), smart fitness bands (such as the Garmin HRM-Dual, Premium Heart Rate Monitor, Wireless Strap and Sensor) that go on the chest and various other wearable technology are used to provide real-time data about a person's heart rate, calories burned, steps taken, sleep quality, VO_2 (Volume of Oxygen) max estimation, stress levels, hydration estimates, blood oxygen levels, bone density, fat percentage estimation and various other aspects of health including estimated age. All this information can both help a person with their fitness and health goals, and/or overload the person leading to anxiety and decreased motivation. As with most parts of this book, it is useful to talk to a trained professional before attempting to understand all this new data.

Wearable technologies can also include mixed reality (augmented reality), virtual reality (such as KAT Walk Personal VR Treadmill) and the gamification of fitness with data from the wearable technology being sent to a computer or output device, with the person winning achievement related goals and badges, often in a software format.

There are now thousands of online and mobile phone apps that provide people with free and premium advice regarding health and fitness including example programs. These websites and apps can be helpful for most people but run the risk of safety. The websites and apps often have a safety message somewhere on their program; however, this is often used for legal reasons. It is best to have a friend who understand fitness training, or a professional explore the website or app with you prior to use. However, there are some websites that encourage online communities and some online communities that can train together using their phone's camera. This allows for social connection and can allow for some live feedback about the techniques, weight, etc.

AI (Artificial Intelligence) is also being used with elite athletes to improve outcomes, and there are some basic versions available to the general public. The AI programs can be used to create personalised workout routines, improve technique, measure in real time strengths or weaknesses of the person's ability and even predict potential injuries and plateaus. Smart clothing involves the use of AI combined with specially designed clothing and wearable sensors that help to assess technique and movement and can be used to provide real-time feedback. However, AI is still a new area in the fitness world and should continue to be monitored.

There are also many devices utilising elements light therapy, heat therapy, sound therapy etc., that might improve the physical recovery following training. However, there is the risk of pop-science (using a tiny amount of science to make large and often unsubstantiated claims) being used to sell products that might not do anything.

Lastly, there is a growing field of custom nutrition and DNA-based nutrition programs. Everyone's food needs are different, and our genetics and environment can influence these needs. Speaking to a trained nutritionist is a good start but not everyone can afford this. As a result, large companies have begun appearing internationally and offer custom nutrition plans based on the genetic data you pay money to provide them. There are benefits to this, but the risks are still not fully understood and can include ethical risks such as your genetic data being sold, as well as using pop-science again to make promises that can't yet be substantiated.

Key Points & Relevant Personal/Professional Experiences

Fitness Exercises – Pilates, Gym, Calisthenics and Yoga

Exercise Overview

Here I will focus on exercises I have used or taught, will briefly discuss programming ideas, and will include some exercise visuals. There are many variations of exercises, some exercises can share the same name, and some exercises are called different names dependent on their historic origins and who taught the exercise. As stated earlier, I will be drawing from my own experiences so there may be some discrepancy in the name of certain exercises. There are many variations I have left out of the book, mainly because there are too many to include, and with the right base knowledge, the human imagination could think of an almost unlimited number of variations that took advantage of planes of movement, equipment differences, speed, muscle control, etc. Everyone is different in their fitness goals, journey etc. and this section is a list of exercise ideas and not exercise prescription. However, there may be many exercises in this section that may benefit you but, check with your own GP or fitness provider if you are unsure.

One area that is often forgotten when people begin their fitness or movement goals, is the awareness of our body. Tools such as a body scan can assist in this understanding of the body. There are examples of exercises found in Pilates, Tai Chi, Qi Gong, Yoga, Circus, AMN Academy and many others that assist in the development of body awareness. The ability to isolate or activate specific muscles or groups of muscles can greatly improve a person's posture, technique, and physical ability when they perform an exercise.

There are many different theories regarding warming up prior to exercise and regarding what stretches are best. Depending on the professional you talk to, there are approximately eight different types of stretches. However, the three basic ways to define a stretch include static stretching, dynamic stretching and mobility stretching. Static stretching is often used at the end of a workout to assist in recovery, dynamic stretching is often used at the start of a workout to assist in warming the body and muscle groups and mobility stretches are often used at the beginning of a workout to assist in joint health.

There are competing ideas about when to exercise. For every study that claims mornings are the best there is a competing study suggesting afternoon and night. To simplify this, exercising in the morning may assist in burning fat throughout the day, may energise a person through the endorphin reward response and may assist in focus and establishing a routine. For some people exercising in the morning is unrealistic as they have difficulty waking early enough before work or study, their body doesn't have enough fuel to burn for the exercise and some people feel more tired throughout the rest of the day when they exercise in the morning. For these people afternoon or even night-time training may be more beneficial. Training at night allows a person to consume enough calories throughout the day to assist in ensuring sufficient training fuel and sleeping soon after a workout may assist in muscle recovery. For some people, training in the afternoon or night is unhelpful as the exercise may "recharge" some people, and therefore negatively impact their sleep. As discussed in different ways throughout this book, everyone has different needs, genetics directly influence what works for the individual and everyone has different exercise related goals, so the best approach is trial and error. Whilst this approach might be difficult and vague, it is often the best way for the individual to find what works for them.

There are also different types of exercises with different and overlapping impacts, that can often work well together and are often suggested/prescribed to be practiced together (during the same workout or during the same week). Aerobic exercises assist in improving cardiorespiratory (circulatory and respiratory systems) endurance and have various forms such as low intensity (walking), medium intensity (light jog) and high intensity (High Intensity Interval Training/HIIT). Aerobic exercises have also been found to improve mitochondrial capacity as well as improving frontal brain functioning. Anerobic exercises help with building and maintaining strength. The force of the muscle contractions such as lifting weights can assist in improving strength, improving self-image, and may assist people with more severe mental health difficulties by lessening the dissociation by helping the person to ground themselves in the present. Resistance exercises help with strength and involves the body's muscles working against a weight from body weight (calisthenics and martial arts), resistance bands and other moving related equipment. Stability exercises assist with core and balance (Pilates) and can assist with improving self-image. Finally, there are energetic type exercises such as Tai Chi, Qi Gong and Yoga that can assist with various physical improvements, mental health improvements and assist people interested in the spiritual aspect of their health.

Pilates Exercises

As with most exercise, it is important to understand what the goal of the exercise of session is. Once the goals are defined, the followings ideas can be helpful when programming a Pilates session – ensure exercises chosen can assist the goal, exercises chosen to assist in gently correcting or supporting any postural issues or imbalances, ensure correct Pilates breathing is practiced, be aware of injury restrictions and if possible, try to include exercises from the frontal, sagittal and transverse planes of motion. Awareness of the body is an important skill to develop and maintain in Pilates, so ensure this mental component of Pilates is including in the training.

List of Pilates Exercises

4 Point Bent 90 degree Leg Lift into Chest

4 Point Bent 90-degree Leg Lift Hold

4 Point Bent 90-degree Leg Lift Pulsing

4 Point Cat

4 Point Cow

4 Point Hamstring Curl

4 Point Hold – Knees in-line with hips, hips are square, wrists in-line with shoulders, activation of transverse abdominus and looking slightly forward.

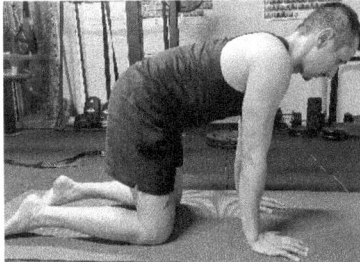

4 Point into Arm Lift (3 Point)

4 Point into Opposite Arm and Leg Lift / Bird Dog - – Knees in-line with hips, hips are square, wrists in-line with shoulders, activation of transverse abdominus and looking slightly forward. Slowly lift the opposite arm and leg and hold, ensuring the hips are still square, knee on ground is still in-line with hips and wrist on ground is still in-line with shoulder.

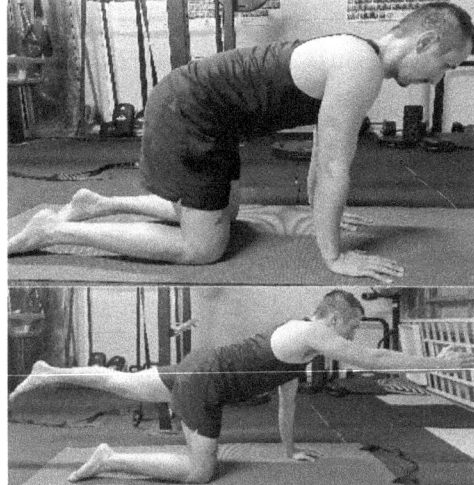

4 Point Knee to Elbow

4 Point Knee to Elbow Variation Hydrant

4 Point Plank

4 Point Straight Leg Lift

4 Point Straight Leg Lift Circles with Heel

4 Point Straight Leg Lift Hold

4 Point Straight Leg Lift Pulse

4 Point Straight Leg Lift to Side

4 Point Straight Leg Toe Tap

4 Point Straight Leg Toe Tap and Slide in

4 Point Straight Leg Toe Tap and Slide to Side

4 Point Thread the Needle

4 Point Triceps Pushup

Adductor Stretch Seated Straight Legs

Back Extension Breaststroke

Back Extension Hold

Back Extension Swimming

Back Extension Variation Dart

Bilateral Femur Circles Supine

Bilateral Overhead Arms Supine on Foam Roller

Bilateral Shoulder Circles Supine on Foam Roller

Bilateral Shoulder Drops Supine on Foam Roller

Bridge

Bridge Variation Lift and Slide

Bridge Variation Single Bent Leg Lift

Bridge Variation Single Straight Leg Lift

Buddha Stretch

Buddha Stretch Supine – feet are hips width or slightly wider than hips width on ground. Spine is neutral. Bring back of hands together, slowly raise arms over face, open up arms, then make a circular motion back to the beginning.

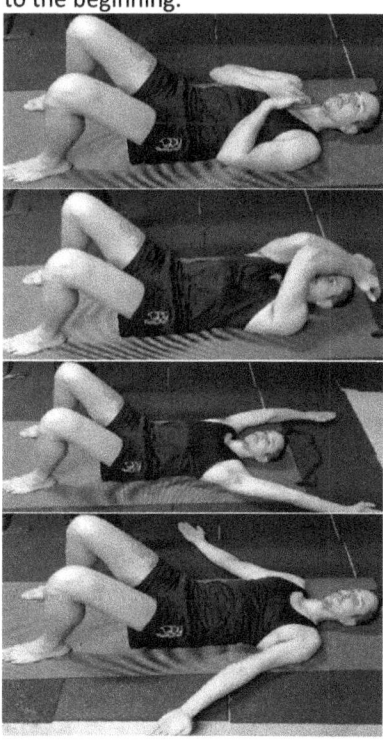

Butterfly Stretch Seated

Calf Raise

Calf Stretch Seated

Calf Stretch Standing

Calf Stretch Variation Tibia Wall Standing

Child's Pose Variation (1 Arm in front, 1 to the side underneath)

Child's Pose Variation (Arms behind)

Child's Pose Variation (Arms in front) – sitting with buttocks on heels. Either gently rest head on the ground and rest arms in front or stretch arms as far forward as possible to add stretch to the latissimus dorsi.

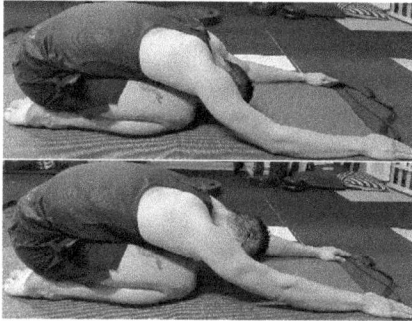

Child's Pose Variation (Lats with Arm Cross Overs)

Cossack Twist

Deadbug Hold Supine

Deadbug Variation Alternating Single Leg Drop

Deadbug Variation Opposite Arm and Leg Alternating – Neutral spine, hands in-line with shoulders, knees in-line with hips, creating an approximate 90-degree angle between the calf muscles and the upper leg. Slowly drop the opposite arm and leg whilst keeping correct posture as stated. Slowly alternate sides.

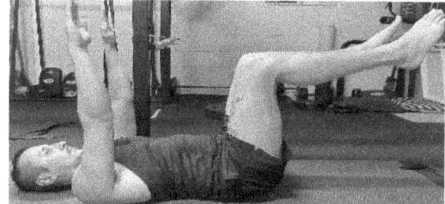

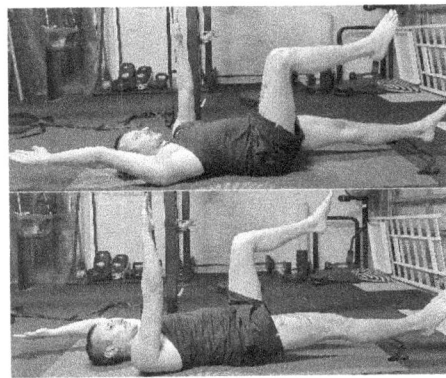

Double Torso Curl/Teaser

Double Torso Hold

Glute Stretch Combo Parts 1-3 – Neutral spine, bring the right ankle to the left leg's quad and hold. Then gently bring the left leg towards face keeping right leg in roughly the same position, and hold. Finally, bring left lg's heel to the right glute and hold. This sequence can be done with the head on the ground, or it can be done with head off the ground, slightly sitting up.

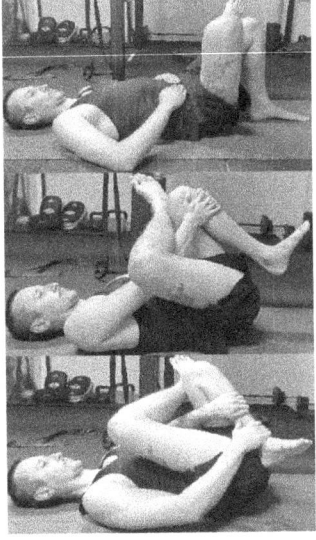

Glute Stretch and Twist

Hamstring Stretch Supine

Hip Flexor Stretch in Supine

Hip Flexor Stretch in Supine 1 Leg

Hula Hoops / Trunk Rotations

Hundreds Supine

Hundreds Variation Bridge

Hundreds Variation Legs Straight and Shoulders off Ground

Hundreds Variation Legs Straight V

Hundreds Variation Tabletop

Hundreds Variation Tabletop Shoulders off Ground

Knees to Chest Relax

Knees to Chest Rocking

Knees to Chest Stretch Variation One Leg Straight

Leg Opening Supine

Leg Opening Supine Variation Heels on Wall

Lunge Stretch Variation

Lunge Stretch Variation Pelvic Lift

Lunge Stretch Variation Pelvic Lift Pulsing Forward

Mermaid Stretch

Mermaid Stretch Easy Variation

Neck Rolls Supine

Pec Stretch Bent Arm

Pec Stretch Straight Arm

Pilates Ring Chest Press

Pilates Ring Leg Raises

Pilates Ring Shoulder Press

Pilates Ring Side Position Pulses

Pilates Ring Squats

Pilates Ring Steering Wheel Front Hold

Pilates Ring Straight Leg Hundreds

Pilates Ring Bridge – Feet slightly wider than hips width, shoulders on the ground, activating transverse abdominus, Pilates ring in-between legs, and gently squeeze ring with thighs and hold the position.

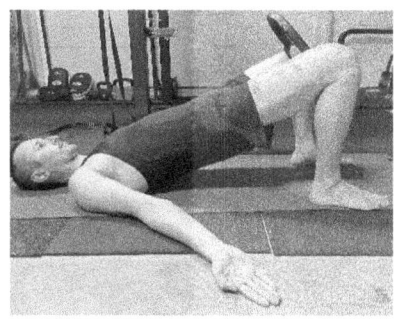

Pilates Ring V-sit-up

Pilates Ring V-sit-up Hold

Plank

Prone Leg Stretch

Quad Stretch Standing

Quad Stretch Standing Variation Pelvic Lift

Rear Tabletop Hold Legs Straight

Rear Tabletop Variation Glute Pulses Legs Straight

Rear Tabletop Variation Leg Lift Legs Straight

Rear Tabletop Hold Legs Bent

Rear Tabletop Variation Glute Pulses Legs Bent

Rear Tabletop Variation Leg Lift Legs Bent

Scapula Dips

Scapula Pushups

Scapula Squeeze and Release Supine

Shoulder Circles Seated

Shoulder Circles Standing

Shoulder Circles Supine

Side Band Walk

Side Position Clam

Side Position Flying Clams

Side Position Inner Thigh Lift

Side Position Kick to Front

Side Position Side Kick

Side Position Straight Leg Heel Alphabet

Side Position Straight Leg Heel Circles

Side Position Straight Leg Hold – Hips in-line, bottom leg on the ground trying to have bottom foot in-line with hips, head either gently on bicep or gently in hand. Top leg up off ground, top foot slightly rotated to assist in gluteus Medius activation and hold top leg up.

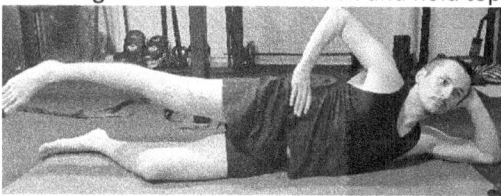

Side Position Straight Leg Pulse

Side Position Straight Leg Top Leg Hold, Bottom Leg Pulse

Side Position Straight Leg Double Pulse

Side/Oblique Knees Plank

Side/Oblique Plank Hand

Single Leg Circles

Single Leg Circles Variation Bottom Leg Straight

Spine Curls Supine

Spine Rolldown and Rollup Standing – Standing feet parallel, shoulder gently pulled back, chin gently touching chest. Slowly roll down as close to vertebra at a time as possible, until finger touch ground. Then slowly roll back to standing.

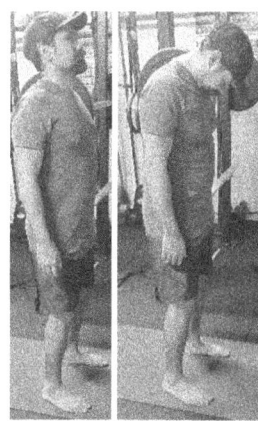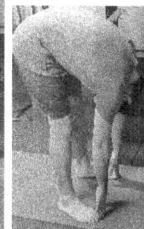

Spine Rolldown Variation into Plank and Rollup Standing

Spine Rolldown Variation into Pushup and Rollup Standing

Spine Rolldown Variation into Shin Hug and Rollup Standing

Spine Rollup and Rolldown Arms to Ceiling

Spine Rollup and Rolldown Assisted (Hands on Hamstrings)

Spine Rollup and Rolldown Wrist to Knees

Spine Rollup and Rolldown Weighted

Spiral Stretch Seated

Starfish Relaxation

Tabletop Hold Supine - Neutral spine, knees in-line with hips, creating an approximate 90-degree angle between the calf muscles and the upper leg, and Hold.

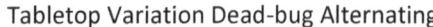

Tabletop Variation Dead-bug Alternating

Tabletop Variation Dead-bug Hold.

Tabletop Variation Straight Leg Circles

Tabletop Variation One Leg Drop to Toe Touch

Tabletop Variation One Leg Drop to Toe Touch and Slide

Tabletop Variation One Leg Straight

Tabletop Variation Touch Toes

Tabletop Variation Touch Opposite Outside Foot

Tabletop Variation Open-Close

Triceps Overhead Stretch

Wall Slide/Angels

Windmills

Windmills ½

Gym

Writing a training program is difficult and writing one for use at a gym can sometimes be more difficult. Some people prefer to train their whole body, while others prefer to train specific muscle groups. As with all programming, identifying the goal is the most important first step. After this identifying fitness level baselines is important and can include how many minutes per kilometre, how many seconds per 100 metres, one rep max weight, the number of reps, etc., ensuring good technique throughout. As a very basic idea, if the goal is endurance smaller weights with more repetitions is used, and when size (hypertrophy) is the goal, more weight with less repetitions are used. However, there are many different ideas available, so training within a realistic, safe, consistent manner should form the foundations of the training and training with a goal in mind and for enjoyment allows for longer term success.

The person's goals will or at least should determine how they train. Most gyms have large weight machines known as pin machines or cable machines and often these can be ideal for beginners as it allows a person to learn the basics whilst lessening the risk of injury. Most large gym equipment also contains stickers on them explaining what the machine can be used for, and some contain pictures of what muscles are used. Some basic tips that people can follow when training at the gym include – trying to train three to four times per week (this can include small training sessions, all the way to larger training sessions; it can include individual training or group training); if training upper body weights then performing vertical pull exercises such as the chin-up prior to horizontal pull exercises such as the row, and training horizontal push exercises such as chest press prior to vertical push exercises such as shoulder press; and if training lower body weights then it is recommended to train the squat movement pattern first, then the leg flexion movement pattern such as a leg machine curl, then a lunge movement pattern, and finally finishing with a hip hinge movement pattern such as a Romanian deadlift.

The primary reason for training vertical pull exercises first is the rhomboids are used for stabilising (better technique) the vertical pull, and if horizontal pull exercises are completed first, then the rhomboid muscle is fatigued, leading to poorer technique and increased risk of injury during the vertical pull. The primary reason for training horizontal push exercises first is the vertical push exercises can exhaust the deltoids and triceps which can negatively impact chest activation during the horizontal push exercises. A lot of the above information is also transferable to training for sports and calisthenics.

List of Gym Equipment Exercises

Agility Ladder Grapevine

Agility Ladder Sprint

Back Extension Hold Variation Weighted

Balance Board Burpees (Hands on board)

Balance Board Mountain Climbers

Balance Board Plank

Balance Board Plank Jacks

Balance Board Pushup – Start from a plank position with hands either side of the board. Then slowly yourself until either stomach or chest touches board. Then slowly raise self-back into plank position.

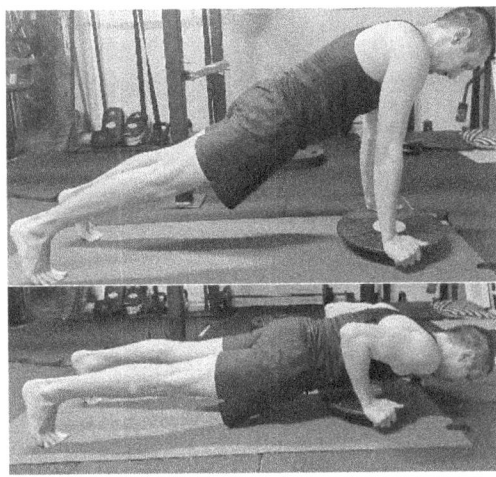

Balance Board Single Leg Squat

Balance Board Squat

Barbell Bench Press

Barbell Bench Press Variation Dead-stop

Barbell Bent Over Row

Barbell Bent Over Row Variation Single Arm

Barbell Bent Over Row Variation Snatch Grip

Barbell Bent Over Row Variation Tripod Row

Barbell Bent Over Row Variation Yates Row

Barbell Bicep Curl

Barbell Cuban Press

Barbell Cuban Rotation

Barbell Deadlift – There are several variations in Deadlift form, but this will focus on the basics or beginner interpretation. Start with either the bar only or a light weight either side. Gently squeeze shoulder blades and activate rest of core. As you lift the bar, keep core activated and press through the heels. Once at the top, slowly lower the bar until approximately shin height, maintaining strong posture throughout. Then, as you lift the bar back to standing, keep core activated once again and press through heels. During the movement keep a slight bend in the knees also known as a soft joint, so the hamstrings can still be activated, whilst minimising knee hyperextension.

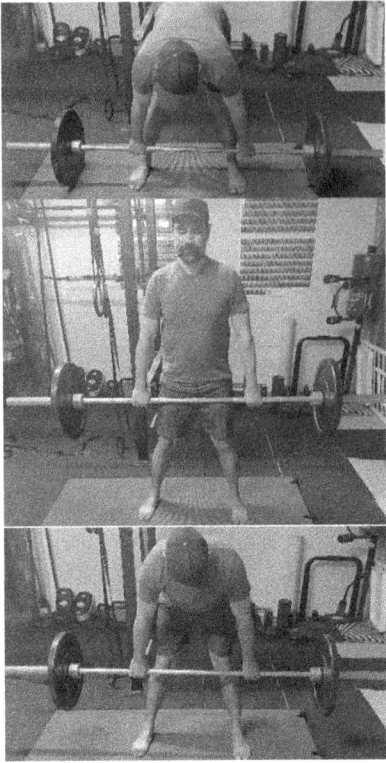

Barbell Deadlift Variation Handle Addition

Barbell Deadlift Variation Single Leg

Barbell Deadlift Variation Wide/Snatch Grip

Barbell Front Squat

Barbell Hip Thrusts

Barbell Lunges

Barbell Overhead Squat

Barbell Rear Squat

Barbell Rollouts

Barbell Shoulder Press Standing

Barbell Skull Crushers

Barbell Squat Variation Hack Squat

Barbell Squat Variation Handle Hack Squat

Barbell T-Bar Row

Barbell Tripod Row

Bench Jump-Overs Hands on Bench

Bench Piriformis Stretch Standing

Bench Pullover Supine Plate Weight

Bench Triceps Dip

Box Jump-Overs

Box Jumps – Start with feet approximately hips width apart. Then use the momentum of your arms to assist in jumping higher. As you land, try to minimise the sound by activating your glute and leg muscles and slowly land into a squat position.

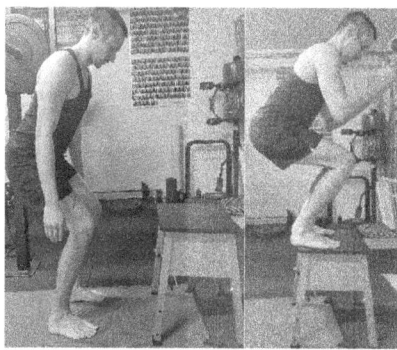

Box Jumps Variation Side Jumps

Box Step-Ups

Butterfly Stretch Seated Variation Loaded/with Weights

Cable Machine Chest Fly

Cable Machine Chest Press

Cable Machine Delt Fly

Cable Machine External Rotation

Cable Machine Face Pulls

Cable Machine Internal Rotation

Cable Machine Leg Curl Prone

Cable Machine Leg Curls Seated

Cable Machine Leg Press

Cable Machine Leg Raises

Cable Machine Palloff Press

Cable Machine Seated Lat Pulldowns

Cable Machine Seated Lat Pulldowns Variation Close Grip

Cable Machine Seated Lat Pulldowns Variation Underhand Grip

Cable Machine Seated Rows

Cable Machine Seated Rows Variation Close Grip

Cable Machine Shoulder Press

Cable Machine Single Arm Lat Pulldown

Cable Machine Single Arm Row

Cable Machine Triceps Overhead

Cable Machine Triceps Pushdown

Dumbbell Bench Chest Press

Dumbbell Bench Chest Press Variation Deadstop

Dumbbell Bench Chest Press Variation One Arm One Weight – Feet either on ground or on support bar to assist in neutral spine. Start with arm almost straight (slight bend in elbow/soft joint). Slowly lower weight until either elbow or weight is in-line with the bench, dependent on strength level, weight, and training goal. Slowly raise again to starting position and repeat until repetitions are complete, then change sides.

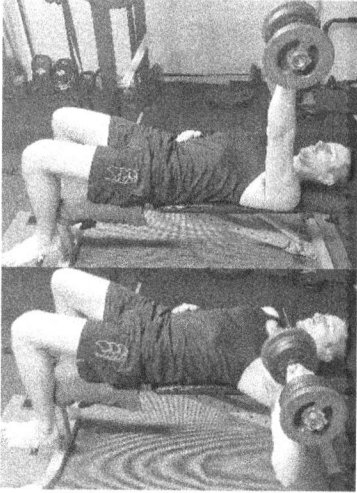

Dumbbell Bench Chest Press Variation One Arm Two Weights

Dumbbell Bench Pullover Supine

Dumbbell Bent Over Row Both Hands

Dumbbell Bent Over Row Variation Both Hands Reverse Grip

Dumbbell Bent Over Row Variation Single Arm

Dumbbell Bent Over Row Variation Single Arm with Bench

Dumbbell Bicep Curl

Dumbbell Bicep Curl Variation Hammer

Dumbbell Chest Fly

Dumbbell Cuban Press

Dumbbell Cuban Rotation

Dumbbell Decline Bench Chest Press

Dumbbell External Rotation

Dumbbell Flys Standing

Dumbbell Flys Standing Bent-Over

Dumbbell Front Raises Seated

Dumbbell Front Raises Standing

Dumbbell Front Raises Standing Bent-Over

Dumbbell Incline Bench Chest Press

Dumbbell Incline Bench Y-T-W

Dumbbell Incline Prone Cuban Press into Y

Dumbbell Internal Rotation

Dumbbell Leaning Lat Pulses

Dumbbell Leaning Lat Raise Hold

Dumbbell Lunges

Dumbbell Rear Delt Fly

Dumbbell Seated Forearm Curl

Dumbbell Shoulder Press Seated

Dumbbell Shoulder Press Standing

Dumbbell Shoulder Press Variation Single Arm Seated

Dumbbell Shoulder Press Variation Single Arm Standing

Dumbbell Side Raises Standing

Dumbbell Side Raises Standing Bent-Over

Dumbbell Skull Crushers

Dumbbell Triceps Kickbacks

Dumbbell Triceps Overhead

Dumbbell Tripod Row

Elliptical Trainer

Fit Ball Decline Plank Forearms

Fit Ball Decline Plank Hands

Fit Ball Incline Plank Forearms

Fit Ball Incline Plank Hands

Fit Ball Leaning Plank Bounce

Fit Ball Leaning Shin Swim

Fit Ball Prone Knees to Chest

Fit Ball Seat

Fit Ball Seat Variation Balance, Feet off Ground

Fit Ball Seiza (shins on Fit Ball) – Shins on ball, glutes on heels, activate your core, find your balance point, and hold position.

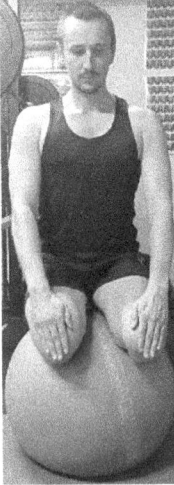

Fit Ball Sit-ups

Fit Ball Toes to Hands Throw Sit-ups

Fit Ball V-Sit-ups

Foam Roller Calf Release

Foam Roller Core Activation

Foam Roller Forearm Release

Foam Roller Gluteal Release

Foam Roller Hamstring Release

Foam Roller Hip Flexor Release

Foam Roller Hip Flexor Release Bent Leg

Foam Roller ITB Release

Foam Roller Knee Raise

Foam Roller Knee Raise Arms to Ceiling Hold

Foam Roller Overhead Arms Supine

Foam Roller Piriformis Release

Foam Roller Quadricep Release

Foam Roller Thoracic Extension

Foam Roller Tibialis Release

Goblet Squat

Good Mornings

Heavy Rope Climb Double/Unilateral Rope Climb

Heavy Rope Climb Double/Unilateral Rope Variation L-Sit

Heavy Rope Climb Single Rope

Heavy Rope Climb Single Rope Variation L-Sit

Hexagon Agility Test

Indoor Bike

Kettle Bell Standing Overhead Hold

Kettle Bell Standing Overhead Shoulder Press

Kettle Bell Standing Overhead Walking

Kettle Bell Turkish Swing

Kettle Bell Walking Forearm Extensor Pulses – Hold kettle Bell in fingertips, then slowly raise fingers into a fist like shape, then slowly extend finger.

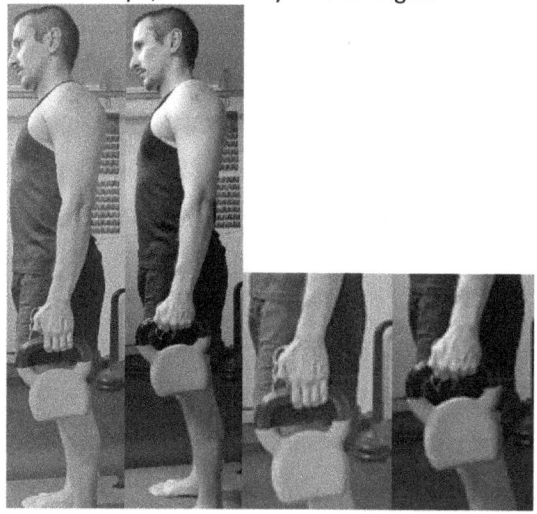

Kettlebell Farmer's Walk / Suitcase Walk

Leg Press Machine 45 degrees

Machine Preacher Curl

Seated Good Mornings

Zercher Barbell Squat

Zercher Barbell Walk

Body Weight, Calisthenics & Gymnastic Rings

Programming tips for writing Calisthenics programs will be using a log of information from the AMN academy holistic health course. The first idea that should be incorporated in calisthenic related training is incorporating locked joints in isometric holds. Traditionally the fitness industry has taught us that locking joints is wrong and dangerous. However, it is now believed that locking joints is only dangerous when lifting heavier weights. When practicing body weight movements, it is recommended to lock joints as long as the person doesn't have any pre-existing injuries. This locking of the joints can increase strength output via strengthening the connective tissue.

Correct or normal range of motion is the healthy range of motion completed during a body weight exercise without negatively impacting posture. For example, a handstand should be done with 180 degrees range of motion with a healthy strong posture. Flexibility also allows for healthier range of motion and easier strength output.The last relevant aspect is body awareness. Body awareness allows for healthier movement, greater muscle activation and muscle control, and better technique. This can improve with body and brain related training as well as longer-term practice of body weight exercises.

When programming calisthenics and gymnastic rings the definition of core strength may be different to the way it is traditionally referred to in gym related fitness circles. Core strength in calisthenics can include the legs, all the way through to the rhomboids and latissimus dorsi muscles. This should be remembered, as doing a day focusing on only the abdominal muscles may be contraindicated. Instead focusing on specific holds, movement patterns or whole-body related training is recommended.

List of Body Weight, Calisthenics & Gym Rings Exercises

Abdominal Wheel Rollouts Full

Abdominal Wheel Rollouts Kneeling

Abdominal Wheel Unilateral Rollouts

Abdominal Wheel Unilateral Rollouts Kneeling – Start in a kneeling plank-like position with hands on rollers. Then slowly lower the body down as the arms straighten away from the body. Lower self as low as safe, then slowly pull body back into starting position.

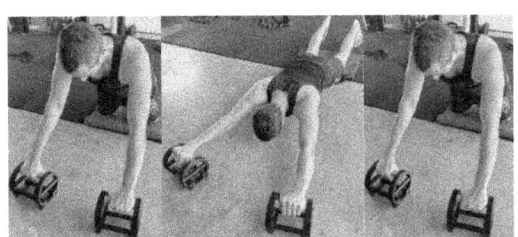

AMN Academy Barrel Rolls

AMN Academy Hamstring Stretch Variation Foot Angled and Extended

AMN Academy Hamstring Stretch Variation Foot Flexed

AMN Academy Resistance Band Figure 8's

AMN Academy Resistance Band Load Stretch

AMN Academy Spiral Stretch

Ankle Circles

Arm Circles with Bar/Pole Standing

Arm Circles with Bar/Pole Standing Bent Over

Arm Circles with Resistance Band Standing / Shoulder Dislocations

Arm Circles with Resistance Band Standing Bent Over

Arm Circles with Thumb Rotation

Arm Side Raises

Back Extension Variation Mission Impossible

Back Extension Variation Superman

Back Leg Scale

Back Lever

Back Lever Variation Advanced Tuck

Back Lever Variation Legs Bent

Back Lever Variation Legs Bent Straddle

Back Lever Variation Straight Legs Straddle

Back Lever Variation Tuck

Backward Shoulder Roll

Bear Crawl

Burpees

Burpees Variation Advanced Military / Pushup and Tuck Jump

Burpees Variation Beginner Military / Pushup

Burpees Variation Burpee and Squat

Burpees Variation Devil Maker

Burpees Variation Hip Thrust

Burpees Variation Sprawl / Wide Base

Calf Raise Standing Variation Tibia Raise

Calf Raises Standing

Candlestick

Candlestick Weight Assisted

Cardio Weighted Boxing Cross

Cardio Weighted Boxing Hook

Cardio Weighted Boxing Jab

Cardio Weighted Boxing Uppercut

Chest Dip

Chicken Wing Seated Stretch

Child's Pose Variation Incline Bench Neutral Grip

Chin Tuck

Chin-up – Start with palms facing towards face. Slowly raise the body until either your chin or chest reach the bar. Then slowly lower the body to start position.

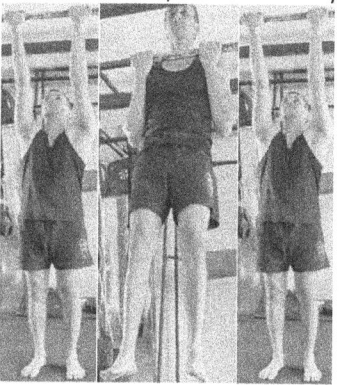

Chin-up Variation Clap Above Bar

Chin-up Variation Concentric

Chin-up Variation Eccentric

Chin-up Variation Eccentric Weighted

Chin-up Variation Headbangers

Chin-up Variation L-Sit

Chin-up Variation Typewriter

Chin-up Variation Weighted

Circus Aerial Human Flag – Similar to the Human flag, the top hand will be pulling as the bottom arm pushes. Since it is on a moving pole, shoulder and core control will be more difficult.

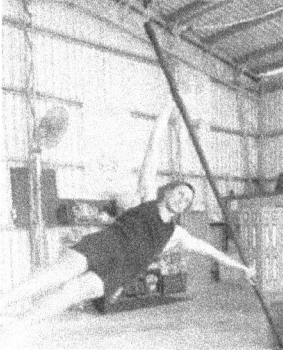

Circus Aerial Trapeze Bar Hang / Bat Hang – The bar will be behind the knees, and hamstrings will be flexed.

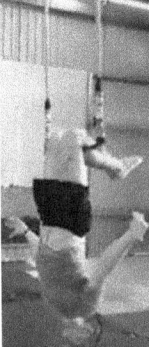

Circus Aerial Trapeze Bar Sit-ups / Bat Hang Sit-ups – From the Bat Hang position, the core will be used to pull the body towards the bar as the hands reach for the rope. Once the rope is held in the hands, slowly lower self to continue repetitions. To finish, the person will be seated on top of the trapeze bar.

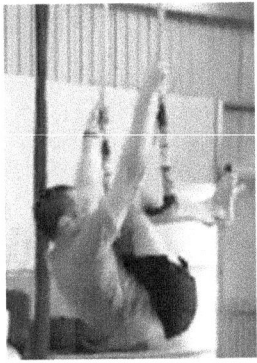

Crab Walk

Cross Arm Stretch

Cross Over Crunches

Crunches

Dead Hang – Set up as if a pull-up was going to be completed. Slowly lift legs off ground as shoulder blades are squeezed, and tense/activate the leg muscles. Hold position for as long as is safe, often up to a minute. Then slowly lower the body so feet are comfortably on ground.

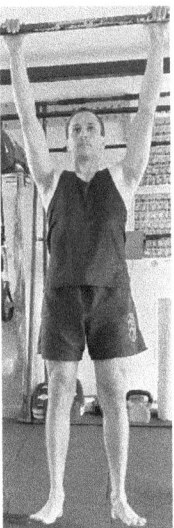

Dead Hang Variation False Grip

Dead Hang Variation Knees Lift and Hold

Dead Hang Variation Knees to Chest

Dead Hang Variation L-Sit

Dead Hang Variation Scapula Squeeze

Dead Hang Variation Scapular Shoulder Circles

Dead Hang Variation Single Arm

Dead Hang Variation Straight Leg Lift

Dead Hang Variation Straight Leg Lift Toes to Bar

Dead Hang Variation Under Hand Grip

Dead Hang Variation Windscreen Wipers

Deadman Squats

Decline Plank Medicine Ball

Decline Plank Wall

Decline Plank Weight Stack or Step

Dish Hold

Dish Rocks

Dragon Flag

Dragon Flag Negatives

External Rotations Band

Figure 8 Head Circles Standing

Finger Hand Extensor Pulses

Forearm Stretch

Forearm Stretch Reverse

Forearm Stretch Variation Palm Closed Fingers Down

Forearm Stretch Variation Palm Open Fingers Down

Forward Shoulder Roll

Frog Jumps

Frog Stand

Frog Stand Variation High Frogger

Frog Stretch Hips Flat

Frog Stretch Hold

Frog Stretch Rocking

Frog Stretch Side Stretch

Front Leg Scale

Front Lever

Front Lever Variation Advanced Single Leg Lever

Front Lever Variation Advanced Tuck Lever

Front Lever Variation Band Assisted on Hips

Front Lever Variation One Leg Bent

Front Lever Variation Single Leg Lever

Front Lever Variation Tabletop Lever

Front Lever Variation Tuck Lever

Glute Hamstring Martin St Louise Nordic Lifts

Glute Hamstring Raises

Gymnastic Ring Static Hold Variation Arms away from Body Palms Facing Back (Moderate)

Gymnastic Ring Static Hold Variation Bicep Hold (Moderate)

Gymnastic Ring Static Hold Variation Palms Facing Body (Easiest)

Gymnastic Rings Back Lever

Gymnastic Rings Basket Stretch Hold

Gymnastic Rings Chest Dip

Gymnastic Rings Front Lever

Gymnastic Rings German Hang – Often used as a warmup or progression on the way to the 'Skin the cat' exercise. Begin as if a 'Skin the cat' was going to be completed. Stop when body has rotated through the gap between the arms. Hold position for as long as safe, then if safe to do so, slowly release grip.

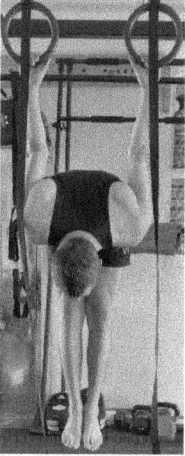

Gymnastic Rings Inverted Deadlifts

Gymnastic Rings Inverted Hold

Gymnastic Rings Inverted Pullups

Gymnastic Rings Inverted Splits

Gymnastic Rings Knees Hold

Gymnastic Rings L-Sit Hold

Gymnastic Rings Plank

Gymnastic Rings Pullups Chinup Grip

Gymnastic Rings Pullups Neutral Grip

Gymnastic Rings Pullups Wide Grip

Gymnastic Rings Pushup

Gymnastic Rings Pushup Decline

Gymnastic Rings Pushup Arrows

Gymnastic Rings Scarecrow

Gymnastic Rings Skin the Cat Bent Legs

Gymnastic Rings Skin the Cat Straight Leg

Gymnastic Rings Supinated Pullups

Gymnastic Rings Supine Rows

Gymnastic Rings Upside Hold – Start sitting under the rings. Then slowly lift and rotate body until the body is upside down. Trying to visualise/hold a straight line from toes through pelvis to shoulders. Head can be looking forward or slightly looking towards toes.

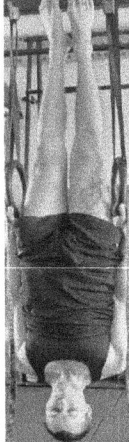

Gymnastic Rings Y-T-W

Hamstring Static Stretch Variation Hips Closed (Slight Twist)

Hamstring Static Stretch Variation Hips Square/Inline

Hamstring Static Stretch Variation Open Hips

Hamstring Supine Figure 8 Stretches Band/Towel

Hand Grip Trainer Squeeze

Handstand Hold Variation Offset

Handstand Hold Variation Single Arm Wall Assisted

Handstand Hold Wall Assisted

Handstand Progression AMN Academy

Handstand Progression Shoulder Width Stance Bent Arm Lift

Handstand Progression Shoulder Width Stance Straight Arm Lift

Handstand Progression Wide Stance Bent Arm Lift

Handstand Progression Wide Stance Straight Arm Lift

Handstand Pushups Wall Assisted

Handstand Variation Offset Wall Pushups

Hanging Hip Hiker – Begin from normal pullup position. Often this will be with hands slightly wider than shoulder width. Then slowly release on hand and allow legs to move to side. Hold position.

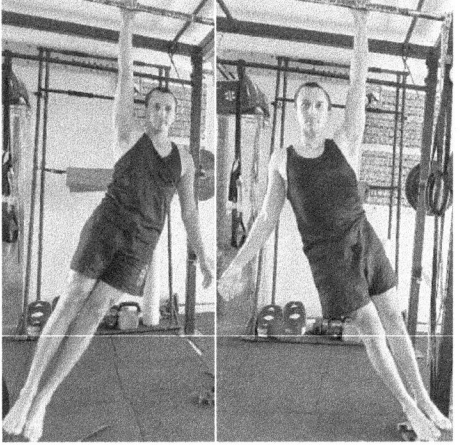

Hanging Leg Raises Variation Legs Bent

Hanging Leg Raises Variation Straight Leg

Hanging L-Sit Hold

Hanging Pike Stretch

Hanging Wind Screen Wipers

Headstand Straight Legs

Headstand Variation Forearm Base

Headstand Variation Knees Bent

Headstand Variation Single Leg Straight

Headstand Variation Tripod Base

High Knees

Hindu Squat

Hip Hurdles

Hip Hurdles Reverse

Hollow Body Hold

Hollow Body Rocks

Hops

Human Flag Chamber Hold Regression

Human Flag Double Bent Knees

Human Flag Hug Regression Hug Pole – Top arm will wrap around pole. Bottom arm will be bent and have side of body resting on triceps. Both hands will be doing a variation of a pistol grip.

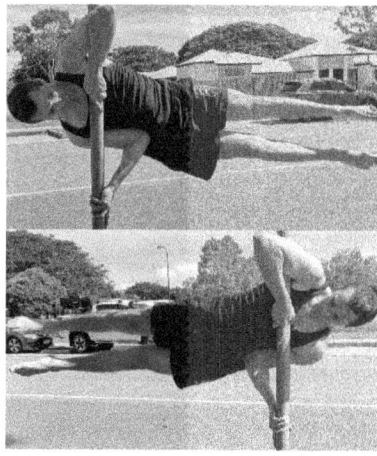

Human Flag Single Bent Knee

Human Flag Support Press Regression

Human Flag Vertical Hold Regression

Human Flag – Gently squeeze shoulder blades, top hand will pull body weight as bottom hand pushes into pole. Once in position the whole body from the neck to the toes should be activated to hold one solid position. Bottom hand will normally be a pistol grip.

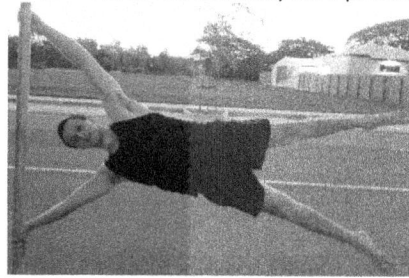

Ice Cream Makers

Incline Bench DB "Y" Hold Stretch

Incline Mountain Climbers

Incline Plank

Incline Plank Medicine Ball

Incline Plank Weight Stack or Step

Internal Rotations Band

Inverted Deadlifts on Bar

Jogging

Knee Circles Standing Feet Together

Knee Circles Standing Single Leg

Lateral Bounds

Lateral Hops

Latissimus Dorsi Static Stretch

Low Arm Pectoralis Major Stretch Standing

Lunge Stretch Variation Pelvic Lift with Weight Above Head

Lunge Stretch Variation Pelvic Lift with Weight Above Head Pulsing Forward

Lunge Stretch Variation Thread the Needle

Lunges

Lunges Plyometric Variation 180 Rotation

Lunges Plyometric Variation Leg Stay Same

Lunges Plyometric Variation Legs Alternate

Lunges Variation Incline Front Leg

Lunges Variation Petersen Inspired Lunge, also known as ATG Lunge

Lunges Variation Walking

Medicine Ball Slams

Medicine Ball Walking Lunges

Medicine Ball Walking Lunges Variation Overhead

Mountain Climbers

Muscle Up Negatives

Muscle Ups

Neck Soft Nods/Deep Neck Flexor Stretches Supine

NFL Inspired Agility Test

Open-Close Supine

Pendulum Supine

Planche Regression ½ Legs

Planche Regression Bent Arm – Start by having elbows in-line with edge of midsection. Slowly lift legs simultaneously off ground. Midsection is gently resting on triceps and elbows.

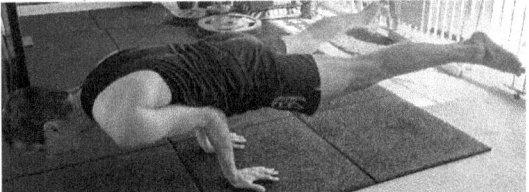

Planche Variation Band Assisted

Planche Variation Box Hold

Planche Variation Frog

Planche Variation Pushup

Planche Variation Straddle

Planche Variation Tuck

Planche Variation Tuck Swing

Plank Forearms

Plank Hands

Plank Variation Alternating Knees to Ribs

Plank Variation Hip Tap

Plank Variation Jacks

Plank Variation Kick

Plank Variation Romper Stompers

Plank Variation Shoulder Tap

Plank Variation Towel Slides

Plank Variation Wrist Tap

Plank Walk

Plank Walk Variation on Hand Blades

Plate Weight Overhead Abdominal Twist Seated

Plate Weight Standing Truck Driver

Plate Weight Steering Wheel Variation Bent Over

Plate Weight Steering Wheel Variation Front Raise Position

Plate Weight Steering Wheel Variation Overhead

Prone Quad Stretch Single Leg

Prone T

Prone T Variation Standing

Prone W

Prone W Variation Standing

Prone Y

Prone Y Variation Standing

Pullup Variation ½ Pullup/Inverted Rows

Pullup Variation 3 Step Pause

Pullup Variation 90 Degree Hold – Set up for the normal pullup position. Often this will be with hands slightly wider than shoulder width. Slowly pullup body upwards until the forearms and elbow crease make an approximately 90-degree angle. Hold position for as long as is safe, then slowly lower body down to starting position.

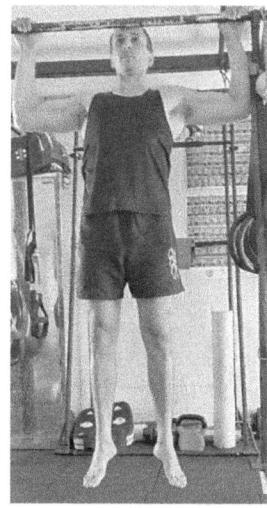

Pullup Variation Archer

Pullup Variation Clap Above Bar

Pullup Variation Commander Close Grip

Pullup Variation Commander Shoulder Width Grip

Pullup Variation Concentric

Pullup Variation Eccentric

Pullup Variation Eccentric Weighted

Pullup Variation False Grip

Pullup Variation Headbangers

Pullup Variation L-Posture

Pullup Variation L-Sit

Pullup Variation Over-Under

Pullup Variation Prison Style

Pullup Variation Single Arm

Pullup Variation Single Arm – Band Assisted with one arm

Pullup Variation Single Arm Arm-Assisted Chinup Grip

Pullup Variation Single Arm Hold– Band Assisted with one arm

Pullup Variation Switch Grip

Pullup Variation Thumbless Grip

Pullup Variation Tuck Front Lever

Pullup Variation Typewriter

Pullup Variation Weighted

Pullup Variation Weighted Chinups

Pullup Variation with Towel – Start with a strong towel over the bar. Grip the towel in each hand and slowly raise body upwards until face is in-line with hands. Briefly hold, then slowly lower body to start position.

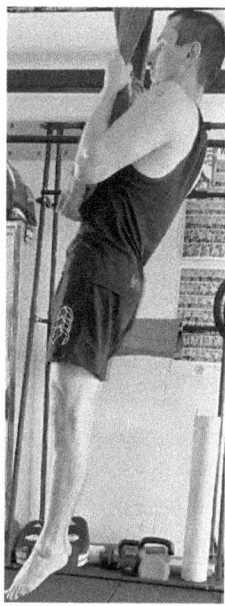

Pullups

Pushup On Knees

Pushup Row Dumbbell

Pushup Variation 'T' / Arrow Medicine Ball

Pushup Variation 'Y' Medicine Ball

Pushup Variation Bicep – Start with fingers pointing towards toes. If possible, begin with wrists in line with shoulders. Slowly lower chest towards ground as low as is safe. Then slowly raise back to start position.

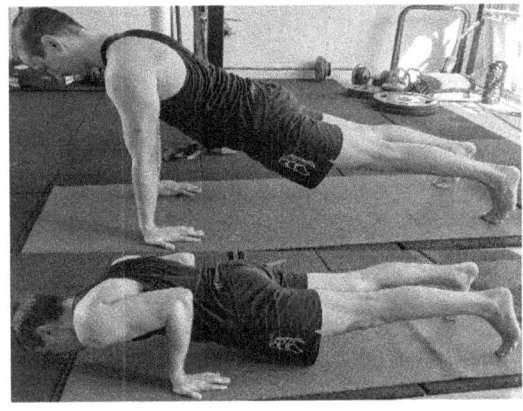

Pushup Variation Chest Tap

Pushup Variation Clap

Pushup Variation Diamond Pushup

Pushup Variation Eccentric Phase

Pushup Variation Gecko

Pushup Variation Pike/Shoulder Pushup

Pushup Variation Pseudo Planche Pushup

Pushup Variation Pseudo Superman

Pushup Variation Semi-Circles

Pushup Variation Single Arm

Pushup Variation Single Arm

Pushup Variation Single Arm Eccentric, Both Arms Concentric

Pushup Variation Sky Diver Hold

Pushup Variation Sky Diver Slide

Pushup Variation Spiderman

Pushup Variation Tiger Bend – Here I have done the easier variation for starting. Hands are in-line with face, and elbows are pulled in. While keeping hands and wrists on ground, slowly lift body until in pull hands plank position. Then slowly lower back to start. To increase difficulty, start with hands further away from face.

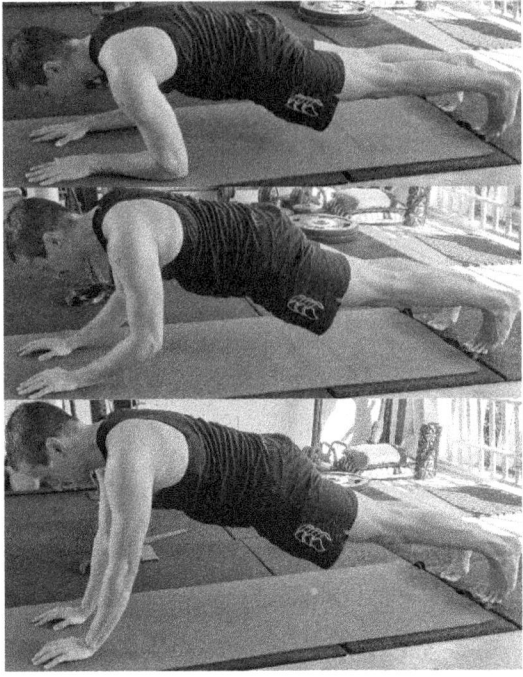

Pushup Variation Tiger Bend Incline

Pushup Variation Tiger Bend on Knees

Pushup Variation Triceps

Pushup Variation Wide Grip

Pushups

Pushups Variation Offset

Pushups Variation Parallette Depth

Quadricep Flex

Quadricep Flex Seated Variation Leg Raise

Quadricep Stretch Hold

Quadratus Lumborum Stretch Hold Variation Feet parallel and angled Left

Quadratus Lumborum Stretch Hold Variation Feet parallel and angled Right

Quadratus Lumborum Stretch Hold Variation Feet parallel and Straight

Quadrupe Hold

Quadrupe Kick Through

Reclining Twist

Reclining Twist Weighted

Resistance Band Chest Pull-apart

Resistance Band Overhead Pull-apart

Resistance Band Standing Delt Fly

Resistance Band Triceps Pushdown

Rhomboid Pushups

Russian Twist

SCM Neck Stretch

Seated Abdominal Twist

Seated Half Frog Stretch Hold

Seated Leg Raises

Seated Pike Hold

Seated Pike Lifts

Seated Pike Pulses

Seated Pike Stretch Nose to Shin

Seated Straddle Lifts

Seated Straddle Variation Extensions

Seiza Hold

Seiza to Lunge to Standing

Shoulder Circles with Arm Straight (Like a Train)

Side Bends

Side Bends Variation Leg Crossed in Front

Side Stepping

Side/Oblique Plank

Side/Oblique Plank Variation Forearm

Side/Oblique Plank Variation Knee to Elbow

Side/Oblique Plank Variation Star Hold

Side/Oblique Plank Variation Star Pulse

Side/Oblique Plank Variation

Side-lying Shoulder External Rotation Variation with Dumbbell

Single Bar Chest Dip

Single Bar Chest Dip Hold

Single Bar Chest Dip Variation Korean Dip

Single Bar Chest Dip Variation Underhand Grip (chinup grip)

Single Bar Chest Dip Variation Underhand Grip (chinup grip)

Single Leg Calf Raise Standing

Single Leg Calf Raise Standing Variation Tibia Raise

Single Leg Squat

Single Leg Squat Variation Band Assisted

Single Leg Squat Variation Dragon Pistol Squat

Single Leg Squat Variation Dragon Pistol Squat Assisted

Single Leg Squat Variation Pistol Squat

Single Leg Squat Variation Pistol Squat Assisted – The resistance band is to assist in form and strength building until the person is ready to attempt the exercise without the assistance. Slowly lower the body as one leg slowly moves in front of the body. Finish once the glutes are as close to the squatted heel as possible. Slowly raise back to start, ensuring the resistance bands are used secondary as needed. The amount of arm activation will depend on how much assistance the leg needs in lowering and raising safely.

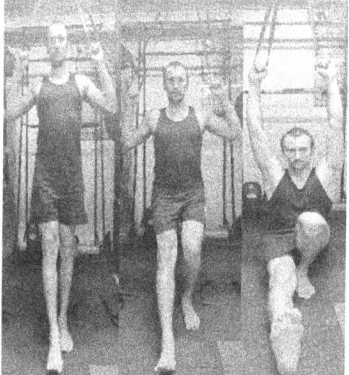

Sit-up

Sit-up Variation Bicycle

Skipping with Rope

Slackline Walking

Sleeper Stretch

Sliding Wall Squat

Speed Punching Straight Punch

Sprinting

Squat Jacks

Squat Pulses

Squat Pulses/Slides Wall Assisted

Squat Seat

Squat Seat Variation Calm Raise

Squat Seat Variation Wall Assisted

Squat Seat Variation Wall Assisted & Weighted

Squat Variation Kicks

Squat Variation Shrimp Squat Elevated

Squat Variation Side Lunge Squat

Squat Variation Sissy Squat

Squats

Squats Variation Close Squats

Standing Lever Over ITB Stretch

Standing Plyometric Hamstring/Leg Swing Variation Straight Leg up and down

Standing Plyometric Hamstring/Leg Swing Variation Straight Leg up and Bent Leg down

Standing Plyometric Side Leg Swing

Standing Shoulder External Rotation 90 degrees Abduction Variation with Dumbbell

Star Jumps

Tai Chi Ankle Warm Up Stretches

Thoracic Mobilisation Supine Horizontal Variation with Arm Stretch

Toe Lifts 4 Small Toes

Toe Lifts Big Toe

Toe Side Lift 4 Small Toes

Toe Side Lift Big Toe

Toe Touch Standing

Toe Touch Standing Variation One Leg in Front

Torso Twist

Trap Stretch Standing

Tuck Jumps

V-Sit-up – Start with hands and feet straight and core activated. Slowly lift upper and lower body towards the top at a similar rate. Then slowly lower back to start position.

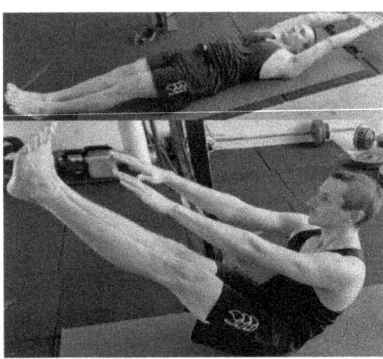

V-Sit-up Hold

V-Sit-up Variation (Head-Shoulders-Knees)

V-Sit-up Variation Side V-Ups

V-Sit-up Variation Single Leg

V-Sit-up Variation Straddle

V-Sit-up Variation X-Up

Waiter Stretch Standing

Weighted Bench Pull Overs

Weighted Plank

Weighted Pullups

Wide Squat Seat

Wide Squat Seat Variation with Calm Raise

Wide Squat Towel Slides

Wood Chops Standing

Wrist Warmup Variation Back of Hand on Ground Fingers Backward, Sidewards Pulsing

Wrist Warmup Variation Fingers Forward, Forward Pulsing

Yoga

As a Yoga student, I will not include programming tips in this section. There are various types of yoga practice, different goals, etc., and I believe a student of yoga suggesting programming tips would be ethically incorrect.

List of Yoga and Yoa Inspired Exercises

2 Prasarita Padottanasana Variations

3 Pigeon Pose Stretch Variations

5 Star Squat Malasana

Bhujapidasana

Bhujapidasana Shoulder Prep

Bow Quad Stretch Standing

Buddha Prayer Deep Squat – Start in a low wide squat. Gentle squeeze shoulder blades as the elbows gently push into the inside thighs. The hands will gently touch forming the prayer-like position with the hands. Hold the position.

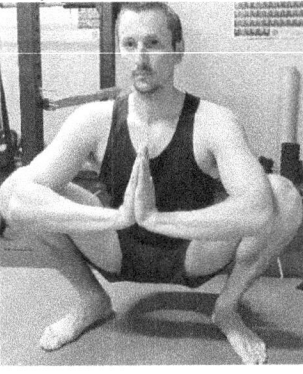

Buddha Squat Bows

Child's Pose Variation (Arms by side)

Crow Pose Bakasana

Downward-Facing Dog

Eagle Garudasana

Elevate Leg Position Legs Together

Elevate Leg Positive Legs Apart Variation

Firefly Prep Standing

Firefly Tittibhasana Resistance Band Assisted

Five Star Squat

Half Moon Sequence

Half Moon Sequence Triangle Hold Standing

Headpull

High Lunge Hold

Knee to Ankle Pose – Agnistambhasana – Sit with left leg on ground making an approximately 60-degree bend between the knee and the hamstring. Then place the right leg on top of the left leg. Hold position, until time to swap legs.

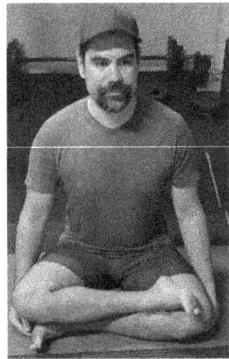

Knee to Ear / Karnapidasana

Lizard Pose Utthan Pristhasana

Low Lunge Stretch Variation

Plow Pose / Halasana

Separate Leg

Separate Leg Head to Knee

Single Leg Straight Leg Hold (Toes in Fingers)

Supta Padangusthasana

Supta Padangusthasana Variation Leg Across the Body

Supta Padangusthasana Variation Leg Open

Tiger Pushup

Triangle

Upavista Konasana

Upward-Facing Dog/Cobra

Utthita Hasta Padangustahasana Standing

Key Points & Relevant Personal/Professional Experiences

Deidentified Case Studies regarding Western and Eastern Integrated Care

Person 1

The following Case Study was completed following the person's life journey regarding stomach pain. This case study was largely written by the person themselves and was included as it demonstrated the strengths and weaknesses of both the Western and Eastern approaches, as well as reasons for integrating both. As will be seen, in real life the line between 'Western' and 'Eastern' blurs, but best outcomes include both. At the request of the person providing the case study, they have been deidentified.

"All my life I've had issues with gut pain. Usually though, it's very short lived and seemed like it was easily explained by something I had eaten and never caused me much mind at all. The amount of pain following these incidents were intense, but I always just figured that's how it was for everyone with gut pain. Besides, a problem that only appears randomly every few months hardly seems like a pattern. At least that's what I thought was true.

Unfortunately for me in 2020 I noticed that the pain seemed to be happening more often. While initially I attributed it to something simple like getting older, I just couldn't shake a bad feeling about it. Towards the end of the year, I found that I had gotten a sore throat, unremarkable in any other context, I found that this one lasted for over a month. Worried, I asked my GP to investigate it but there didn't seem to be much of an explanation. This continued until one day it suddenly stopped. This might have been a cause for celebration for me, but unfortunately soon after the gut pain got even worse and more frequent to the point of being daily. Terrified, I had asked a new GP to help me figure it out. A long series of tests later I was found to have increasingly worse levels of inflammation in my gut and put on a schedule towards the end of 2021 for scopes and biopsies to see what was going wrong.

When I received the results, there was a significant stricture between my large and small intestine and that the biopsies unfortunately confirmed that I was now suffering from a condition called Crohn's Disease. Shortly after my diagnosis I was offered the standard course of treatment for this disease which was encapsulated by an ever-increasing schedule of immunomodulating drugs designed to suppress responses from the immune system.

I was sceptical because no medical professional at that point could offer me a clear understanding of the mechanisms upon which Crohn's Disease functioned, and the treatment plan seemed only to treat symptoms, with no belief that there was a cure for this condition. Initially, I began treatment with a corticosteroid, which didn't even help with the symptoms, but did manage to buy me more time for private research.

In a desperate bid for more time after that I also tried enteral therapy, which involved weeks of a liquid only diet. I was happy to do anything that avoided chronic use of powerful drugs for the rest of my life. Unfortunately, that *didn't help with the symptoms, but it had given me the time to find information about a small team of researchers working with the goal of creating a vaccine for Crohn's Disease.*

This new information had opened several doors for me into my understanding of the disease. If there was a vaccine being developed, then did this mean I was fighting some kind of virus?

With some more digging I learnt that the researchers believed it was a bacteria at the root of Crohn's, called Mycobacterium Avium subspecies Paratuberculosis (or MAP for short). This would turn out to be the same bacteria implicated in the well-known Johne's Disease, which shares very similar symptom profiles with Crohn's but in cattle instead (only it's much harder to detect in humans). This research went on for myself and got deeper all the while my condition was getting worse. Constant pain, agonising flares, a bad reaction to just about any food I ate, an overwhelming and randomly affecting fatigue and psychological strain were a day-to-day problem that seemed to ever increase in pressure. I had lost a lot of weight too, dropping 20 kg in only six weeks. Everything became more difficult.

Eventually I found that there was a treatment called AMAT being offered by a private clinic in New South Wales called the Centre for Digestive Diseases (CDD). Their treatment worked under the same pretence that MAP was the driving factor in Crohn's, and involved using a powerful selection of antibiotics for weeks at a time and supplementing with extremely high daily doses of vitamin D. I had read that this treatment worked better in individuals who had avoided the traditional course of immunomodulators so I decided that before any other treatment I would at least try that.

I discussed it with the head of Gastroenterology at my hospital and was told on no uncertain terms that their research was "junk science" and that if I didn't act soon with a traditional therapy that I would be looking at an unavoidable surgery. I still decided to go ahead with it and with referral in hand in late 2022 I went to the CDD in New South Wales, who very quickly set me up on AMAT therapy with an enormous disclaimer on the side effects of these drugs. While a little scared I still agreed. For 24 weeks I took the powerful antibiotics and astonishingly found that after the first day my symptoms seemed to vanish. Fully aware of the placebo effect I gave it more time and dreaded feeling the return of the pain I had felt pre-treatment. Weeks went by and nothing came out to haunt me. I was clear and rapidly feeling better and more awake. When I was finally tested again in December, I received the best news I could hope for. That the tests were returning normal calprotectin ranges (a measurement of gut inflammation). I was overjoyed but soon learnt that it wasn't the end of my treatment.

Another more interesting treatment lay ahead for me. A microbiome transplant was the next step. This involved taking the bacteria that formed the gut microbiome from a donor and transplanting it into my own gut, which at this point was very damaged by the long-term application of antibiotics. The theory was that a healthy microbiome would help to prevent the re-establishment of an MAP infection and as I understood it there were other patients who had gone into long term remission that way. I agreed and in April 2023 I underwent a procedure and began a course of home infusions for about 26 weeks.

Additionally, I was asked to change my diet to something that would help to maintain and nurture my new microbiome, which included a high-fibre diet and supplements like inulin, which were designed to feed the growing bacterial microbiome. It was a pleasant pivot from the often drug-heavy approach that I was used to dealing with, and focused more on how I could work with my own body to overcome disease. I followed the plan as strictly as I could and found that it improved my own health.

Finally, I felt like I was free from a purgatory of perpetually being "treated". Still, it would be foolish to believe that diet alone made this change. The combination of two different approaches, one more pharmaceutical and one more holistic, were required to provide the maximum benefit to me.

At the end of this treatment, I was monitored again, and my calprotectin was acceptably low, as is the case for my tests in 2024. While I'm not out of the woods yet and believe I won't be until there's a viable vaccination against MAP, I find that I'm symptom free and healthy without needing any further drugs at all."

Person 2

The following case study was completed by a person managing joint pain long term. Again, this case study was largely written by the person themselves and was included as it demonstrated the strengths and weaknesses of both the Western and Eastern approaches, as well as reasons for integrating both. As will be seen, in real life the line between 'Western' and 'Eastern' blurs, but best outcomes include both. At the request of the person providing the case study, they have been deidentified.

"I had experienced joint pain in both knees since my early teenage years. I had spoken with multiple bulk billing doctors who told me all I needed to do was rest and take anti-inflammatories. This continued for almost five years until I eventually found a "gap-fee" doctor who spent the time to investigate the cause of the inflammation. After a scan and a brief assessment, the doctor concluded I would need surgery and referred me to a knee specialist. I spoke with the specialist who confirmed I would need keyhole surgery on both sides of both knees to "clean up" my knees. Following the successful surgery, I was unable to walk for 12 weeks and was told that there was a large chance I would not be able to do contact or high impact sports again.

I was unhappy with this future prediction so investigated rehabilitation pathways. Several physiotherapists confirmed what the surgeon had said until one physiotherapist pointed me in the right direction. I was given specific exercises to improve mobility but was still advised to restrict the amount of exercise. I then spent the following ten years researching and completing short courses in exercise until I was able to find a balance. I also spoke with several dieticians and nutritionists who gave advise on what foods to eat to maintain a healthy weight (and to help maintain muscle growth).

By having the surgery, improving my nutrition, and finally finding exercises that improved my joint health and mobility, I am now able to perform most of the contact and high impact exercises I was once able to do. Although the quantity has been reduced. I still have to complete regular exercises (known as prehab exercises) as part of my warm up and continue to make healthy life choices."

Appendix/References

Formal References

1. Abel, J. L., & Larkin, K. T. (1990). Anticipation of performance among musicians: Physiological arousal, confidence, and state-anxiety. Psychology of music, 18(2), 171-182.
2. Abrahamson, E., & Langston, J. (2017). Making Sense of Human Anatomy and Physiology A Learner-Friendly Approach.
3. Academis, N. (2005). Dietary reference intakes for energy, carbohydrates, fiber, fat, fatty acids, cholesterol, protein, and amino acids., *Vol. 5.*, National Academy Press
4. Acebedo, A. (2012). Phenomenological analysis of the transformational experience of self in Ashtanga Vinyasa Yoga practice. Institute of Transpersonal Psychology.
5. Acid, P. Fact Sheet for Health Professionals". National Institutes of Health [Internet]. Available: https://ods.od.nih.gov/factsheets/PantothenicAcid, HealthProfessional.
6. Ackerman, D. (1991). A natural history of the senses. Vintage.
7. Ackerman, S. (1992). Discovering the brain.
8. Adams, A. (1973). Ninja: The Invisible Assassins. Ohara Publications Inc.
9. Aisbett, B. (2013). Fixing It: The Complete Survivor's Guide to Anxiety-Free Living. Harper Collins Inc.
10. Akinrodyoye, M. A., & Lui, F. (2020). Neuroanatomy, Somatic Nervous System
11. Albert, P. R. (2010). Epigenetics in mental illness: Hope or hype?. *Journal of psychiatry & neuroscience: JPN, 35*(6), 366.
12. Alberts, B. (2002). Molecular biology of the cell 4th edition. (No Title).
13. Alexander, P. (1994). It Could Be Allergy and It Can Be Cured
14. Ambrose, S. A., Bridges, M. W., DiPietro, M., Lovett, M. C., & Norman, M. K. (2010). How learning works: Seven research-based principles for smart teaching. John Wiley & Sons.
15. American Psychiatric Association. (2013). Diagnostic and statistical manual of mental disorders (5th ed.).
16. American Psychological Association. (2015). Guidelines for clinical supervision in health service psychology. *The American Psychologist, 70*(1), 33-46. https://doi.org/10.1037/a0038112
17. Anderson, Lorin W., and David R. Krathwohl, eds. 2001. A Taxonomy for Learning, Teaching, and Assessing: A Revision of Bloom's Taxonomy of Educational Objectives. New York: Addison Wesley Longman, Inc.
18. Andersson, L., King, R., & Lalande, L. (2010). Dialogical mindfulness in supervision role-play. Counselling and *Psychotherapy Research, 10*(4), 287-294. https://doi.org/10.1080/14733141003599500
19. Anderton, B. H. (2002). Ageing of the brain. Mechanisms of ageing and development, 123(7), 811-817.
20. Arden, J. B. (2010). Rewired Your Brain: Think Your Way to a Better Life. Wiley.
21. Armitage, C. J. (2009). Is there utility in the transtheoretical model?. British journal of health psychology, 14(2), 195-210.
22. Armstrong, T. (2015). The myth of the normal brain: Embracing neurodiversity. AMA Journal of Ethics, 17(4), 348-352. https://doi.org/10.1001/journalofethics.2015.17.4.msoc1-1504
23. Armstrong, P. (2010). Bloom's Taxonomy. Vanderbilt University Center for Teaching. Retrieved [January, 2024] from https://cft.vanderbilt.edu/guides-sub-pages/blooms- taxonomy/.
24. Armstrong, T. (2009). Multiple intelligences in the classroom. Ascd.
25. Arnow, L. E. (1976). Introduction to Physiological and Pathological Chemistry. Mosby Inc.
26. Aten, J. D., Strain, J. D., & Gillespie, R. E. (2008). A Transtheoretical Model of Clinical Supervision. *Training and Education in Professional Psychology, 2*(1), 1-9. https://doi.org/10.1037/1931-3918.2.1.1
27. Ausubel, D. P. (2012). The acquisition and retention of knowledge: a cognitive view. Springer Science Business Media.
28. Azizan, M. T., Mellon, N., Ramli, R. M., & Yusup, S. (2018). Improving teamwork skills and enhancing deep learning via development of board game using cooperative learning method in Reaction Engineering course. Education for Chemical Engineers, 22, 1-13.
29. Bahr, M. (1996). Structured Group Supervision: A Model for Supervisors of School Psychology Students and Practitioners. Presented at the *Annual National Convention of the National Association of School Psychologists*, Atlanta, GA, March 12-16. https://eric.ed.gov/?id=ED397379
30. Bailie, J. M. (1984). Giant Book of Knowledge. Octopus Publishing Group.
31. Baker, M. (2007). Music moves brain to pay attention. Stanford Study Finds. Retrieved December, 15, 2015.
32. Bandura, A. (1977). Social learning theory. Englewood Cliffs, NJ: Prentice Hall.
33. Barnett, J. E., Erickson Cornish, J. A., Goodyear, R. K., & Lichtenberg, J. W. (2007). Commentaries on the ethical and effective practice of clinical supervision. *Professional Psychology: Research and Practice, 38*(3), 268-275. https://doi.org/10.1037/0735-7028.38.3.268
34. Barret, K. E. (2010). Ganong; s Review of Medical Physiology. USA.
35. Barrett, C. A., Hazel, C. E., & Newman, D. S. (2017). Training confident school-based consultants: The role of course content, process, and supervision. Training and Education in Professional Psychology, 11(1), 41-48. https://doi.org/10.1037/tep0000128
36. Barrett, J., Gonsalvez, C. J., & Shires, A. (2020). Evidence-based practice within supervision during psychology practitioner training: A systematic review. Clinical Psychologist, 24(1), 3-17. https://doi.org/10.1111/cp.12196
37. Bastable, S. B. (2017). *Nurse as educator: Principles of teaching and learning for nursing practice*. Jones & Bartlett Learning, Boston. http://samples.jbpub.com/9781284104448/Sample_CH05_Bastable.pdf
38. Becker, R. O., Selden, G. (1998). The Body Electric: Electromagnetism and The Foundation of life
39. Ben-David, S., Blitzer, J., Crammer, K., Kulesza, A., Pereira, F., & Vaughan, J. W. (2010). A theory of learning from different domains. Machine learning, 79, 151-175.
40. Bennett-Levy, J. (2006). Therapist skills: A cognitive model of their acquisition and refinement. *Behavioural and Cognitive Psychotherapy, 34*(1), 57-78. https://doi.org/10.1017/S1352465805002420
41. Benowicz, R. J. (1983). Vitamins & You. Grosset & Dunlap.

42. Bergquist, W. The New Johari Window III: Interpersonal Relationships and the Locus of Control.
43. Bigger, B. B. (2012). Anita Marie Collins (Doctoral dissertation, The University of Melbourne).
44. Blocher, D. H. (1983). Toward a cognitive developmental approach to counseling supervision. *The Counseling Psychologist,* 11(1), 27-34. https://doi.org/10.1177/0011000083111006
45. Bodri, B., & Newtson, J. (2011) Internal Martial Arts Nei-gong Cultivating Your Inner Energy to Raise Your Martial Arts to the Next Level. Top Shape Publishing.
46. Bohlander, A., Geweniger, V. (2014). Pilates – A Teacher's Manual: Exercises with Mats and Equipment for Prevention and Rehabilitation
47. Bokiev, D., Bokiev, U., Aralas, D., Ismail, L., & Othman, M. (2018). Utilizing music and songs to promote student engagement in ESL classrooms. International Journal of Academic Research in Business and Social Sciences, 8(12), 314–332
48. Bolton, G. & Delderfield, R. (2018). *Reflective practice: Writing and professional development* (5th ed.). Sage Publishing.
49. Bordin, E. S. (1983). A working alliance based model of supervision. The Counselling Psychologist, 11, 35-41.
50. Borghuis, J., Hof, A. L., & Lemmink, K. A. (2008). The importance of sensory-motor control in providing core stability: implications for measurement and training. *Sports Medicine, 38, 893-916.*
51. Borriello, F., Iannone, R., & Marone, G. (2017). Histamine release from mast cells and basophils. Histamine and histamine receptors in health and disease, 121-139.
52. Bowman, P. (2019). Deconstructing martial arts (p. 182). Cardiff University Press.
53. Bradd, P., Travaglia, J., & Hayen, A. (2017). Leadership in allied health: A review of the literature. *Asia-Pacific Journal of Health Management, 12*(1), 17-24.
54. Brannon, L., & Feist, P. (1996). Health Psychology: An Introduction to Behaviour and Health. *Third Edition*. Wadsworth Publishing.
55. Bransford, J. D., & Johnson, M. K. (1972). Contextual prerequisites for understanding: Some investigations of comprehension and recall. Journal of verbal learning and verbal behavior, 11(6),717-726.
56. Brewer, B.C. (2012). Music and learning: Integrating music in the classroom. Johns Hopkins School of Education.
57. Brod, G., Werkle-Bergner, M., & Shing, Y. L. (2013). The influence of prior knowledge on memory: a developmental cognitive neuroscience perspective. Frontiers in behavioral neuroscience, 7, 139.
58. Burgoyne, A. P., Sala, G., Gobet, F., Macnamara, B. N., Campitelli, G., & Hambrick, D. Z. (2016). The relationship between cognitive ability and chess skill: A comprehensive meta-analysis. Intelligence, 59, 72-83.
59. Burkard, A. W., Knox, S., Clarke, R. D., Phelps, D. L., & Inman, A. G. (2014). Supervisors' experiences of providing difficult feedback in cross-ethnic/racial supervision. *The Counseling Psychologist, 42*(3), 314-344. https://doi.org/10.1177/0011000012461157
60. Burnham, T. (2001). Mean Genes: From Sex to Money to Food – Taming Our Primal Instincts. Simon & Schuster.
61. Burton, L., Westen, D., & Kowalski, R. (2006). Psychology: Australian and New Zealand Edition. John Wiley & Sons, Inc.
62. Burton, L., Westen, D., & Kowalski, R. (2008). Psychology 2: Australian and New Zealand Edition. John Wiley & Sons, Inc.
63. Bybee, R. W., Taylor, J. A., Gardner, A., Van Scotter, P., Powell, J. C., Westbrook, A., & Landes, N. (2006). The BSCS 5E instructional model: Origins and effectiveness. Colorado Springs, Co: BSCS, 5(88-98).
64. Calvert, F. L., Crowe, T. P., & Grenyer, B. F. S. (2017). An Investigation of Supervisory Practices to Develop Relational and Reflective Competence in Psychologists. *Australian Psychologist, 52*(6), 467-479. https://doi.org/10.1111/ap.12261
65. Campbell, J. (2000). *Becoming an effective supervisor: A workbook for counselors and psychotherapists.* Routledge.
66. Campbell, J. M. (2006). Essentials of clinical supervision (Vol. 28). John Wiley & Sons.
67. Cantillon, P., & Sargeant, J. (2008). Giving feedback in clinical settings. *British Medical Journal (International Edition), 337*(a1961), 1292–1294.
68. Carey, N. (2012). Epigenetics Revolution: How Modern Biology is Rewriting our Understanding of Genetics, Disease and Inheritance. Icon Books.
69. Carr, S. C., & Thompson, B. (1996). The effects of prior knowledge and schema activation strategies on the inferential reading comprehension of children with and without learning disabilities. Learning Disability Quarterly, 19(1), 48-61.
70. Carr, M., Borkowski, J. G., & Maxwell, S. E. (1991). Motivational components of underachievement. Developmental Psychology, 27(1), 108.
71. Carroll, M. (2009). From mindless to mindful practice: On learning reflection in supervision. *Psychotherapy in Australia, 15*(4), 38-
72. Carroll, M. (2010). Levels of reflection: On learning reflection. *Psychotherapy in Australia, 16*(2), 24-31.
73. Carroll, M. (2010). Supervision: Critical reflection for transformational learning (Part 2). *The Clinical Supervisor, 29*(1), 1-19. https://doi.org/10.1080/07325221003730301
74. Case-Smith, J., Weaver, L. L., & Fristad, M. A. (2014). A systematic review of sensory processing interventions for children with autism spectrum disorders. *Autism: The International Journal of Research and Practice*.
75. Cattaneo, L., & Rizzolatti, G. (2009). The mirror neuron system. Archives of neurology, 66(5), 557-560.
76. Center for Substance Abuse Treatment [CSAT]. (2009). Clinical supervision and professional development of the substance abuse counselor. *Treatment Improvement Protocol (TIP) Series*, No. 52. Rockville, MD, USA: Substance Abuse and Mental Health Services Administration [SAMHSA]. https://www.ncbi.nlm.nih.gov/books/NBK64845/
77. Ch'oe, H. (1998). Hap Ki Do: The Korean Art of Self Defense.
78. Chamberlain, T., & Smith, C. (2018). Shaping supervisory working alliance from a distance. *The Journal of Counselor Preparation and Supervision*, 11(2), 2.
79. Chang, T. I., Park, H., Kim, D. W., Jeon, E. K., Rhee, C. M., Kalantar-Zadeh, K., ... & Han, S. H. (2020). Polypharmacy, hospitalization, and mortality risk: a nationwide cohort study. Scientific reports, 10(1), 18964.
80. Chaplan, J. P. (1970). Dictionary of Psychology. Dell Publishing.
81. Chaurasia, B. D. (2004). Human anatomy (p. 53). New Delhi, India: CBS Publisher.
82. Cheetham, G., & Chivers, G. (1998). The reflective (and competent) practitioner: A model of professional competence which seeks to harmonise the reflective practitioner and competence-based approaches. *Journal of European Industrial Training, 22*(7), 267-276. https://doi.org/10.1108/03090599810230678

83. Chen, N., Xia, X., Qin, L., Luo, L., Han, S., Wang, G., ... & Wan, Z. (2016). Effects of 8-Week Hatha Yoga Training on Metabolic and Inflammatory Markers in Healthy, Female Chinese Subjects: A Randomized Clinical Trial. BioMed research international, 2016(1), 5387258.
84. Chen, W., & Zhao, J. (2022). Open the Black-box of "Informational Learning Style": Discussions Based-on Don Ihde's Phenomenology of Technology. Journal of East China Normal University (Educational Sciences), 40(10), 100.
85. Cheng, G., & Chau, J. (2016). Exploring the relationships between learning styles, online participation, learning achievement and course satisfaction: An empirical study of a blended learning course. British Journal of Educational Technology, 47(2), 257–278. https://doi.org/10.1111/bjet.12243
86. Chia, M. (1986). Iron Shirt Chi Kung I: Once a Martial Art, Now the Practice that Strengthens the Internal Organs, Roots Oneself Solidly, and Unifies Physical, Mental, and Spiritual Health. Universal Tao Publications.
87. Cho, S. H. (1969). Self-Defense Karate. Stravon Educational Press.
88. Christ, S. (2013). 20 Surprising, Science-backed Health Benefits of Music. USA Today. Gannett, 17.
89. Chutkan, R. (2016). Microbiome Solution: A radical new way to heal your body from the inside out. Scribe Publications.
90. Clarke, G., Stilling, R. M., Kennedy, P. J., Stanton, C., Cryan, J. F., & Dinan, T. G. (2014). Minireview: gut microbiota: the neglected endocrine organ. Molecular endocrinology, 28(8), 1221-1238.
91. Clark, R. (2012). Pressure-point Fighting: A Guide to the Secret Heart of Asian Martial Arts. Tuttle Publishing.
92. Cohen, M. J. (1993). Integrated ecology: The process of counseling with nature. The Humanistic Psychologist, 21(3), 277-295.
93. Cohen, M., J., Schreiner, R. (2007). Reconnecting with Nature: Finding wellness through restoring your bond with the Earth.
94. Collins, A. (2009). A boy's music ecosystem. Male voices: Stories of boys learning through making music.
95. Collins, A. (2014). Neuroscience, music education and the pre-service primary (elementary) generalist teacher. International Journal of Education & the Arts, 15(5).
96. Cook, R. M., McKibben, W. B., & Wind, S. A. (2018). Supervisee perception of power in clinical supervision: The Power Dynamics in Supervision Scale. Training and Education in Professional Psychology, 12(3), 188-195. https://doi.org/10.1037/tep0000201
97. Cooper, C. L., & Cartwright, S. (1994). Healthy mind; healthy organization: A proactive approach to occupational stress. Human Relations, 47, 455-471.
98. Cooper, G. M., & Adams, K. (2022). The cell: a molecular approach. Oxford University Press.
99. Cooper, E. L. (2003). Neuroimmunology of autism: a multifaceted hypothesis. International journal of immunopathology and pharmacology, 16(3), 289-292.
100. Coulson, D., & Harvey, M. (2013). Scaffolding student reflection for experience-based learning: A framework. Teaching in Higher Education, 18(4), 401-413.
101. Cowan, N. (2008). What are the differences between long-term, short-term, and working memory?. Progress in brain research, 169, 323-338.
102. Cramer, H., Quinker, D., Pilkington, K., Mason, H., Adams, J., & Dobos, G. (2019). Associations of yoga practice, health status, and health behavior among yoga practitioners in Germany—Results of a national cross-sectional survey. Complementary Therapies in Medicine, 42, 19-26.
103. Crawford, S., & Stucki, L. (1990). Peer review and the changing research record. Journal of the American Society for Information Science, 41(3), 223-228.
104. Crudelli, C. (2008). The Way of the Warrior. Dorling Kindersley Ltd.
105. Cruise, T. K. (2018). Supervision: Feedback and Evaluation. Communique, 47(1), 4-6.
106. Cummins, A. (2016). Samurai and Ninja: The Real Story Behind the Japanese Warrior Myth that Shatters the Bushido Mystique. Tuttle Publishing.
107. Curtis, D. F., Elkins, S. R., Duran, P., & Venta, A. C. (2016). Promoting a climate of reflective practice and clinician self-efficacy in vertical supervision. Training and Education in Professional Psychology, 10(3), 133-140. https://doi.org/10.1037/tep0000121
108. D'Souza, C., (n.d.)., Good Health Through Spices, Herbs and Indian Dishes
109. Dapretto, M., Davies, M.S., Pfiefer, J.H., Scott, A.A., Sigman, M., Bookheimer, S.Y., Iacoboni, M. (2006). Understanding Emotions in Others: Mirror Neuron Dysfunction in Children with Autism Spectrum Disorders. Nature Neuroscience, 9(1), 28–30.
110. Dattilio, F. M. (2015). The self-care of psychologists and mental health professionals: A review and practitioner guide. Australian Psychologist, 50(6), 393–399. https://doi.org/10.1111/ap.12157
111. Davey, B. (1983). Think aloud: Modeling the cognitive processes of reading comprehension. Journal of reading, 27(1), 44-47.
112. Davis Jr, G. E., & Lowell, W. W. (2006). Solar Cycles and their relationship to human disease and adaptability. Medical hypotheses, (67(3), 447-461.
113. Dawson, M., Phillips, B., & Leggat, S. G. (2013). Effective clinical supervision for regional allied health professionals: the supervisor's perspective. Australian Health Review, 37(2), 262-267.
114. De Stefano, J., Hutman, H., & Gazzola, N. (2017). Putting on the face: A qualitative study of power dynamics in clinical supervision. The Clinical Supervisor, 36(2), 223-240. https://doi.org/10.1080/07325223.2017.1295893
115. Deane, F. P., Gonsalvez, C., Blackman, R., Saffioti, D., & Andresen, R. (2015). Issues in the Development of e-supervision in Professional Psychology: A Review. Australian Psychologist, 50(3), 241-247. https://doi.org/10.1111/ap.12107
116. Delany, C. & Watkin, D. (2009). A study of critical reflection in health professional education: 'learning where others come from.' Advances in Health science Education, 14, 411-429. https://doi.org/10.1007/s10459-008-9128-0
117. Demarin, V., & MOROVIĆ, S. (2014). Neuroplasticity. Periodicum biologorum, 116(2), 209-211.
118. Devdas, L. (2015). Evaluation Feedback Process in Supervision Using Critical Events Model [Unpublished doctoral dissertation]. Lehigh University. https://preserve.lehigh.edu/cgi/viewcontent.cgi?article=3572&context=etd
119. Dewar, G. C. (2003). Innovation and social transmission in animals: A cost-benefit model of the predictive function of social and nonsocial cues. University of Michigan.
120. Dezelic, M. (2013). Window of tolerance – trauma/anxiety related responses: Wielding the comfort zone for increased flexibility

121. Dickson, J. M., Moberly, N. J., Marshall, Y., & Reilly, J. (2011). Attachment style and its relationship to working alliance in the supervision of British clinical psychology trainees. *Clinical Psychology & Psychotherapy*, 18(4), 322-330. https://doi.org/10.1002/cpp.715
122. Dietrich, K., & Bidart, M. G. (2021). Hatha yoga improves psychophysiological responses of college students in both indoor and outdoor environments. OBM Integrative and Complementary Medicine, 6(4), 1-14.
123. Dochy, F., Gijbels, D., Segers, M., & Van, D. B. P. (2021). Theories of workplace learning in changing times. ProQuest Ebook Central. https://ebookcentral.proquest.com
124. Doidge, N. (2008). The Brain that Changes Itself: Stories of Personal Triumph from the Frontiers of Brain Science.
125. Dollard, M. F. (1996). Work stress: Conceptualisations and implications for research methodology and workplace intervention. PhD dissertation. Whyalla, South Australia: Work & Stress Research Group, University of South Australia.
126. Dompe, C., Moncrieff, L., Matys, J., Grzech-Leśniak, K., Kocherova, I., Bryja, A., ... & Dyszkiewicz-Konwińska, M. (2020). Photobiomodulation—underlying mechanism and clinical applications. *Journal of clinical medicine*, 9(6), 1724.
127. Doran, G.T. (1981) There's a SMART Way to Write Management's Goals and Objectives. Journal of Management Review, 70, 35-36.
128. Doss, C. J., Steiner, E. D., & Hamilton, L. S. Teacher Perspectives on Social and Emotional Learning in Massachusetts.
129. Driscoll, J., & Teh, B. (2001). The potential of reflective practice to develop individual orthopaedic nurse practitioners and their practice. *Journal of Orthopaedic Nursing, 5*(2), 95-103.
130. Drucker, P. F., (1954). "The Practice of Management". New York: Elsevier, : 109-110.
131. Ducat, W. H., & Kumar, S. (2015). A systematic review of professional supervision experiences and effects for allied health practitioners working in non-metropolitan health care settings. *Journal of Multidisciplinary Healthcare, 8*, 397-407. https://doi.org/10.2147/JMDH.S84557
132. Duff, C. T., & Shahin, J. (2010). Conflict in Clinical Supervision: Antecedents, Impact, Amelioration, and Prevention. *Alberta Counsellor*, 31(1), 3.
133. Duplechain, R., Reigner, R., & Packard, A. (2008). Striking differences: The impact of moderate and high trauma on reading achievement. Reading Psychology, 29(2), 117-136.
134. Duțu, R., & Butucescu, A. (2019). On the Link between Transformational Leadership and Employees' Work Engagement: The Role of Psychological Empowerment. *Psychology of Human Resources Journal, 17*(2), 76–87. https://doi.org/10.24837/pru.v17i2.291
135. Easley, T., & Horne, S. (2016). The Modern Herbal Dispensatory: A Medicine-Making Guide
136. Eight Ways framework. (2009). NSW Department of Education initiative. https://www.8ways.online/
137. Ellis, M. V. (2017). Narratives of harmful clinical supervision. *The Clinical Supervisor*, 36(1), 20-87. https://doi.org/10.1080/07325223.2017.1297752
138. Ellis, M. V., Berger, L., Hanus, A. E., Ayala, E. E., Swords, B. A., & Siembor, M. (2014). Inadequate and Harmful Clinical Supervision: Testing a Revised Framework and Assessing Occurrence. *The Counseling Psychologist*, 42(4), 434-472. https://doi.org/10.1177/0011000013508656
139. Elshakry, M. (2010). When science became Western: Historiographical reflections. Isis, 101(1), 98-109.
140. Falender, C. A. & E. P. Shafranske (2017). Competency-based clinical supervision: status, opportunities, tensions, and the future. *Australian Psychologist, 52*(2), 86-93.
141. Falender, C. A. (2014). Clinical supervision in a competency-based era. *South African Journal of Psychology*, 44(1), 6-17. https://doi.org/10.1177/0081246313516260
142. Falender, C. A. (2018). Clinical supervision-the missing ingredient. *The American psychologist*, 73(9), 1240-1250. https://doi.org/10.1037/amp0000385
143. Falender, C. A., & Shafranske, E. P. (2014). Clinical Supervision: The State of the Art. Journal of Clinical *Psychology, 70*(11), 1030-1041. https://doi.org/10.1002/jclp.22124
144. Falender, C. A., & Shafranske, E. P. (2017). Competency-based Clinical Supervision: Status, Opportunities, Tensions, and the Future. *Australian Psychologist, 52*(2), 86-93. https://doi.org/10.1111/ap.12265
145. Falender, C. A., & Shafranske, E. P. (2017b). Supervision essentials for the practice of competency-based supervison. American Psychological Association.
146. Falender, C. A., Cornish, J. A. E., Goodyear, R., Hatcher, R., Kaslow, N. J., Leventhal, G., . . . Grus, C. (2004). Defining competencies in psychology supervision: A consensus statement. *Journal of Clinical Psychology, 60*(7), 771-785. https://doi.org/10.1002/jclp.20013
147. Falender, C. A., Cornish, J. A. E., Goodyear, R., Hatcher, R., Kaslow, N. J., Leventhal, G., Shafranske, E., Sigmon, S. T., Stoltenberg, C., & Grus, C. (2004). Defining competencies in psychology supervision: A consensus statement. *Journal of Clinical Psychology, 60*(7), 771-785. https://doi.org/10.1002/jclp.20013
148. Falender, C. A., Falender, C. A., Shafranske, E. P., & Shafranske, E. P. (2012). The Importance of Competency-based Clinical Supervision and Training in the Twenty-first Century: Why Bother? *Journal of Contemporary Psychotherapy, 42*(3), 129-137. https://doi.org/10.1007/s10879-011-9198-9
149. Falender, C. A., Shafranske, E. P., & Ofek, A. (2014). Competent clinical supervision: Emerging effective practices. *Counselling Psychology Quarterly*, 27(4), 393-408.
150. Falender, C.A. & Shafranske, E.P. (2014), Clinical supervision: The state of the art. *Journal of Clinical Psychology, 70*, 1030-1041.
151. Feldenkrais, M. (1985). The potent self: A guide to spontaneity. Harper & Row.
152. Feldenkrais, M. (1987). Awareness Through Movement: Health Exercises for Personal Growth. Penguin Handbooks
153. Feldenkrais, M. (2011). Embodied wisdom: The collected papers of Moshé Feldenkrais. North Atlantic Books.
154. Felder, R. M., & Soloman, B. A. (2000). *Learning styles and strategies*. https://www.andrews.edu/services/ctcenter/career-center/learning-styles-strategies/learning-styles-and-strategies.pdf
155. Felder, R.M., & Soloman, B. A. (1997). *Index of Learning Styles questionnaire*. https://www.webtools.ncsu.edu/learningstyles/
156. Figley, C.R. (1995). Compassion fatigue: Coping with secondary traumatic stress disorder in those who treat the traumatized. New York: Brummer/Mazel.
157. Finkelstein, H., & Tuckman, A. (1997). Supervision of psychological assessment: A developmental model. *Professional Psychology: Research and Practice*, 28(1), 92-95. https://doi.org/10.1037//0735-7028.28.1.92

158. Fook, J. (2006). *Beyond reflective practice: reworking the 'critical' in critical reflection*. Keynote paper presented at Professional Lifelong Learning: beyond reflective practice, a one-day conference held at Trinity and All Saints College, Leeds, 3 July. http://www.leeds.ac.uk/educol/documents/155665.pdf
159. Fook, J. (2015). Reflective practice and critical reflection. In J. Lishman (Ed.), *Handbook for practice learning in social work and social care: Knowledge and theory* (3rd ed., pp. 440-454).
160. Foran, L. M. (2009). Listening to music: Helping children regulate their emotions and improve learning in the classroom. Educational Horizons, 88(1) 51-58.
161. Forehand, M. (2005). Bloom's taxonomy: Original and revised. Emerging perspectives on learning, teaching, and technology, 8, 41-44.
162. Fortuna, L. R., & Vallejo, Z. (2015). Treating co-occurring adolescent PTSD and addiction: Mindfulness-based cognitive therapy for adolescents with trauma and substance-abuse disorders. New Harbinger Publications.
163. Fourlanos, S., Dotta, F., Greenbaum, C. J., Palmer, J. P., Rolandsson, O., Colman, P. G., & Harrison, L. C. (2005). Latent autoimmune diabetes in adults (LADA) should be less latent., *Diabetologia, 48*, 2206-2212.
164. Fox, K. C., Nijeboer, S., Dixon, M. L., Floman, J. L., Ellamil, M., Rumak, S. P., Sedleimer, P., & Christoff, K. (2014). Is meditation associated with altered brain structure? A systematic review and meta-analysis of morphometric neuroimaging in meditation practitioners. *Neuroscience & Biobehavioral Reviews, 43*, 48-73. https://doi.org/10.1016/j.neubiorev.2014.03.016
165. Fragkos, K. C. (2016). Reflective practice in healthcare education: an umbrella review. *Education Sciences, 6*(3), 27.
166. Freeberg, L. (2009). Discovering Biological Psychology. Cengage Learning.
167. Freire, P. (2005). *Pedagogy of the Oppressed* (30th Anniversary). New York, NY: Continuum. https://commons.princeton.edu/inclusivepedagogy/wp-content/uploads/sites/17/2016/07/freire_pedagoy_of_the_oppresed_ch2-3.pdf
168. Frensch, P. A. (1998). One concept, multiple meanings: On how to define the concept of implicit learning. In M. A. Stadler & P. A. Frensch (Eds.), *Handbook of implicit learning* (pp. 47–104). Sage Publications, Inc.
169. Freshwater, D., Taylor, B. J., & Sherwood, G (2008). *International Textbook of Reflective Practice in Nursing*. Blackwell Publishing.
170. Friedlander, M. L. (2015). Use of relational strategies to repair alliance ruptures: How responsive supervisors train responsive psychotherapists. Psychotherapy, 52(2), 174-179. https://doi.org/10.1037/a0037044
171. Frieze, S. (2015). How Trauma Affects Student Learning and Behaviour. BU Journal of Graduate Studies in Education, 7(2), 27-34.
172. Gallese, V. (2006). Intentional attunement: A neurophysiological perspective on social cognition and its disruption in autism. Brain Research, 1079(1), 15-24
173. Gardner, H. (1993). Multiple intelligences: The theory in practice. Basic books.
174. Gardner, H., & Hatch, T. (1989). Educational implications of the theory of multiple intelligences. Educational researcher, 18(8), 4-10.
175. Garg, G., Bhati, S., & Kataria, S. The role of wild plants and herbs in restoring holistic health and fighting the infections borne by the epidemic COVID-19.
176. Garrett, R. H., & Grisham, C. M. (2016). Biochemistry. Cengage Learning.
177. Gasiorowicz, S., & Langacker, P. (2022). Elementary Particles in Physics.
178. Gaskins, R., Jennings, E., Thind, H., Becker, B., & Bock, B. (2014). Acute and cumulative effects of vinyasa yoga on affect and stress among college students participating in an eight-week yoga program: A pilot study. International journal of yoga therapy, 24(1), 63-70.
179. Gates, N. J. & C. I. Sendiack (2017). Neuropsychology Supervision: Incorporating Reflective Practice. *Australian Psychologist, 52*(3): 191-197.
180. Geiger, G., Cattaneo, C., Galli, R., Pozzoli, U., Lorusso, M. L., Facoetti, A., & Molteni, M. (2008). Wide and diffuse perceptual modes characterize dyslexics in vision and audition. Perception, 37(11), 1745-1764.
181. Gerber, A. S., Green, D. P., Kaplan, E. H., Shapiro, I., Smith, R. M., & Massoud, T. (2014). The illusion of learning from observational research. Field experiments and their critics: Essays on the uses and abuses of experimentation in the social sciences, 9-32.
182. Ghaye, T., & Lillyman, S. (2006). *Learning journals and critical incidents: Reflective practice for health care professionals*. Quay books.
183. Gibbs, G. (1988). *Learning by doing: A guide to teaching and learning methods*. Further Education Unit.
184. Gimbert, B. G., Miller, D., Herman, E., Breedlove, M., & Molina, C. E. (2023). Social emotional learning in schools: The importance of educator competence. Journal of Research on Leadership Education, 18(1), 3-39.
185. Goldstein, E. B. (2014). Cognitive psychology: Connecting mind, research and everyday experience. Cengage Learning.
186. Goleman, D. (1996). Emotional Intelligence: Why it can matter more than IQ. Bloomsbury Publishing.
187. Goleman, D., & Boyatzis, R. (2008). Social intelligence and the biology of leadership. *Harvard Business Review, 86*(9), 74-81. http://files-au.clickdimensions.com/aisnsweduau-akudz/files/inteligencia-social-y-biologia-de-un-lider.pdf
188. Gonsalvez, C. J., & Crowe, T. P. (2014). Evaluation of psychology practitioner competence in clinical supervision. *American Journal of Psychotherapy*, 68(2), 177-193. https://doi.org/10.1176/appi.psychotherapy.2014.68.2.177
189. Gonsalvez, C. J., & McLeod, H. J. (2008). Toward the science-informed practice of clinical supervision: The Australian context. *Australian Psychologist*, 43(2), 79-87. https://doi.org/10.1080/00050060802054869
190. Gonsalvez, C. J., Wahnon, T., & Deane, F. P. (2017). Goal-setting, Feedback, and Assessment Practices Reported by Australian Clinical Supervisors. *Australian Psychologist, 52*(1), 21-30. https://doi.org/10.1111/ap.12175
191. Gonzalez, M. F., & Aiello, J. R. (2019, January 28). More than meets the ear: Investigating how music affects cognitive task performance. Journal of Experimental Psychology: Applied. Advance online publication. http://dx.doi.org/10.1037/xap0000202
192. Goodman, F. (2015). Karate, Aikido, Ju-jitso & Judo. Anness Publishing.
193. Goodyear, R. K., & Bernard, J. M. (1998). Clinical supervision: Lessons from the literature. *Counselor Education and Supervision, 38*(1), 6-22. https://doi.org/10.1002/j.1556-6978.1998.tb00553.x
194. Goodyear, R., Lichtenberg, J.W., Bang, K. & Gragg, J.B. (2014). Ten changes psychotherapists typically make as they mature into the role of supervisor. *Journal of Clinical Psychology*, 70(11), 1042-1050.
195. Gormally, C., Brickman, P., Hallar, B., & Armstrong, N. (2009). Effects of inquiry-based learning on students' science literacy skills and confidence. International journal for the scholarship of teaching and learning, 3(2), 16.

196. Grabara, M. (2017). Hatha yoga as a form of physical activity in the context of lifestyle disease prevention. Polish Journal of Sport and Tourism, 24(2), 65-71.
197. Graesser, A. C. (2009). *Inaugural Editorial for Journal of Educational Psychology* (Vol. 101, Issue 2, pp. 259–261). American Psychological Association.
198. Gray, D. E. (2007). Towards a systemic model of coaching supervision: Some lessons from psychotherapeutic and counselling models. *Australian Psychologist*, 42(4), 300-309. https://doi.org/10.1080/00050060701648191
199. Green, T. A. (2010). Martial arts of the world: an encyclopedia of history and innovation (Vol. 2). Abc-Clio.
200. Green, T. A. (2010). Martial arts of the world: an encyclopedia of history and innovation (Vol. 1). Abc-Clio.
201. Greenberg, G. (2014). How new ideas in physics and biology influence developmental science. Research in Human Development, 11(1), 5-21.
202. Greene, R. (2013). Mastery. Penguin.
203. Greensfelder, L. (2009). Study Finds Brain Hub That Links Music, Memory and Emotion. UC Davis. Science & Technology. February, 23.
204. Grimmer-Somers, K., Milanese, S., & Chipchase, L. (2011). *Research into Best Practices in e-Learning for Allied Health clinical education and training*. Brisbane: Clinical Education and Training Queensland. https://pdfs.semanticscholar.org/8ca2/5e279bd94fa45e178848199fb362e3f2dcda.pdf
205. Grus, C. L. (2013). The Supervision Competency: Advancing Competency-Based Education and Training in Professional Psychology. *The Counseling Psychologist*, 41(1), 131-139. https://doi.org/10.1177/0011000012453946
206. Guiffrida, D. A. (2005). The emergence model: An alternative pedagogy for facilitating self-reflection and theoretical fit in counseling students. *Counselor Education and Supervision, 44*(3), 201-213. https://doi.org/10.1002/j.1556-6978.2005.tb01747.x
207. Guiffrida, D. A. (2015). *Constructive clinical supervision in counseling and psychotherapy*. Routledge.
208. Hadjistavropoulos, H., Kehler, M., & Hadjistavropoulos, T. (2010). Training Graduate Students to be Clinical Supervisors: A Survey of Canadian Professional Psychology Programmes. *Canadian Psychology/Psychologie Canadienne*, 51(3), 206-212. https://doi.org/10.1037/a0020197
209. Hall, J. E., & Hall, M. E. (2020). Guyton and Hall textbook of medical physiology e-Book. Elsevier Health Sciences.
210. Hall, J., Kasujja, R. & Oakes, P. Clinical supervision for clinical psychology students in Uganda: an initial qualitative exploration. Int J Ment Health Syst 9, 24 (2015). https://doi.org/10.1186/s13033-015-0016-8
211. Halli-Tierney, A. D., Scarbrough, C., & Carroll, D. (2019). Polypharmacy: evaluating risks and deprescribing. *American family physician, 100*(1), 32-38.
212. Hamasaki, H. (2020). Effects of diaphragmatic breathing on health: a narrative review. *Medicines, 7*(10), 65.
213. Hambrick, D. Z., Campitelli, G., & Macnamara, B. N. (Eds.). (2017). The science of expertise: Behavioral, neural, and genetic approaches to complex skill. Routledge.
214. Hamilton, H., & Rose, M. B., (1984). Cardiovascular Disorders. Lippincott Williams & Wilkins.
215. Hanfstingl, B., Arzenšek, A., Apschner, J., & Gölly, K. I. (2021). Assimilation and accommodation. European Psychologist.
216. Harbottle, L., & Schonfelder, N. (2008). Nutrition and Depression: A review of the evidence. *Journal of Mental Health, 17*(6), 576-587.
217. Hari, J. (2016). Chasing the Scream: The First and Last Days of the War on Drugs. Bloomsbury Publishing.
218. Harmon-Jones, E., Harmon-Jones, C., & Levy, N. (2015). An action-based model of cognitive-dissonance processes. Current Directions in Psychological Science, 24(3), 184-189.
219. Harris, N., Case, E., & Sheppard, H. (2018). Predoctoral internship training: Psychology intern perspectives on an internship rotation targeting supervision competency development. *The Clinical Supervisor, 37*(2), 278-297. https://doi.org/10.1080/07325223.2017.1421110
220. Harrison, S. D. (2007). Where have the boys gone? The perennial problem of gendered participation in music. British Journal of Music Education, 24(3), 267-280.
221. Hatcher, R. L. (2015). Interpersonal competencies: Responsiveness, technique, and training in psychotherapy. *The American Psychologist*, 70(8), 747-757. https://doi.org/10.1037/a0039803
222. Hattie, J. (2011). *Which strategies best enhance teaching and learning in higher education in empirical research in teaching and learning?* (Eds D. Mashek and E.Y. Hammer). https://doi.org/10.1002/9781444395341.ch8
223. Hayes S.C., Strosahl K.D., Bunting K., Twohig M., Wilson K.G. (2004) What is Acceptance and Commitment Therapy? In S. C. Hayes & K. D. Strosahl (Eds.), *A Practical Guide to Acceptance and Commitment Therapy*. Springer, Boston, MA.
224. Heidenstam, D., Kramer, A., Midgley, R., Sturrock., et. al. (1984). Human Body. Galley Press.
225. Henderson, P. (2018). *A Different Wisdom: Reflections on Supervision Practice: Guide to Supervision*. Routledge.
226. Hendrickx, S. (2010). The adolescent and adult neuro-diversity handbook: Asperger's syndrome, ADHD, dyslexia, dyspraxia, and related conditions. Jessica Kingsley Publishers.
227. Heppner, P. P., & Roehlke, H. J. (1984). Differences among supervisees at different levels of training: Implications for a developmental model of supervision. *Journal of Counseling Psychology, 31*(1), 76-90. https://doi.org/10.1037/0022-0167.31.1.76
228. Hernández, P. (2008). The Cultural Context Model in Clinical Supervision. *Training and Education in Professional Psychology*, 2(1), 10-17. https://doi.org/10.1037/1931-3918.2.1.10
229. Hersh, D., Worrall, L., Howe, T., Sherratt, S., & Davidson, B. (2011). SMARTER goal setting in aphasia rehabilitation. Aphasiology, 26(2), 220–233. https://doi.org/10.1080/02687038.2011.640392
230. Hewson, D. & Carroll, M. (2016). *Reflective Supervision Toolkit*. MoshPit Publishing.
231. Hill, H. R. M., Crowe, T. P., & Gonsalvez, C. J. (2016). Reflective dialogue in clinical supervision: A pilot study involving collaborative review of supervision videos. *Psychotherapy Research*, 26(3), 263-278. https://doi.org/10.1080/10503307.2014.996795
232. Hmelo-Silver, C. E., Duncan, R. G., & Chinn, C. A. (2007). Scaffolding and achievement in problem-based and inquiry learning: a response to Kirschner, Sweller, and. Educational psychologist, 42(2), 99-107.
233. Ho, D. W., & Whitehill, T. (2009). Clinical supervision of speech-language pathology students: Comparison of two models of feedback. *International Journal of Speech-Language Pathology, 11*(3), 244-255. https://doi.org/10.1080/17549500902795468
234. Ho'o, M. (2004). Tai Chi Chun. Black Belt Magazine Video.

235. Honey, P. & Mumford, A. (1992). *The manual of learning styles* (3rd Edn.). Honey Publications.
236. Hossain, A., Habibullah-Al-Mamun, M., Nagano, I., Masunaga, S., Kitazawa, D., & Matsuda, H. (2022). Antibiotics, antibiotic-resistant bacteria, and resistance genes in aquaculture: risks, current concern, and future thinking. Environmental Science and Pollution Research, 1-22.
237. Huber, J. R. (2016). Strength-based clinical supervision: A positive psychology approach to clinical training. *Journal of Marital and Family Therapy, 42*(2), 363.
238. Hulse, D., & Robert, T. (2014). Preplanning for feedback in clinical supervision: enhancing readiness for feedback exchange. *The Journal of Counselor Preparation and Supervision, 6*(2), 4. https://doi.org/10.7729/62.1091
239. Iversen, S., Kupfermann, I., & Kandel, E. R. (2000). Emotional states and feelings. Principles of neural science, 4, 982-997.
240. Iwanicki, S., & Peterson, C. (2017). An Exploratory Study Examining Current Assessment Supervisory Practices in Professional Psychology. *Journal of Personality Assessment*, 99(2), 165-174. https://doi.org/10.1080/00223891.2016.1228068
241. Jackson, M. A., Verdi, S., Maxan, M. E., Shin, C. M., Zierer, J., Bowyer, R. C., ... & Steves, C. J. (2018). Gut microbiota associations with common diseases and prescription medications in a population-based cohort. Nature communications, 9(1), 2655.
242. Jacob. S. W., & Francone, C. A. (1974). Structure and Function in Man. Saunders, Ken & Georgie.
243. Jaycox, L. H., Langley, A. K., Stein, B., Wong, M., Sharma, P., Scott, M., & Schonlau, M. (2009). Support for students exposed to trauma: A pilot study. School Mental Health, 1(2), 49-60.
244. Jehaman, I., Yulianty, M., Karo-karo, T. M., & Harahap, F. R. (2023). Benefits of yin yoga and plank exercise on weight loss in overweight adolescents. Jurnal Pengmas Kestra (Jpk), 3(1), 115-120.
245. Jensen, P. S., Mrazek, D., Knapp, P. K., Steinberg, L., Pfeffer, C., Schowalter, J., & Shapiro, T. (1997). Evolution and revolution in child psychiatry: ADHD as a disorder of adaptation. Journal of the American Academy of Child & Adolescent Psychiatry, 36(12), 1672-1681.
246. Jessop, T., & Maleckar, B. (2016). The influence of disciplinary assessment patterns on student learning: a comparative study. Studies in Higher Education, 41(4), 696-711. https://doi.org/10.1080/03075079.2014.943170
247. Johns C. (2017). *Becoming A Reflective Practitioner* (5th. Edn). Blackwell Science Ltd, London, UK.
248. Johns, C. (1995). Framing learning through reflection within Carper's fundamental ways of knowing in nursing. *Journal of Advanced Nursing, 22*(2), 226-234.
249. Johnson, W. B., Barnett, J. E., Elman, N. S., Forrest, L., & Kaslow, N. J. (2013). The competence constellation model: A communitarian approach to support professional competence. *Professional Psychology: Research and Practice, 44*(5), 343-354. https://doi.org/10.1037/a0033131
250. Johnson, W. B., Skinner, C. J., & Kaslow, N. J. (2014). Relational Mentoring in Clinical Supervision: The Transformational Supervisor. *Journal of Clinical Psychology*, 70(11), 1073-1081. https://doi.org/10.1002/jclp.22128
251. Justice, N., Murphy, J. M., & Newman, D. S. (2018). A Deliberate Framework for Supervision in School Psychology. *Communique, 47*(2), 8-11.
252. Kaminoff, L., & Matthews, A. (2021). Yoga anatomy. Human Kinetics.
253. Kangos, K. A., Ellis, M. V., Berger, L., Corp, D. A., Hutman, H., Gibson, A., & Nicolas, A. I. (2018). American Psychological Association Guidelines for Clinical Supervision: Competency-Based Implications for Supervisees. *The Counseling Psychologist, 46*(7), 821-845. https://doi.org/10.1177/0011000018807128
254. Kapp, S. K., Gillespie-Lynch, K., Sherman, L. E., & Hutman, T. (2013). Deficit, difference, or both? Autism and neurodiversity. Developmental Psychology, 49(1), 59–71. https://doi.org/10.1037/a0028353
255. Karpicke, J. D. (2012). Retrieval-based learning: Active retrieval promotes meaningful learning. Current Directions in Psychological Science, 21(3), 157-163.
256. Katzir, T., Hershko, S., & Halamish, V. (2013). The effect of font size on reading comprehension on second and fifth grade children: Bigger is not always better. PloS one, 8(9), e74061.
257. Keil, M. S. (2016). *Mindfulness in clinical supervision: Impacts on the working alliance and supervisees' perceptions of self-efficacy* [Doctoral dissertation, Azusa Pacific University]. ProQuest Dissertations Publishing. https://search-proquest-com.elibrary.jcu.edu.au/docview/1800556808?pq-origsite=summon
258. Kendall, E., Murphy, P., O'Neill, V., & Bursnall, S. (2000). Occupational stress: Factors that contribute to its occurrence and effective management. Centre for Human Services, Griffith University.
259. Kelly, R. (2007). MD, The Human Antenna: Reading the Language of the Universe in the Songs of Our Cells.
260. Kendroud, S., Fitzgerald, L. A,. Murray, I., & Hanna, A. (2021). Physiology, Nociceptive pathways.
261. Kennedy, E.-K., Keaney, C., Shaldon, C., & Canagaratnam, M. (2018). A relational model of supervision for applied psychology practice: professional growth through relating and reflecting. *Educational Psychology in Practice, 34*(3), 282-299. https://doi.org/10.1080/02667363.2018.1456407
262. Khalsa, S. B., Cohen, L., McCall, T., Telles, S., & Cramer, H. (2024). The principles and practice of yoga in health care. Jessica Kingsley Publishers.
263. Kılavuz, Y. (2005). The effect of 5E learning method based on constructivist approach to the understanding of the concepts related to acids and bases of 10th graders. Post graduate Thesis, Institute of Science, Ankara.
264. Kimball, D. R., & Holyoak, K. J. (2000). Transfer and expertise. The Oxford handbook of memory, 109-122.
265. Kleingeld, A., van Mierlo, H., & Arends, L. (2011). "The Effect of Goal Setting on Group Performance: A Meta-analysis," Journal of Applied Psychology 96, no. 6: 1,289-1,304.
266. Knowles, M. S. (1984). *Andragogy in Action. Applying Modern Principles of Adult education*. Jossey-Bass.
267. Koenig, H. G., & Cohen, H. J. (2002). Psychosocial factors, immunity, and wound healing. The link between religion and health: Psychoneuroimmunology and the faith factor, 124-136.
268. Koga, R. (2004). Practical Aiki-Do Volume 1. DVD. Black Belt Magazine Video.
269. Kolb, D. (2007). *The Kolb learning style inventory*. Hay Resources Direct.
270. Kolb, D. (2015). *Experiential learning: Experience as the source of learning and Development*. Pearson Education Press.
271. Kolb, D. A. (1984). *Experience as the source of learning and development*. Prentice Hall.

272. Kolb, D. A., Boyatzis, R. E., & Mainemelis, C. (2001). Experiential learning theory: Previous research and new directions. In R. J. Sternberg & L.-F. Zhang (Eds.), *Perspectives on Thinking, Learning, and Cognitive Styles* (pp. 227-247). Lawrence Erbaum Associates.
273. Koruk, S., & Kara, A. (2019). Supervision Models in Psychological Counseling. Eskişehir Osmangazi Üniversitesi Sosyal Bilimler Dergisi, 20, 51-63. https://doi.org/10.17494/ogusbd.548256
274. Kouka, N. (2009). Psychiatry for Medical Students and Residents. USA.
275. Kozlowski, J. M., Pruitt, N. T., DeWalt, T. A., & Knox, S. (2014). Can boundary crossings in clinical supervision be beneficial? *Counselling Psychology Quarterly, 27*(2), 109-126. https://doi.org/10.1080/09515070.2013.870123
276. Kraemer Tebes, J., Matlin, S. L., Migdole, S. J., Farkas, M. S., Money, R. W., Shulman, L., & Hoge, M. A. (2011). Providing Competency Training to Clinical Supervisors Through an Interactional Supervision Approach. *Research on Social Work Practice*, 21(2), 190-199. https://doi.org/10.1177/1049731510385827
277. Kristenson, S. (2002). Alternatives to SMART goals. Found at www.developgoodhabits.com/
278. Krogh, A. (1922). The anatomy and physiology of capillaries. Yale University Press.
279. Kruk, R., Sumbler, K., & Willows, D. (2008). Visual processing characteristics of children with Meares–Irlen syndrome. Ophthalmic and Physiological Optics, 28(1), 35-46.
280. Kuiper, R. A., & Pesut, D. J. (2004). Promoting cognitive and metacognitive reflective reasoning skills in nursing practice: self-regulated learning theory. *Journal of advanced nursing, 45*(4), 381-391.
281. Kuipers, P., Pager, S., Bell, K., Hall, F., & Kendall, M. (2013). Do structured arrangements for multidisciplinary peer group supervision make a difference for allied health professional outcomes? *Journal of Multidisciplinary Healthcare, 6*, 391-397. https://doi.org/10.2147/JMDH.S51339
282. Ladany, N., Mori, Y., & Mehr, K. E. (2013). Effective and Ineffective Supervision. *The Counseling Psychologist*, 41(1), 28-47. https://doi.org/10.1177/0011000012442648
283. Lam, P., & Miller, M. (2006). Teaching Tai Chi Effectively: Simple and Proven Methods to Make Tai Chi Accessible to Everyone
284. Lane, S. J., Mailloux, Z., Schoen, S., Bundy, A., May-Benson, T. A., Parham, L. D., ... & Schaaf, R. C. (2019). Neural foundations of ayres sensory integration®. *Brain sciences, 9*(7), 153.
285. Larsson Sköld, M., Aluan, M., Norberg, J., Carlsson, J., Örebro, u., & Institutionen för juridik, p. o. s. a. (2018). To fail psychotherapy training: Students' and supervisors' perspectives on the supervisory relationship. European *Journal of Psychotherapy & Counselling*, 20(4), 391-410. https://doi.org/10.1080/13642537.2018.1529688
286. LaTrobe University. (2013, April 17). *Field Placement 1st Supervision Session Roleplay* [Video]. YouTube. https://youtu.be/saCn4nmLuKo
287. Lawson, A. E., & Karplus, R. (2002). The learning cycle. In A love of discovery: Science education—The second career of Robert Karplus (pp. 51-76). Dordrecht: Springer Netherlands.
288. Leach, R. M., Rees, P. J., & Wilmshurst, P. (1998). Hyperbaric oxygen therapy. *Bmj, 317*(7166), 1140-1143.
289. Ledet, L., Esparza, C. K., & Peloquin, S. M. (2005). The conceptualization, formative evaluation, and design of a process for student professional development. The American Journal of Occupational Therapy, 59(4), 457-466. https://doi.org/10.5014/ajot.59.4.457
290. Lee, B., & Uyehara, M. (2007). Bruce Lee's Fighting Method: Advanced Techniques. Ohara Publications, Incorporated.
291. Lee, B., & Uyehara, M. (2007). Bruce Lee's Fighting Method: Self-Defense Techniques. Ohara Publications, Incorporated.
292. Lee, B., & Uyehara, M. (2007). Bruce Lee's Fighting Method: Skill in Techniques. Ohara Publications, Incorporated.
293. Lee, J. L., Nader, K., & Schiller, D. (2017). An update on memory reconsolidation updating. Trends in cognitive sciences, 21(7), 531-545.
294. Lenz, A. S., & Smith, R. L. (2010). Integrating Wellness Concepts within a Clinical Supervision Model. *The Clinical Supervisor*, 29(2), 228-245.
295. Lépine, F. (2006). Qi-Gong and Kuji-In: A Practical Guide to an Oriental Esoteric Experience.
296. Lertola, J., Park, A. (2002). Anatomy of Anxiety: What triggers it and how the body responds., Time Magazine
297. Levine, J. A. (2002). Non-exercise activity thermogenesis (NEAT). Best Practice & Research Clinical Endocrinology & Metabolism, 16(4), 679-702.
298. Levitin, D. J. (2006). This is your brain on music: The science of a human obsession. Penguin.
299. Li, D., Duys, D. K., & Granello, D. H. (2019). Interactional patterns of clinical supervision: using sequential analysis. *Asia Pacific Journal of Counselling and Psychotherapy*, 10(1), 70-92. https://doi.org/10.1080/21507686.2018.1553791
300. Lieberman, M., & Peet, A. (2018). Marks' Basic Medical Biochemistry: A Clinical Approach.
301. Liese, B. S., & Esterline, K. M. (2015). Concept mapping: A supervision strategy for introducing case conceptualization skills to novice therapists. *Psychotherapy*, 52(2), 190-194. https://doi.org/10.1037/a0038618
302. Link, N., Chou, L., & Kasturia, S. (2011). The anatomy of martial arts: an illustrated guide to the muscles used in key kicks, strikes & throws. (No Title).
303. Little, J. (2016). *The warrior within: The philosophies of Bruce Lee*. Chartwell Books.
304. Littrell. J. M.. Lee-Borden, N.. & Lorenz, J. A. (1979). A developmental framework for counseling supervision. Counselor Education and Supervision, 19, 119-136.
305. Lizzio, A., Stokes, L., & Wilson, K. (2005). Approaches to learning in professional supervision: Supervisee perceptions of processes and outcome. *Studies in Continuing Education, 27*(3), 239-256. https://doi.org/10.1080/01580370500376622
306. Lloyd-Price, J., Abu-Ali, G., & Huttenhower, C. (2016). The healthy human microbiome. Genome medicine, 8, 1-11.
307. Lohman, D. F., & Lakin, J. M. (2011). Intelligence and reasoning. The Cambridge handbook of intelligence, 419-441.
308. London, M., Smither, J. W., & Adsit, D. J. (1997). Accountability: The achilles' heel of multisource feedback. *Group & Organization Management*, 22(2), 162–184. https://doi.org/10.1177/1059601197222003
309. Louth, S., Wheeler, K., Jamieson-Proctor, R., & Sanderson, T. (2023). Stoking the Fires of Pre-service Educators through Aboriginal and Torres Strait Islander Ways of Learning. International Journal of Educational Innovation and Research, 2(2), 104-113.
310. Low, S. (2011). Overcoming Gravity; A Systemic Approach to Gymnastics and Bodyweight Strength
311. Lu, D., Suetani, S., Cutbush, J., & Parker, S. (2019). Supervision contracts for mental health professionals: a systematic review and exploration of the potential relevance to psychiatry training in Australia and New Zealand. *Australasian Psychiatry*, 27(3), 225-229. https://doi.org/10.1177/1039856219845486

312. Luders, E., & Toga, A. W. (2010). Sex differences in brain anatomy. Progress in brain research, 186, 2-12.
313. Luft, J., & Ingham, H. (1961). The johari window. Human relations training news, 5(1), 6-7.
314. Luo, S., Valencia, C. A., Zhang, J., Lee, N. C., Slone, J., Gui, B., ... & Huang, T. (2018). Biparental inheritance of mitochondrial DNA in humans. Proceedings of the National Academy of Sciences, 115(51), 13039-13044.
315. Maddux, R. E., Daukantaité, D., & Tellhed, U. (2018). The effects of yoga on stress and psychological health among employees: An 8-and 16-week intervention study. Anxiety, Stress, & Coping, 31(2), 121-134.
316. Maltz, Maxwell., Furey, M. (2015). Psycho-Cybernetics: Updated and Expanded. Souvenir Press, UK.
317. Mann, K., Gordon, J., & MacLeod, A. (2009). Reflection and reflective practice in health professions education: a systematic review. *Advances in Health Sciences Education, 14*(4), 595-621.
318. Mantle, S. (2001). The seven learning styles. Teaching/Learning Methods and Skills-Pedagogy.
319. Marchesi, J. R., & Ravel, J. (2015). The vocabulary of microbiome research: a proposal. *Microbiome, 3*, 1-3.
320. Marino, M., Jamal, Z., & Zito, P. M. (2018). Pharmacodynamics.
321. Martin, G. N., Carlson, N. R., & Buskist, W. (2010). Psychology. *Fourth Edition*. Pearson Education.
322. Martin, P., Baldock, K., Kumar, S., & Lizarondo, L. (2019b). Factors that contribute to high-quality clinical supervision of the rural allied health workforce: lessons from the coalface. *Australian Health Review, 43*(6), 682-688. https://doi.org/10.1071/AH17258
323. Martin, P., Copley, J., & Tyack, Z. (2014). Twelve tips for effective clinical supervision based on a narrative literature review and expert opinion. *Medical teacher, 36*(3), 201-207.
324. Martin, P., Kumar, S., Lizarondo, L., & Baldock, K. (2019a). Debriefing about the challenges of working in a remote area: A qualitative study of Australian allied health professionals' perspectives on clinical supervision. *PLOS ONE, 14*(3). https://doi.org/10.1371/journal.pone.0213613
325. Maslach, C. & Jackson, S.E. (1981). The measurement of experienced burnout. Journal of Organizational Behavior, 2(2): 99-113. https://doi.org/10.1002/job.4030020205
326. Maslach, C., Jackson, S. E., & Leiter, M. P. (1996). Maslach burnout inventory manual (3rd ed.). Consulting Psychologists Press.
327. Maslach, C. (2008). Preventing burnout and building engagement. International Journal of Psychology, 43(3-4), 714–714.
328. Maslach, C. (2011). Burnout and engagement in the workplace: New perspectives. The European Health Psychologist, 13(3), 44-47.
329. McCann, T. (2011). *An evaluation of the effects of a training programme in Trauma Release Exercises on quality of life* (Master's thesis, University of Cape Town).
330. McEwen, B. Allostasis and Allostatic Load: Implications for Neuropsychomarmacology. Neuropsychopharmacology, 22, 108–124 (2000). https://doi.org/10.1016/S0893-133X(99)00129-3
331. McGrath, P. (2004). The burden of RA RA positive: survivors' and hospice patients' reflection on maintaining a positive attitude to serious illness. Support Care Cancer, 12, 25-33.
332. McLaughlin, A. C., & Byrne, V. E. (2020). A fundamental cognitive taxonomy for cognition aids. Human Factors, 62(6), 865-873.
333. McMahon, A. (2014). Four guiding principles for the supervisory relationship. Reflective Practice, 15(3), 333-346. https://doi.org/10.1080/14623943.2014.900010
334. McMahon, A., & Errity, D. (2014). From new vistas to life lines: Psychologists' satisfaction with supervision and confidence in supervising. *Clinical Psychology & Psychotherapy, 21*(3), 264-275. https://doi.org/10.1002/cpp.1835
335. Medina, J. (2009). Brain Rules: 12 Principles for Surviving and Thriving at Work, Home and School. Pear Press.
336. Melegrito, J. (2008). Philippine Fighting Arts. DVD. Black Belt Magazine Video.
337. Merizzi, A. (2019). Clinical supervision in older adult mental health services. *Working with Older People*, 23(4), 241-250. https://doi.org/10.1108/WWOP-09-2019-0024
338. Metz, A. E., Boling, D., DeVore, A., Holladay, H., Liao, J. F., & Vlutch, K. V. (2019). Dunn's model of sensory processing: an investigation of the axes of the four-quadrant model in healthy adults. *Brain sciences, 9*(2), 35.
339. Miller, T. W., Miller, J. M., Burton, D., Sprang, R., & Adams, J. (2005). Telehealth: A model for clinical supervision in allied health. *Internet Journal of Allied Health Sciences and Practice, 1*(2), 6. https://doi.org/ 10.1037/0735-7028.36.2.173
340. Miller, W. R., & Rollnick, S. (2012). Motivational interviewing: Helping people change. Guilford press.
341. Mills, M., Martino, W., & Lingard, B. (2007). Getting boys' education 'right': The Australian Government's Parliamentary Inquiry Report as an exemplary instance of recuperative masculinity politics. British journal of sociology of education, 28(1), 5-21.
342. Milne, D. (2007). An empirical definition of clinical supervision. *British Journal of Clinical Psychology, 46*(4), 437-447. https://doi.org/10.1348/014466507X197415
343. Milner, C. E. (2008). Functional Anatomy for Sport and Exercise: Quick Reference
344. Mol, S. (2001). Classical fighting arts of Japan: A complete guide to Koryū Jūjutsu. Kodansha International.
345. Moran, A. M., Coyle, J., Pope, R., Boxal, D., Nancarrow, S. A., & Young, J. (2014). Supervision, support and mentoring interventions for health practitioners in rural and remote contexts: An integrative review and thematic synthesis of the literature to identify mechanisms for successful outcomes. *Human Resources for Health, 12*, 10-40. https://doi.org/10.1186/1478-4491-12-10
346. Moran, D. J., & Ming, S. (2023). Finding your why and finding your way: An acceptance and commitment therapy workbook to help you identify what you care about and reach your goals. New Harbinger Publications.
347. Morris, E. M. J.& L. Bilich-Eric (2017). A framework to support experiential learning and psychological flexibility in supervision: SHAPE. *Australian Psychologist, 52*(2), 104-113.
348. Mottron, L. (2011). The power of autism. Nature, 479(7371), 33-35.
349. Mukhalalati, B. A., & Taylor, A. (2019). Adult learning theories in context: A quick guide for healthcare professional educators. *Journal of Medical Education and Curricular Development, 6*, 1-10. https://doi.org/10.1177/2382120519840332
350. Murchie, G. (1999). The seven mysteries of life: an exploration in science & philosophy. Houghton Mifflin Harcourt.
351. Musacchia, G., Sams, M., Skoe, E., and Kraus, N. 2007. Musicians have enhanced subcortical auditory and audiovisual processing of speech and music. Proc. Natl. Acad. Sci. U.S.A. 104:15894–8.
352. Myers, T. W. (2020). Anatomy Trains: Myofascial Meridians for Manual Therapists and Movement Professionals

353. Nakamura, M., Imaoka, M., & Takeda, M. (2021). Interaction of bone and brain: osteocalcin and cognition. International Journal of Neuroscience, 131(11), 1115-1123.
354. Nancarrow, S. A., Wade, R., Moran, A., Coyle, J., Young, J., & Boxall, D. (2014). Connecting practice: a practitioner centred model of supervision. *Clinical Governance: An International Journal*, 19(3), 235-252.
355. Nassif, C., Nassif, C., Schulenberg, S. E., Hutzell, R. R., & Rogina, J. M. (2010). Clinical supervision and logotherapy: Discovering meaning in the supervisory relationship. *Journal of Contemporary Psychotherapy*, 40(1), 21-29. https://doi.org/10.1007/s10879-009-9111-y
356. Nelson, M. L., Barnes, K. L., Evans, A. L., & Triggiano, P. J. (2008). Working with conflict in clinical supervision: Wise supervisors' perspectives. *Journal of Counseling Psychology*, 55(2), 172-184. https://doi.org/10.1037/0022-0167.55.2.172
357. Nestler, E. J., Peña, C. J., Kundakovic, M., Mitchell, A., & Akbarian, S. (2016). Epigenetic basis of mental illness. *The Neuroscientist*, 22(5), 447-463.
358. Neumann, K., D. (2023). Your Complete Guide to the Body Chakras., https://www.forbes.com/health/body/body-chakras-guide/
359. Nishikawa, T., & Motter, A. E. (2016). Symmetric states requiring system asymmetry. Physical review letters, 117(11), 114101.
360. Nishioka, H., & West, J. R. (2007). The Judo Textbook: In Practical Application. Black Belt Books.
361. Noonan, W. C., & Moyers, T. B. (1997). Motivational interviewing. Journal of Substance Misuse, 2(1), 8-16.
362. Northouse, P. G. (2013). *Leadership: Theory and practice* (6th ed.). SAGE.
363. Novak, J. R., Robinson, L. P., & Korn, L. E. (2021). What MFTs should know about nutrition, psychosocial health, and collaborative care with nutrition professionals. *Journal of Marital and Family Therapy*, 00, 1-21. https://doi.org/10.1111/jmft.12540
364. Oberman, L. M., & Ramachandran, V. S. (2007). The simulating social mind: The role of the mirror neuron system and simulation in the social and communicative deficits of autism spectrum disorders. Psychological Bulletin, 133(2), 310-327.
365. Oceana. (2007). Human Body: A comprehensive guide to the wonders of the body. Quantum Publishing Ltd.
366. Odendaal, J. S. (2000). Animal-assisted therapy—magic or medicine? *Journal of psychosomatic research*, 49(4), 275-280.
367. O'Donovan, A., et al. (2011). Towards best practice supervision of clinical psychology trainees. *Australian Psychologist*, 46(2), 101-112. https://doi.org/10.1111/j.1742-9544.2011.00033.x
368. Oleg, Y. (2015). Interdisciplinary Aspects of Learning: Physics and Psychology. Universal Journal of Educational Research, 3(11), 810-814.
369. Oleson, K. C., Poehlmann, K. M., Yost, J. H., Lynch, M. E., & Arkin, R. M. (2000). Subjective overachievement: Individual differences in self-doubt and concern with performance. Journal of Personality, 68(3), 491-524.
370. On, F. R., Jailani, R., Norhazman, H., & Zaini, N. M. (2013, March). Binaural beat effect on brainwaves based on EEG. In 2013 IEEE 9th International Colloquium on Signal Processing and its Applications (pp. 339-343). IEEE.
371. Orchowski, L., Evangelista, N. M., & Probst, D. R. (2010). Enhancing supervisee reflectivity in clinical supervision: A case study illustration. *Psychotherapy: Theory, Research, Practice, Training*, 47(1), 51. https://doi.org/10.1037/a0018844
372. Oren, G. K. (2012). Anatomy of Fitness: Yoga.
373. Oyama, M. (1967). Vital Karate. Japan Publications Trading Co.
374. Page, A., & Stritzke, W. (2014). *Clinical Psychology for Trainees: Foundations of Science-Informed Practice* (2nd ed.). Cambridge University Press. https://doi.org/10.1017/CBO9781139857109
375. Pailoor, S., & Mahato, S. P. (2024). Effect of Yoga Practice on Lung Capacity in Adolescent Girls. Indian Journal of YOGA Exercise & Sport Science and Physical Education, 21-25.
376. Pan, S. C., & Rickard, T. C. (2018). Transfer of test-enhanced learning: Meta-analytic review and synthesis. Psychological bulletin, 144(7), 710.
377. Pandey, K. R., Naik, S. R., & Vakil, B. V. (2015). Probiotics, prebiotics and synbiotics-a review. Journal of food science and technology, 52, 7577-7587.
378. Patrick, R. P., & Ames, B. N. (2015). Vitamin D and the omega-3 fatty acids control serotonin synthesis and action, part 2: Relevance for ADHD, bipolar disorder, schizophrenia, and impulsive behaviour. *The FASEB Journal*, 29(6), 2207-2222.
379. Pattie, S. (2023). My Eclectic Human Body: Eclectic Knowledge Journey. Ingram Content Group Australia Pty Ltd.
380. Pattie, S. (2024). Learning: Understanding Oneself and Improving How We Learn. Ingram Content Group Australia Pty Ltd.
381. Peale, N. V. (1990). The Power of Positive Thinking. Ebury Press.
382. Pearce, N., Beinart, H., Clohessy, S., & Cooper, M. (2013). Development and validation of the supervisory relationship measure: A self-report questionnaire for use with supervisors. *British Journal of Clinical Psychology*, 52(3), 249-268. https://doi.org/10.1111/bjc.12012
383. Peborde, S. & Pokorny, L. (n.d.). Review of Leadership Models. https://static1.squarespace.com/static/5796bb93d2b857facb720cde/t/57d9fdb6d2b85760483044a8/1473904056710/LeadershipGroupProjecthandout+SPeborde+LPokorny.pdf
384. Peeck, J., Van den Bosch, A. B., & Kreupeling, W. J. (1982). Effect of mobilizing prior knowledge on learning from text. Journal of Educational Psychology, 74(5), 771.
385. Perlmutter, D., & Loberg, K. (2014). Grain Brain: The Surprising Truth About Wheat, Carbs, and Sugars – Your Brain's Silent Killers. Hodder & Stoughton.
386. Pert, C. B. (2010). Molecules of emotion: The science behind mind-body medicine. Simon and Schuster.
387. Plomin, R., & Rowe, D. C. (1977). A twin study of temperament in young children. The Journal of Psychology, 97(1), 107-113.
388. Poole, David C.; Kano, Yutaka; Koga, Shunsaku; Musch, Timothy I. (March 2021). "August Krogh: Muscle capillary function and oxygen delivery". Comparative Biochemistry and Physiology Part A: Molecular & Integrative Physiology. 253: 110852. doi:10.1016/j.cbpa.2020.110852. PMC 7867635. PMID 33242636
389. Popper, K. (2005). The logic of scientific discovery. Routledge.
390. PosNER, G. J., Strike, K. A., Hewson, P. W., & Gertzog, W. A. (1982). Toward a theory of conceptual change. Science education, 66(2), 211-227.
391. Powell, D. J. (2006). *Clinical supervision in alcohol and drug abuse counseling: Principles, models, methods* (Rev. ed.). John Wiley & Sons.
392. Preston, A. R., & Eichenbaum, H. (2013). Interplay of hippocampus and prefrontal cortex in memory. Current biology, 23(17), R764-R773.
393. Pribram, K., & Gill, M. (1976). Freud's 'Project' Re-Assessed. Hutchinson & Co. Publishers.

394. Proctor, B. (1986). *Supervision: A cooperative exercise in accountability*. In: M. Marken & M. Payne (Eds.), Enabling and ensuring: Supervision in practice (pp. 21–34). National Youth Bureau and Council for Education and Training in Youth and Community Work.
395. Psychology Board of Australia (2020a). *Codes guidelines and policies*. Author. https://www.psychologyboard.gov.au/Standards-and-Guidelines/Codes-Guidelines-Policies.aspx
396. Psychology Board of Australia. (2013). *Guidelines for supervisors and supervisor training providers.* https://www.psychologyboard.gov.au/standards-and-guidelines/codes-guidelines-policies.aspx
397. Psychology Board of Australia. (2015-2019). *Registration standards: mandatory and psychology standards under National Law.* https://www.psychologyboard.gov.au/Standards-and-Guidelines/Registration-Standards.aspx
398. Psychology Board of Australia. (2018). *Guidelines for supervisors.* Author. https://www.psychologyboard.gov.au/documents/default.aspx?record=WD18%2f25494&dbid=AP&chksum=h5glqx6YFDTJqi3ihdaGlw%3d%3d
399. Psychology Board of Australia. (2018). *Guidelines for supervisors.* https://www.psychologyboard.gov.au/documents/default.aspx?record=WD18%2f25494&dbid=AP&chksum=h5glqx6YFDTJqi3ihdaGlw%3d%3d
400. Ptak, C., & Petronis, A. (2022). Epigenetic approaches to psychiatric disorders. *Dialogues in clinical neuroscience*.
401. Purves, D., Augustine, G. J., et. al. (2004). Neuroscience: Third Edition., Sinauer Associates.
402. Quail, M., Brundage, S. B., Spitalnick, J., Allen, P. J., & Beilby, J. (2016). Student self-reported communication skills, knowledge and confidence across standardised patient, virtual and traditional clinical learning environments. *BMC Medical Education*, 16(1), 73-85.
403. Quigley, E. M. (2013). Gut bacteria in health and disease. Gastroenterology & hepatology, 9(9), 560.
404. Radey, M & Figley, C.R. (2007). The social psychology of compassion. Clinical Social Work Journal, 35, 207-214.
405. Rakovshik, S. G., McManus, F., Vazquez-Montes, M., Muse, K., & Ougrin, D. (2016). Is supervision necessary? Examining the effects of internet-based CBT training with and without supervision. *Journal of Consulting and Clinical Psychology*, 84(3), 191-199. https://doi.org/10.1037/ccp0000079
406. Ram, B. (2009). The 8 Limbs of Yoga: Pathway to Liberation. Lotus Press.
407. Randall, J. M., Matthews, R. T., and Stiles, M. A. (1997). Resonant frequencies of standing humans. *Ergonomics, 40(9), 879-886*
408. Rauscher, F. H., Shaw, G. L., and Ky, K. N. 1995. Listening to Mozart enhances spatial-temporal reasoning: towards a neurophysiological basis. Neurosci. Lett. 185:44–7
409. Reinisch, S., Höller, J., & Maluschka, A. (2012). The Secrets of Kyusho-Pressure Point Fighting. Meyer & Meyer Verlag.
410. Rim, J. B., & Sheya, J. (2005). Traditional Hapkido Volume 2. DVD. Black Belt Magazine Video.
411. Robert M. Sapolsky: Award for Distinguished Scientific Contributions (2013). American Psychologist, 68(8), 613–615. https://doi.org/10.1037/a0034773
412. Roche, A. M., Todd, C. L., & O'Connor, J. (2007). Clinical supervision in the alcohol and other drugs field: An imperative or an option? *Drug and Alcohol Review*, 26(3), 241–249. https://doi.org/10.1080/09595230701247780
413. Roe, R. A. (2002). What makes a competent psychologist? *European Psychologist*, 7(3), 192-203. https://doi.org/10.1027//1016-9040.7.3.192
414. Roediger, H. L., & Butler, A. C. (2011). The critical role of retrieval practice in long-term retention. Trends in cognitive sciences, 15(1), 20-27.
415. Romans, J. S. C., & Worthen, V. E. (1989). Comment on developmental models of supervision. *Professional Psychology: Research and Practice*, 20(6), 363-363. https://doi.org/10.1037/h0092790
416. Roney, A & Cooper, C. (1997). Professionals on workplace stress: The essential facts. Chichester:John Wiley and Sons.
417. Rosko, L., Smith, V. N., Yamazaki, R., & Huang, J. K. (2019). Oligodendrocyte bioenergetics in health and disease. The Neuroscientist, 25(4), 334-343.
418. Rowland, C. A. (2014). The effect of testing versus restudy on retention: a meta-analytic review of the testing effect. Psychological bulletin, 140(6), 1432.
419. Ruiz-Martín, H., & Bybee, R. W. (2022). The cognitive principles of learning underlying the 5E Model of Instruction. International journal of STEM Education, 9(1), 21.
420. Saarikallio, S., and Erkkila, J. (2007). The role of music in adolescents' mood regulation. Psychology of Music. 35 (1), 88-109.
421. Saddawi-Konefka, D., Baker, K., Guarino, A., Burns, S. M., Oettingen, G., Gollwitzer, P. M., & Charnin, J. E. (2017). Changing resident physician studying behaviors: A randomized, comparative effectiveness trial of goal setting versus use of WOOP. Journal of graduate medical education, 9(4), 451-457.
422. Sadock, B. J., Sadock, V. A., & Ruiz, P. (2015). Kaplan & Sadock's Synopsis of Psychiatry: Behavioural Sciences/Clinical Psychiatry. *Eleventh Edition*.
423. Sakai, J. (2020). How synaptic pruning shapes neural wiring during development and, possibly, in disease. Proceedings of the National Academy of Sciences, 117(28), 16096-16099.
424. Santrock, J. W. (2010). Life-Span Development. McGraw-Hill Higher Education.
425. Sari, O., Purnawati, S., & Wahyuni, N. (2022). Yin yoga improves sleep quality more than Vinyasa yoga on female office workers with mild to moderate insomnia during the COVID-19 pandemic. International Journal of Research in Medical Sciences, 10(9), 1.
426. Saxena, P. (2015). Johari Window: An effective model for improving interpersonal communication and managerial effectiveness. SIT Journal of Management, 5(2), 134-146.
427. Scaer, R. (2011). The Body Bears the Burden: Trauma, Dissociation, and Disease.
428. Scarff, C. E., Bearman, M., Chiavaroli, N., & Trumble, S. (2019). Keeping mum in clinical supervision: private thoughts and public judgements. *Medical Education*, 53(2), 133-142. https://doi.org/10.1111/medu.13728
429. Schauer, E., & Elbert, T. (2010). The psychological impact of child soldiering. *Trauma rehabilitation after war and conflict: Community and individual perspectives*, 311-360.
430. Schlaug, G. 2009. "Music, musicians, and brain plasticity," in Oxford Handbook of Music Psychology, eds S. Hallam, I. Cross and M. Thaut (Oxford: Oxford University Press), 197–207.

431. Schön, D. A. (1991). *The reflective practitioner: How professionals think in action*. Arena. Ashgate Publishing.
432. Schön, D.A. (1983). The Reflective Practitioner: How Professionals Think in Action. Basic Books.
433. Schumacher, J. A., Williams, D. C., Burke, R. S., Epler, A. J., Simon, P., & Coffey, S. F. (2018). Competency-based supervision in motivational interviewing for advanced psychology trainees: Targeting an a priori benchmark. *Training and Education in Professional Psychology, 12*(3), 149-153. https://doi.org/10.1037/tep0000177
434. Schunk, D. (2016). Learning theories: An educational perspective. Pearson.
435. Schweitzer, R. D., & Witham, M. (2018). The supervisory alliance: Comparison of measures and implications for a supervision toolkit. *Counselling and Psychotherapy Research, 18*(1), 71-78. https://doi.org/10.1002/capr.12143
436. Sender, R., Fuchs, S., & Milo, R. (2016). Are we really vastly outnumbered? Revisiting the ratio of bacterial to host cells in humans. Cell, 164(3), 337-340.
437. Sertić, H., Čorak, S., & Segedi, I. (2016). APPLICABLE RESEARCH IN JUDO.
438. Shafique, M. (2015). Are we doomed not to reach our goals despite how optimistic we are?. Read on LinkedIn.
439. Shafique, M. (2015). Pursuit vs End Result – What's more Important?. Read on LinkedIn.
440. Shafique, M. (2015). The Fear of Failing and How to Reclaim It. Read on LinkedIn.
441. Shafique, M. (2015). The origin of Goal-Setting. Read on LinkedIn.
442. Shapiro, F., Wesselmann, D., & Mevissen, L. (2017). Eye movement desensitization and reprocessing therapy (EMDR). Evidence-based treatments for trauma related disorders in children and adolescents, 273-297.
443. Shea, S. E., Goldberg, S., & Weatherston, D. J. (2016). A community mental health professional development model for the expansion of reflective practice and supervision: Evaluation of a pilot training series for infant mental health professionals. *Infant Mental Health Journal, 37*(6), 653-669.
444. Shekelle, P. G., Cook, I. A., Miake-Lye, I. M., Booth, M. S., Beroes, J. M., & Mak, S. (2018). Benefits and harms of cranial electrical stimulation for chronic painful conditions, depression, anxiety, and insomnia: a systematic review. *Annals of internal medicine, 168*(6), 414-421.
445. Shultz, L. A. S., Pedersen, H. A., Roper, B. L., & Rey-Casserly, C. (2014). Supervision in Neuropsychological Assessment: A Survey of Training, Practices, and Perspectives of Supervisors. *The Clinical Neuropsychologist, 28*(6), 907-925. https://doi.org/10.1080/13854046.2014.942373
446. Siegel, D. J. (1999). The Developing Mind. New York: Guilford.
447. Simpson-Southward, C., Waller, G., & Hardy, G. E. (2017). How do we know what makes for "best practice" in clinical supervision for psychological therapists? A content analysis of supervisory models and approaches. *Clinical Psychology & Psychotherapy, 24*(6), 1228-1245. https://doi.org/10.1002/cpp.2084
448. Sinicki, A. (2022). The Protean Performance System: SuperFunctional Training 2.
449. Sitler, H. C. (2009). Teaching with awareness: The hidden effects of trauma on learning. Clearing House: A Journal of Education Strategies, Issues, and Ideas, 82(3), 119-124.
450. Sköld, M. L., Aluan, M., Norberg, J., Carlsson, J. (2018). To fail psychotherapy training: Students' and supervisors' perspectives on the supervisory relationship. *European Journal of Psychotherapy & Counselling, 20*(4), 391-410. https://doi.org/10.1080/13642537.2018.1529688
451. Snowdon, D. A., Sargent, M., Williams, C. M., Maloney, S., Caspers, K., & Taylor, N. F. (2019). Effective clinical supervision of allied health professionals: a mixed methods study. *BMC Health Services Research, 20*(1), 2-11. https://doi.org/10.1186/s12913-019-4873-8
452. Snyder, A. N. Mirror Neurons and Their Effects on Social-Emotional Learning. Medford Public Schools.
453. Snyder, D. M. (1990). On the relation between psychology and physics. The Journal of Mind and Behavior, 1-17.
454. Sophia. (2022). Shito Ryu: A Complete list of Shito Ryu Kata with Videos., https://www.karatephilosophy.com/category/kata/shito-ryu/.
455. Spence, S.H., Wilson, J., Kavanagh, D., Strong, J. & Worrall, L. (2001). Clinical supervision in four mental health professions: A review of the evidence. *Behaviour Change, 18*, 135–155.
456. Sperling, A. P. (1992). Psychology Made Simple. Butterworth- Heinemann Limited.
457. Stampi, C. (1989). Polyphasic sleep strategies improve prolonged sustained performance: a field study on 99 sailors. Work & Stress, 3(1), 41-55.
458. Stampi, C. (1992). Evolution, chronobiology, and functions of polyphasic and ultrashort sleep: main issues. Why we nap: evolution, chronobiology, and functions ofpolyphasic and ultrashort sleep, 1-20.
459. Staples-Bradley, L. K., Duda, B., & Gettens, K. (2019). Student self-disclosure in clinical supervision. *Training and Education in Professional Psychology, 13*(3), 216-221. https://doi.org/10.1037/tep0000242
460. Stevens, B., Hyde, J., Knight, R., Shires, A., & Alexander, R. (2017). Competency-based training and assessment in Australian postgraduate clinical psychology education. *Clinical Psychologist, 21*(3), 174-185. https://doi.org/10.1111/cp.12061
461. Stillman, J., Anderson, L., Arellano, A., Wong, P. L., Berta-Avila, M., Alfaro, C., & Struthers, K. (2013). Putting PACT in context and context in PACT: Teacher educators collaborating around program-specific and shared learning goals. Teacher Education Quarterly, 40(4), 135-157.
462. Strickler, A., Valenti, M. W., & Mihalo, J. R. (2018). Mechanisms for building working alliances in clinical supervision. *Clinical Social Work Journal, 46*(4), 361-373. https://doi.org/10.1007/s10615-018-0684-3
463. Strutt, A., MacDonald, B., & Stinson, J. (2019). A-06 The Culturally Expressive and Responsive (CER) Supervision Model in Neuropsychology. *Archives of Clinical Neuropsychology, 34*(6), 865-865. https://doi.org/10.1093/arclin/acz034.06
464. Sull, D & Escobari. (2005). "Success Against the Odds: What Brazilian Champions Teach Us About Thriving in Unpredictable Markets" (Rio de Janeiro and Cambridge, Massachusetts: Editora Campus.
465. Sull, D., & Sull, C. (2018). With Goals, FAST Beats SMART. *The Strategic Agility Project / Research Highlights*.
466. Sull, D., Kang H., Thompson, N., and Hu, L. (2018). "Trade-offs in Firm Culture? Nope, You Can Have It All," MIT Sloan School of Management working paper.
467. Sumner, A. T. (2008). Chromosomes: organization and function. John Wiley & Sons.

468. Sun, H. H., Meng, J., & Yan, K. (Eds.). (2020). The Book of Chinese Medicine, Volume 1: The Timeless Science of Balance and Harmony for Modern Life (Vol. 1). Cambridge Scholars Publishing.
469. Sweeney, J., & Creaner, M. (2014). What's not being said? Recollections of nondisclosure in clinical supervision while in training. *British Journal of Guidance & Counselling, 42*(2), 211-224. https://doi.org/10.1080/03069885.2013.872223
470. Świątczak, B. (2019). Francisco Varela's Vision of the Immune System.
471. Taghvaei, E., & Miasnikova, T. I. (2024). Current Trends in Fitness Development.
472. Taylor, D. & Hamdy, H. (2013) Adult learning theories: Implications for learning and teaching in medical education, AMEE Guide No. 83. *Medical Teacher, 35*(11), e1561-e1572. https://doi.org/10.3109/0142159X.2013
473. Temmerman, N. (2006). Improving school music education: We all have a part to play. Professional Educator, 5(1), 34-39.
474. Tenger, B. (1978). Self-Defense: Nerve Centres & Pressure Points for Karate, Jujutsu, and Atemi-Waza
475. Thomas, G. B. B., & Thomas, M. F. S. (1967). The Biology of Man. Hulton Educational Publications.
476. Trangucci, K. A. (2013). *The supervisory working alliance and self-efficacy of school psychology graduate interns* [Doctoral dissertation, Forham University]. Proquest. https://search.proquest.com/docview/1357146958
477. Trumbo, P., Schlicker, S., Yates, A. A., & Poos, M. (2002). Dietary reference intakes for energy, carbohydrate, fiber, fat, fatty acids, cholesterol, protein and amino acids. (Commentary). Journal of the American dietetic association, 102(11), 1621-1631.
478. Tubbs, R. S., Riech, S., Verma, K., Chern, J., Mortazavi, M., & Cohen-Gadol, A. A. (2011). China's first surgeon: Hua Tuo (c. 108–208 AD). Child's Nervous System, 27, 1357-1360.
479. Ulrich, R. S. (1984). View through a window may influence recovery from surgery. science, 224(4647), 420-421.
480. Uttal, W. R. (2014). Time, Space, and Number in Physics and Psychology (Psychology Revivals). Psychology Press.
481. Van Assche, M. (2012). The Thymus Gland.
482. Van der Kolk. B. A. (2015). The Body Keeps the Score: Mind, Brain and Body in the Transformation of Trauma. Penguin Books.
483. Vanderstukken, A., Schreurs, B., Germeys, F., Van den Broeck, A., & Proost, K. (2019). Should supervisors communicate goals or visions? The moderating role of subordinates' psychological distance. *Journal of Applied Social Psychology, 49*(11), 671-683. https://doi.org/10.1111/jasp.12626
484. Vandette, M.-P., & Gosselin, J. (2019). Conceptual models of clinical supervision across professions: A scoping review of the professional psychology, social work, nursing, and medicine literature in Canada. *Canadian Psychology/Psychologie Canadienne, 60*(4), 302-314. https://doi.org/10.1037/cap0000190
485. Vannucci, M. J., Whiteside, D. M., Saigal, S., Nichols, L., & Hileman, S. (2017). Predicting Supervision Outcomes: What is Different about Psychological Assessment Supervision? *Australian Psychologist, 52*(2), 114-120. https://doi.org/10.1111/ap.12258
486. Váradi, J. (2022). A review of the literature on the relationship of music education to the development of socio-emotional learning. Sage Open, 12(1), 21582440211068501.
487. Vasilev, V., Meridth, S., & Ryabko, M. (2006). Let Every Breath: Secrets of the Russian Breath Masters.
488. Verweij, K. J., Mosing, M. A., Zietsch, B. P., & Medland, S. E. (2012). Estimating heritability from twin studies. Statistical human genetics: methods and protocols, 151-170.
489. Vidyadharan, V., & Tharayil, H. M. (2019). Learning disorder or learning disability: Time to rethink. Indian Journal of Psychological Medicine, 41(3), 276-278.
490. Vineyard, M. (2007). How you stand, how you move, how you live: Learning the Alexander Technique to explore your mind-body connection and achieve self-mastery. Da Capo Lifelong Books.
491. Vivanti, G., & Rogers, S. J. (2014). Autism and the mirror neuron system: Insights from learning and teaching. Philosophical Transactions of the Royal Society B: Biological Sciences, 369(1644), 20130184.
492. Vogel, W., Baker, R. W., & Lazarus, R. S. (1958). The role of motivation in psychological stress. The Journal of Abnormal and Social Psychology, 56(1), 105-122. https://doi.org/10.1037/h0040719
493. Wallbank, S., & Wonnacott, J. (2015). The integrated model of restorative supervision for use within safeguarding. *Community Practitioner, 88*(5), 41-45.
494. Walsh, W. J. (2014). Nutrient power: Heal your biochemistry and heal your brain. Simon and Schuster.
495. Ward, C. C., & House, R. M. (1998). Counseling supervision: A reflective model. *Counselor Education and Supervision, 38*(1), 23-33. https://doi.org/10.1002/j.1556-6978.1998.tb00554.x
496. Warren, M. P. (1983). Effects of undernutrition on reproductive function in the human. Endocrine Reviews, 4(4), 363 - 377.
497. Washburne, J. N. (1936). The definition of learning. *Journal of Educational Psychology, 27*(8), 603–611. https://doi.org/10.1037/h0060154
498. Wasik, B. H., & Fishbein, J. E. (1982). Problem solving: A model for supervision in professional psychology. *Professional Psychology, 13*(4), 559-564. https://doi.org/10.1037/0735-7028.13.4.559
499. Watkins Jr, C. E., & Watkins Jr, C. E. (2012). Psychotherapy supervision in the new millennium: Competency-based, evidence-based, particularized, and energized. *Journal of Contemporary Psychotherapy, 42*(3), 193-203. https://doi.org/10.1007/s10879-011-9202-4
500. Watkins, J. C. E. (2014). The supervisory alliance: a half century of theory, practice, and research in critical perspective. *American Journal of Psychotherapy, 68*(1), 19-55. https://doi.org/10.1176/appi.psychotherapy.2014.68.1.19
501. Waugh, A., & Grant, A. (2014). Ross & Wilson Anatomy and physiology in health and illness E-book. Elsevier Health Sciences.
502. Wenzel, K., & Reinhard, M. A. (2021). Does the end justify the means? Learning tests lead to more negative evaluations and to more stress experiences. Learning and Motivation, 73, 101706.
503. Wessels, T. M. (2012). Evaluating a session- punitive vs. reflective. *Journal of Genetic Counseling, 21*(2), 241. https://doi.org/10.1007/s10897-011-9456-8
504. Westefeld, J. S. (2009). Supervision of psychotherapy: Models, issues, and recommendations. *The Counseling Psychologist, 37*(2), 296-316. https://doi.org/10.1177/0011000008316657
505. Wheeler, D. (2005). A taxonomy for learning, teaching and assessing.
506. While, A. E. (1994). Competence versus performance: which is more important? Journal of Advanced Nursing, 20(3), 525-531. https://doi.org/10.1111/j.1365-2648.1994.tb02391.x

507. White, H. A., & Shah, P. (2011). Creative style and achievement in adults with attention-deficit/hyperactivity disorder. Personality and individual differences, 50(5), 673-677.
508. Wikinson, J. (1999). Implementing reflective practice. *Nursing Standard (through 2013), 13*(21), 36-40. https://search.proquest.com/docview/219802785?accountid=16285
509. Wiley, M. V. (2011). Filipino martial culture. Tuttle Publishing.
510. Willey, J. M., Sherwood, L. M., & Woolverton, C. J. (2014). Prescott's microbiology. McGraw-Hill.
511. Williams, J., Whiten, A., Suddendorf, T., & Perrett, D. (2001). Imitation, mirror neurons and autism. Neuroscience & Biobehavioral Reviews, 25(4), 287-295.
512. Williams, T. R., & Raney, S. (2020). Relational cultural supervision enhances the professional development of postdoctoral residents of color in health service psychology. *Journal of Psychotherapy Integration, 30*(1), 140-146. https://doi.org/10.1037/int0000169
513. Wisneski, L., & Anderson, L. (2005). The scientific basis of integrative medicine.
514. Woloshyn, V. E., Paivio, A., & Pressley, M. (1994). Use of elaborative interrogation to help students acquire information consistent with prior knowledge and information inconsistent with prior knowledge. Journal of Educational Psychology, 86(1), 79.
515. Wood, S. J., Allen, N. B., & Pantelis, C. (Eds.). (2009). The neuropsychology of mental illness. Cambridge University Press.
516. Wu, Q., Wang, H., Liu, X., Zhao, Y., & Su, P. (2023). Microglial activation and over pruning involved in developmental epilepsy. Journal of Neuropathology & Experimental Neurology, 82(2), 150-159.
517. Wynn, G. H. (2015). Complementary and alternative medicine approaches in the treatment of PTSD., *Curr Psychiatry Rep.*; 17: 600
518. Yang, C., Ji, J., Lv, Y., Li, Z., & Luo, D. (2022). Application of Piezoelectric Material and Devices in Bone Regeneration. Nanomaterials, 12(24), 4386.
519. Young, E. (2012). Gut Instincts: The secrets of your second brain. *New Scientist, 216 (2895), 38-42*
520. Young, K. (2020). Hey Awesome. Hey Sigmund Publishing.
521. Zehr, E. P. (2008). Becoming Batman: The Possibility of a Superhero. The Johns Hopkins University Press.
522. Zhong, J. J., Timofeevich, A. (2008). Training Methods of 72 Arts of Shaolin
523. Zorga, S. (2002). Supervision: the process of life-long learning in social and educational professions. *Journal of interprofessional care, 16*(3), 265–276. https://doi.org/10.1080/13561820220146694
524. Zoughari, K. (2010). The Ninja: Ancient Shadow Warriors of Japan. Berkeley Books.

Relevant Course/Degree/CPD References

525. AMN Academy Student.
526. Bachelor of Psychology group Honours – James Cook University.
527. Calisthenics Student.
528. Certificate 3, 4, Master Trainer – Australian Institute of Fitness.
529. Diploma Counselling – TAFE North.
530. Arielle Schwartz – PESI Australia – Complex Trauma Treatment.
531. Bessel van der Kolk – PESI – Online Certificate regarding 'Rewiring the Brain: Neurofeedback.
532. Black Dog Institute – REACH Facilitator Training.
533. Blue Knot Foundation – A Three-Phased Approach – 'Working Therapeutically with Complex Trauma Clients'.
534. Community Training Australia – Workshop for 'Body Therapies'.
535. Community Training Australia – Workshop for 'Understanding Grief and Loss'.
536. Comorbidity Guidelines online training – Management of Co-occurring alcohol and other drug and mental health conditions in alcohol and other drug treatment settings.
537. GriffinOT – Sensory Processing Aware Level 1.
538. GriffinOT – Sensory Processing Aware Level 2.
539. GriffinOT – Sensory Processing Aware Level 3.
540. Headspace online training – Developmental Disorders in Young People.
541. Insight Alcohol and other drug training and workforce development Queensland – Modules 1-6.
542. Jennifer Sweeton – PESI Australia – PTSD Trauma treatment – EMDR, CBT and Somatic-Based Interventions.
543. Jon Kabat-Zinn – PESI – Online Certificate regarding 'Mindfulness, Healing and Transformation: The Pain and the Promise of Befriending the Full Catastrophe.
544. Leslie Korn – PESI – Online Certificate regarding 'Nutrition for Mental Health'.
545. Linda Curran – PESI – Online Certificate regarding 'Master Clinician Series The Adverse Childhood Experiences Study.
546. Mental Health First Aid Australia – Standard Mental Health First Aid Facilitator fourth edition course.
547. Mental Health First Aid Australia – Webcast 'MHFA Auditory Hallucination Simulation'.
548. Online training NCETA – Ice: Training for Frontline Workers Certificate of Completion modules 1-7.
549. PESI Australia – Autism and Sensory Processing Disorder.
550. PESI Australia – Autism Meltdowns in Children and Adolescents.
551. PESI Australia – High-Functioning Autism.
552. Stephen Porges PhD – PESI Australia – Clinical Applications of the Polyvagal Theory.
553. Advanced Master Herbalist Diploma Online – Centre of Excellence.
554. Yoga for Mental Health – Rewire Therapy.
555. Tai Chi for Arthritis.
556. White Tiger Qi Gong.
557. Trinity System Chinese Medicine Fundamentals.
558. Fascia Foundations Course.
559. 5 Element QiYo Course.
560. Qi Gong for Worry and Anxiety.
561. Yoga Student.
562. Yoga and Physiology Student.

Informal References

563. AMN Academy Holistic Health Coach Course
564. MacroFit Inc. app – Simon Ata program – Project Calisthenics Level 1-3
565. Movement Athlete fitness app – https://themovementathlete.com/
566. PNI Global Awareness – PNI course and Wellness Management information
567. Various Articles by Sifu Anthony Korahais – https://flowingzen.com/
568. Various Articles by Yogapedia - https://www.yogapedia.com/
569. Various GMB Online Articles – https://gmb.io/
570. Various 'Nutrition with Judy' Articles – https://www.nutritionwithjudy.com/
571. Various Onnit Online Articles – https://www.onnit.com/
572. Peter Attia – https://peterattiamd.com/podcast/
573. Various Podcasts and articles by Dr. Rhonda Patrick -www.foundmyfitness.com
574. ArtofOneDojo. (n.d.). Art of One Dojo. YouTube. Retrieved from 2024, from https://www.youtube.com/@ArtofOneDojo/videos
575. AshtonFitness. (n.d.). Ashton Fitness. YouTube. Retrieved 2022-2021, from https://www.youtube.com/@AshtonFitness
576. Aucademy6195. (n.d.). Aucademy. YouTube. Retrieved 2022-2023, from https://www.youtube.com/@aucademy6195
577. Athleanx. (n.d.). Athlean-X. YouTube. Retrieved 2018-2023, from https://www.youtube.com/@athleanx
578. Aucademy6195. (n.d.). Aucademy. YouTube. Retrieved 2022-2023, from https://www.youtube.com/@aucademy6195
579. Blackbelt_magazine. (n.d.). Black Belt Magazine. YouTube. Retrieved from 2012-2023, from https://www.youtube.com/@blackbelt_magazine
580. BudoBrothers. (n.d.). Budo Brothers. YouTube. Retrieved from 2024, from https://www.youtube.com/@BudoBrothers/videos
581. CaptainTepes. (n.d.) Mike Ciardi. YouTube. Retrieved from 2019-2020, from https://www.youtube.com/@CaptainTepes
582. CitizenAthletics. (n.d.). Citizen Athletics. YouTube. Retrieved from 2024, from https://www.youtube.com/@CitizenAthletics/videos
583. CKFAHQ. (n.d.). Henry Sue Circular Tong Long. YouTube. Retrieved from 2018-2021, from https://www.youtube.com/@CKFAHQ
584. ClearMartialArts. (n.d.). Clear's Internal Combat Arts. YouTube. Retrieved from 2015-2021, from https://www.youtube.com/@ClearMartialArts
585. CrashCourse. (n.d.) CrashCourse. YouTube. Retrieved from 2023-2024. https://www.youtube.com/@crashcourse/
586. DifferingMinds. (n.d.). Differing Minds. YouTube. Retrieved from 2023, from https://www.youtube.com/@DifferingMinds
587. Elasticsteel. (n.d.). ElasticSteel. YouTube. Retrieved from 2018-2022, from https://www.youtube.com/@Elasticsteel
588. Everythingwingchun1. (n.d.). Everything Wing Chun. YouTube. Retrieved from 2013-2021, from https://www.youtube.com/@Everythingwingchun1
589. Fightscience. (n.d.). Fight Science. YouTube. Retrieved from 2018-2021, from https://www.youtube.com/@fightscience
590. Fitnessblender. (n.d.). FitnessBlender. YouTube. Retrieved from 2018-2021, from https://www.youtube.com/@fitnessblender
591. FitnessFAQs. (n.d.). FitnessFAQs. YouTube. Retrieved from 2021-2023, from https://www.youtube.com/@FitnessFAQs
592. FlowwithAdee. (n.d.). Adison Briana. YouTube. Retrieved 2020-2021, from https://www.youtube.com/@FlowwithAdee
593. FoundMyFitness. (n.d.). FoundMyFitness. YouTube. Retrieved from 2020-2023, from https://www.youtube.com/@FoundMyFitness
594. Frank_Medrano. (n.d.). Frank Medrano. YouTube. Retrieved from 2018-2022, from https://www.youtube.com/@frank_medrano
595. GarageStrength. (n.d.). Garage Strength. YouTube. Retrieved from 2024, from https://www.youtube.com/@GarageStrength/videos
596. GinaScarangella. (n.d.). Gina Scarangella. YouTube. Retrieved from 2019-2020, from https://www.youtube.com/@GinaScarangella
597. GMBfit. (n.d.). GMB Fitness. YouTube. Retrieved from 2018-2023, from https://www.youtube.com/@gmbfit
598. HowtoADHD. (n.d.). How to ADHD. YouTube. Retrieved from 2022-2023, from https://www.youtube.com/@HowtoADHD
599. Iamcarlpaoli. (n.d.). Carl Paoli. YouTube. Retrieved from 2018-2023, from https://www.youtube.com/@iamcarlpaoli
600. IzzoWingChun. (n.d.). Izzo Wing Chun. YouTube. Retrieved from 2013-2021, from https://www.youtube.com/@IzzoWingChun
601. JeffNippard. (n.d.). Jeff Nippard. YouTube. Retrieved from 2021- 2023, from https://www.youtube.com/@JeffNippard
602. KaratebyJesse. (n.d.). Jesse Enkamp. YouTube. Retrieved from 2022-2023, from https://www.youtube.com/@KARATEbyJesse
603. KarateDojowaKu. (n.d.). Karate Dojo waKu. YouTube. Retrieved from 2024, from https://www.youtube.com/@KarateDojowaKu/videos
604. KevinLeeVlog. (n.d.). Kevin Lee. YouTube. Retrieved from, https://www.youtube.com/@KevinLeeVlog/videos
605. KinoYoga. (n.d.). Kino Yoga. YouTube. Retrieved from 2018-2023, from https://www.youtube.com/@KinoYoga
606. Kurzgesagt. (n.d.) Kurzgesagt – In a Nutshell. YouTube. Retrieved from 2015-2023, from https://www.youtube.com/@kurzgesagt
607. LeagueFitAcademy. (n.d.) League Fit Academy. YouTube. Retrieved 2024. https://www.youtube.com/@leaguefitacademy/
608. LeeWeiland. (n.d.). Lee Weiland. YouTube. Retrieved from 2023, from https://www.youtube.com/@LeeWeiland/videos
609. Livinleggings. (n.d.). Livinleggings. YouTube. Retrieved from 2022-2023, from https://www.youtube.com/@Livinleggings
610. MartialArtsJourney. (n.d.). Martial Arts Journey with Rokas. Youtube. Retrieved from 2023, from https://www.youtube.com/@MartialArtsJourney/videos
611. MovementProjectPT. (n.d.). Movement Project PT. YouTube. Retrieved from 2023-2023, from https://www.youtube.com/@MovementProjectPT
612. Neuroscientificallychallenged. (n.d.). Neuroscientifically Challenged. YouTube. Retrieved from 2021-2022, from https://www.youtube.com/@Neuroscientificallychallenged
613. Nicabm. (n.d.). NICABM. YouTube. Retrieved from 2020-2023, from https://www.youtube.com/@nicabm
614. OfficialBarstarzz. (n.d.). OfficialBarstarzz. YouTube. Retrieved from 2018-2022, from https://www.youtube.com/@OfficialBarstarzz
615. OFFICIALTHENXSTUDIOS. (n.d.). THENX. YouTube. Retrieved from 2019-2022, from https://www.youtube.com/@OFFICIALTHENXSTUDIOS

Relevant Course/Degree/CPD References

525. AMN Academy Student.
526. Bachelor of Psychology group Honours – James Cook University.
527. Calisthenics Student.
528. Certificate 3, 4, Master Trainer – Australian Institute of Fitness.
529. Diploma Counselling – TAFE North.
530. Arielle Schwartz – PESI Australia – Complex Trauma Treatment.
531. Bessel van der Kolk – PESI – Online Certificate regarding 'Rewiring the Brain: Neurofeedback.
532. Black Dog Institute – REACH Facilitator Training.
533. Blue Knot Foundation – A Three-Phased Approach – 'Working Therapeutically with Complex Trauma Clients'.
534. Community Training Australia – Workshop for 'Body Therapies'.
535. Community Training Australia – Workshop for 'Understanding Grief and Loss'.
536. Comorbidity Guidelines online training – Management of Co-occurring alcohol and other drug and mental health conditions in alcohol and other drug treatment settings.
537. GriffinOT – Sensory Processing Aware Level 1.
538. GriffinOT – Sensory Processing Aware Level 2.
539. GriffinOT – Sensory Processing Aware Level 3.
540. Headspace online training – Developmental Disorders in Young People.
541. Insight Alcohol and other drug training and workforce development Queensland – Modules 1-6.
542. Jennifer Sweeton – PESI Australia – PTSD Trauma treatment – EMDR, CBT and Somatic-Based Interventions.
543. Jon Kabat-Zinn – PESI – Online Certificate regarding 'Mindfulness, Healing and Transformation: The Pain and the Promise of Befriending the Full Catastrophe.
544. Leslie Korn – PESI – Online Certificate regarding 'Nutrition for Mental Health'.
545. Linda Curran – PESI – Online Certificate regarding 'Master Clinician Series The Adverse Childhood Experiences Study.
546. Mental Health First Aid Australia – Standard Mental Health First Aid Facilitator fourth edition course.
547. Mental Health First Aid Australia – Webcast 'MHFA Auditory Hallucination Simulation'.
548. Online training NCETA – Ice: Training for Frontline Workers Certificate of Completion modules 1-7.
549. PESI Australia – Autism and Sensory Processing Disorder.
550. PESI Australia – Autism Meltdowns in Children and Adolescents.
551. PESI Australia – High-Functioning Autism.
552. Stephen Porges PhD – PESI Australia – Clinical Applications of the Polyvagal Theory.
553. Advanced Master Herbalist Diploma Online – Centre of Excellence.
554. Yoga for Mental Health – Rewire Therapy.
555. Tai Chi for Arthritis.
556. White Tiger Qi Gong.
557. Trinity System Chinese Medicine Fundamentals.
558. Fascia Foundations Course.
559. 5 Element QiYo Course.
560. Qi Gong for Worry and Anxiety.
561. Yoga Student.
562. Yoga and Physiology Student.

Informal References

563. AMN Academy Holistic Health Coach Course
564. MacroFit Inc. app – Simon Ata program – Project Calisthenics Level 1-3
565. Movement Athlete fitness app – https://themovementathlete.com/
566. PNI Global Awareness – PNI course and Wellness Management information
567. Various Articles by Sifu Anthony Korahais – https://flowingzen.com/
568. Various Articles by Yogapedia - https://www.yogapedia.com/
569. Various GMB Online Articles – https://gmb.io/
570. Various 'Nutrition with Judy' Articles – https://www.nutritionwithjudy.com/
571. Various Onnit Online Articles – https://www.onnit.com/
572. Peter Attia – https://peterattiamd.com/podcast/
573. Various Podcasts and articles by Dr. Rhonda Patrick -www.foundmyfitness.com
574. ArtofOneDojo. (n.d.). Art of One Dojo. YouTube. Retrieved from 2024, from https://www.youtube.com/@ArtofOneDojo/videos
575. AshtonFitness. (n.d.). Ashton Fitness. YouTube. Retrieved 2022-2021, from https://www.youtube.com/@AshtonFitness
576. Aucademy6195. (n.d.). Aucademy. YouTube. Retrieved 2022-2023, from https://www.youtube.com/@aucademy6195
577. Athleanx. (n.d.). Athlean-X. YouTube. Retrieved 2018-2023, from https://www.youtube.com/@athleanx
578. Aucademy6195. (n.d.). Aucademy. YouTube. Retrieved 2022-2023, from https://www.youtube.com/@aucademy6195
579. Blackbelt_magazine. (n.d.). Black Belt Magazine. YouTube. Retrieved from 2012-2023, from https://www.youtube.com/@blackbelt_magazine
580. BudoBrothers. (n.d.). Budo Brothers. YouTube. Retrieved from 2024, from https://www.youtube.com/@BudoBrothers/videos
581. CaptainTepes. (n.d.) Mike Ciardi. YouTube. Retrieved from 2019-2020, from https://www.youtube.com/@CaptainTepes
582. CitizenAthletics. (n.d.). Citizen Athletics. YouTube. Retrieved from 2024, from https://www.youtube.com/@CitizenAthletics/videos
583. CKFAHQ. (n.d.). Henry Sue Circular Tong Long. YouTube. Retrieved from 2018-2021, from https://www.youtube.com/@CKFAHQ
584. ClearMartialArts. (n.d.). Clear's Internal Combat Arts. YouTube. Retrieved from 2015-2021, from https://www.youtube.com/@ClearMartialArts
585. CrashCourse. (n.d.) CrashCourse. YouTube. Retrieved from 2023-2024. https://www.youtube.com/@crashcourse/
586. DifferingMinds. (n.d.). Differing Minds. YouTube. Retrieved from 2023, from https://www.youtube.com/@DifferingMinds
587. Elasticsteel. (n.d.). ElasticSteel. YouTube. Retrieved from 2018-2022, from https://www.youtube.com/@Elasticsteel
588. Everythingwingchun1. (n.d.). Everything Wing Chun. YouTube. Retrieved from 2013-2021, from https://www.youtube.com/@Everythingwingchun1
589. Fightscience. (n.d.). Fight Science. YouTube. Retrieved from 2018-2021, from https://www.youtube.com/@fightscience
590. Fitnessblender. (n.d.). FitnessBlender. YouTube. Retrieved from 2018-2021, from https://www.youtube.com/@fitnessblender
591. FitnessFAQs. (n.d.). FitnessFAQs. YouTube. Retrieved from 2021-2023, from https://www.youtube.com/@FitnessFAQs
592. FlowwithAdee. (n.d.). Adison Briana. YouTube. Retrieved 2020-2021, from https://www.youtube.com/@FlowwithAdee
593. FoundMyFitness. (n.d.). FoundMyFitness. YouTube. Retrieved from 2020-2023, from https://www.youtube.com/@FoundMyFitness
594. Frank_Medrano. (n.d.). Frank Medrano. YouTube. Retrieved from 2018-2022, from https://www.youtube.com/@frank_medrano
595. GarageStrength. (n.d.). Garage Strength. YouTube. Retrieved from 2024, from https://www.youtube.com/@GarageStrength/videos
596. GinaScarangella. (n.d.). Gina Scarangella. YouTube. Retrieved from 2019-2020, from https://www.youtube.com/@GinaScarangella
597. GMBfit. (n.d.). GMB Fitness. YouTube. Retrieved from 2018-2023, from https://www.youtube.com/@gmbfit
598. HowtoADHD. (n.d.). How to ADHD. YouTube. Retrieved from 2022-2023, from https://www.youtube.com/@HowtoADHD
599. Iamcarlpaoli. (n.d.). Carl Paoli. YouTube. Retrieved from 2018-2023, from https://www.youtube.com/@iamcarlpaoli
600. IzzoWingChun. (n.d.). Izzo Wing Chun. YouTube. Retrieved from 2013-2021, from https://www.youtube.com/@IzzoWingChun
601. JeffNippard. (n.d.). Jeff Nippard. YouTube. Retrieved from 2021- 2023, from https://www.youtube.com/@JeffNippard
602. KaratebyJesse. (n.d.). Jesse Enkamp. YouTube. Retrieved from 2022-2023, from https://www.youtube.com/@KARATEbyJesse
603. KarateDojowaKu. (n.d.). Karate Dojo waKu. YouTube. Retrieved from 2024, from https://www.youtube.com/@KarateDojowaKu/videos
604. KevinLeeVlog. (n.d.). Kevin Lee. YouTube. Retrieved from, https://www.youtube.com/@KevinLeeVlog/videos
605. KinoYoga. (n.d.). Kino Yoga. YouTube. Retrieved from 2018-2023, from https://www.youtube.com/@KinoYoga
606. Kurzgesagt. (n.d.) Kurzgesagt – In a Nutshell. YouTube. Retrieved from 2015-2023, from https://www.youtube.com/@kurzgesagt
607. LeagueFitAcademy. (n.d.) League Fit Academy. YouTube. Retrieved 2024. https://www.youtube.com/@leaguefitacademy/
608. LeeWeiland. (n.d.). Lee Weiland. YouTube. Retrieved from 2023, from https://www.youtube.com/@LeeWeiland/videos
609. Livinleggings. (n.d.). Livingleggings. YouTube. Retrieved from 2022-2023, from https://www.youtube.com/@Livinleggings
610. MartialArtsJourney. (n.d.). Martial Arts Journey with Rokas. Youtube. Retrieved from 2023, from https://www.youtube.com/@MartialArtsJourney/videos
611. MovementProjectPT. (n.d.). Movement Project PT. YouTube. Retrieved from 2023-2023, from https://www.youtube.com/@MovementProjectPT
612. Neuroscientificallychallenged. (n.d.). Neuroscientifically Challenged. YouTube. Retrieved from 2021-2022, from https://www.youtube.com/@Neuroscientificallychallenged
613. Nicabm. (n.d.). NICABM. YouTube. Retrieved from 2020-2023, from https://www.youtube.com/@nicabm
614. OfficialBarstarzz. (n.d.). OfficialBarstarzz. YouTube. Retrieved from 2018-2022, from https://www.youtube.com/@OfficialBarstarzz
615. OFFICIALTHENXSTUDIOS. (n.d.). THENX. YouTube. Retrieved from 2019-2022, from https://www.youtube.com/@OFFICIALTHENXSTUDIOS

616. Portaldo. (n.d.). Ido Portal. YouTube. Retrieved from 2020-2023, from https://www.youtube.com/@portaldo
617. PsychAlive. (n.d.). PsychAlive. YouTube. Retrieved from 2021-2022, from https://www.youtube.com/@PsychAlive
618. Psychologyofeating. (n.d.). Institute for the Psychology of Eating. Youtube. Retrieved from 2023, from https://www.youtube.com/@Psychologyofeating
619. Physioevangelist. (n.d.). Physio Evangelist. YouTube. Retrieved from 2023, from https://www.youtube.com/@physioevangelist/videos
620. RealMichaelJaiWhite. (n.d.). Real Michael Jai White. YouTube. Retrieved from 2019-2022, from https://www.youtube.com/@RealMichaelJaiWhite
621. Reflexionyogaonline. (n.d.). Reflexion Yoga. YouTube. Retrieved from 2018-2021, from https://www.youtube.com/@Reflexionyogaonline
622. RenaissancePeriodization. (n.d.). Renaissance Periodization. YouTube. Retrieved from 2023, from https://www.youtube.com/@RenaissancePeriodization/videos
623. SciShow. (n.d.). SciShow. YouTube. Retrieved from 2015-2023, from https://www.youtube.com/@SciShow
624. SenseiSeth. (n.d.). Sensei Seth. YouTube. Retrieved from 2021-2023, from https://www.youtube.com/@SenseiSeth
625. Sidpaulson1. (n.d.). Sid Paulson. YouTube. Retrieved from 2022-2023, from https://www.youtube.com/@sidpaulson1
626. Socialworkact8660. (n.d.). Social Work & ACT. YouTube. Retrieved from 2020-2022, from https://www.youtube.com/@socialworkact8660
627. Strengthcamp. (n.d.). Elliott Hulse's Strength Camp. YouTube. Retrieved from 2021-2023, from https://www.youtube.com/@strengthcamp
628. Strengthoversize. (n.d.). StrengthOVERsize. YouTube. Retrieved from 2020-2021, from https://www.youtube.com/@strengthoversize
629. Synergyfitnessteam1. (n.d.). Synergyfitnessteam. YouTube. Retrieved from 2020-2022, from https://www.youtube.com/@synergyfitnessteam1
630. TEDEd. (n.d.). TED-Ed. Youtube. Retrieved from 2015-2023, from https://www.youtube.com/@TEDEd
631. TheBioneer. (n.d.). The Bioneer. YouTube. Retrieved from 2022-2023, from https://www.youtube.com/@TheBioneer
632. TheKneesovertoesguy. (n.d.). The Kneesovertoesguy. YouTube. Retrieved from 2022-2023, from https://www.youtube.com/@TheKneesovertoesguy
633. TomMorrison. (n.d.). Tom Morrison. YouTube. Retrieved from 2022-2023, from https://www.youtube.com/@TomMorrison
634. Treforall312. (n.d.) TRE FOR ALL. YouTube. Retrieved from 2021-2023, from https://www.youtube.com/@treforall312
635. Warrenerica1. (n.d.) Erica Warren. YouTube. Retried 2023, from https://www.youtube.com/@warrenerica1
636. Westmoretonmartialarts. (n.d.). West Moreton Academy of Martial Arts. YouTube. Retrieved from 2018-2021, from https://www.youtube.com/@Westmoretonmartialarts
637. WillTennyson. (n.d.). Will Tennyson. YouTube. Retrieved from 2024, from https://www.youtube.com/@WillTennyson/videos
638. YiannisChristoulas. (n.d.). Yiannis Christoulas. YouTube. Retrieved 2023. http://www.youtube.com/@YiannisChristoulas
639. Yogabycandace. (n.d.). Candace Cabrera Tavino. YouTube. Retrieved from 2018-202, from https://www.youtube.com/@yogabycandace
640. YogaBody. (n.d.). YogaBody.Official. YouTube. Retrieved from 2023, from https://www.youtube.com/@YogaBody.Official/featured
641. YogaVibes. (n.d.). YogaVibes. YouTube. Retrieved from 2018-2022, from https://www.youtube.com/@YogaVibes
642. ZuzkaLight. (n.d.). Zuzka Light. YouTube. Retrieved from 2018-2022, from https://www.youtube.com/@ZuzkaLight

Previous Influential Professionals

Gym Manager – Donna Hartley

Long Term Personal Training Client – Janelle Fox

Mental Health Facilitator – Philippa Harris

Mental Health Manager – Alison Fairleigh

Mental Health Manager – Cassandra Parry

Personal Training Course Instructor – Rebecca Leddy

Personal Training Manager / Zen Do Kai Karate / BJC Muay Thai Instructor – Marco Vogel

Pilates Mentor – Kat Syzmanski

Psychology Manager – Liezel Gordon

Psychology Manager – Suzy Dormer

Psychology Manager – Alana Bowen

Psychology Supervisor – Gayle Roe

Psychology Supervisor – Kirsten Seymour

Science Teacher / Itosu Shito Ryu Karate Instructor – Murray Burrows

Wing Chun Instructor – Pablo Cardenas

Various other Athletics Volunteers, Fitness Colleagues, Psychology Colleagues, School Coaches and School Teachers

Many partners of the professionals who helped me with my knowledge journey.

www.ingramcontent.com/pod-product-compliance
Lightning Source LLC
Chambersburg PA
CBHW080213040426
42333CB00044B/2651